The Language and Imagery of Coma and Brain Injury

Also available from Bloomsbury

Applying Linguistics in Illness and Healthcare Contexts, edited by Zsófia Demjén
Corpus, Discourse and Mental Health, by Daniel Hunt and Gavin Brookes
Discursive Constructions of the Suicidal Process, by Dariusz Galasiński and Justyna Ziółkowska
Discourses of Men's Suicide Notes, by Dariusz Galasiński
Investigating Adolescent Health Communication, by Kevin Harvey
Sylvia Plath and the Language of Affective States, by Zsófia Demjén

The Language and Imagery of Coma and Brain Injury

Representations in Literature, Film and Media

Matthew Colbeck

BLOOMSBURY ACADEMIC
LONDON • NEW YORK • OXFORD • NEW DELHI • SYDNEY

BLOOMSBURY ACADEMIC
Bloomsbury Publishing Plc
50 Bedford Square, London, WC1B 3DP, UK
1385 Broadway, New York, NY 10018, USA
29 Earlsfort Terrace, Dublin 2, Ireland

BLOOMSBURY, BLOOMSBURY ACADEMIC and the Diana logo are trademarks of Bloomsbury Publishing Plc

First published in Great Britain 2021
Paperback edition published in 2022

Copyright © Matthew Colbeck, 2021

Matthew Colbeck has asserted his right under the Copyright, Designs and Patents Act, 1988, to be identified as Author of this work.

For legal purposes the Acknowledgements on p. vii constitute an extension of this copyright page.

Cover design by Ben Anslow
Cover image: © SCIEPRO/SCIENCE PHOTO LIBRARY / Getty Images

All rights reserved. No part of this publication may be reproduced or transmitted in any form or by any means, electronic or mechanical, including photocopying, recording, or any information storage or retrieval system, without prior permission in writing from the publishers.

Bloomsbury Publishing Plc does not have any control over, or responsibility for, any third-party websites referred to or in this book. All internet addresses given in this book were correct at the time of going to press. The author and publisher regret any inconvenience caused if addresses have changed or sites have ceased to exist, but can accept no responsibility for any such changes.

A catalogue record for this book is available from the British Library.

A catalog record for this book is available from the Library of Congress.

ISBN: HB: 978-1-3500-7779-9
PB: 978-1-3502-3815-2
ePDF: 978-1-3500-7780-5
eBook: 978-1-3500-7781-2

Typeset by Deanta Global Publishing Services, Chennai, India

To find out more about our authors and books visit www.bloomsbury.com and sign up for our newsletters.

Contents

List of figures	vi
Acknowledgements	vii
Introduction	1
1 Contextualizing coma and brain injury: A linguistic, cultural and medical history	13
2 Coma, trauma and the exilic self	37
3 Coma and the katabatic archetype	69
4 Selfhood and the post-coma condition	105
5 Coma, brain injury and lived experience	139
6 Metaphor and narrative prosthesis	159
Notes	191
Bibliography	192
Index	207

Figures

1.1	Still from *The Cabinet of Dr Caligari*, dir. Robert Wiene	22
1.2	Photograph of Price's 'Sleeping Beauty', c. 1950s	23
1.3	The Glasgow Coma Scale	30
2.1	Facsimile of woodcut illustration from Alex Garland's *The Coma*	64
4.1	Image of the ancient symbol of the Ouroboros	118
4.2	Image of the mathematical symbol for Infinity	122
4.3	Photograph 'Anna and I Get Married' by Mark E. Hogancamp	130
6.1	Facsimile of a page from Steph Grant's 'Unremembered Memoirs'	176

Acknowledgements

It has been a long road between the inception of this book and its publication so there are several people I would like to thank who have helped me in this journey. Many thanks to Professor Brendan Stone and Professor Adam Piette for nurturing the project in its earliest stages, and to Professor Sue Vice and Professor Roger Luckhurst for their invaluable advice in developing it further. Thanks also to Professor Neil Roberts for instructive conversations and insights into the life and works of Peter Redgrove.

Thanks to Andrew Wardell and Becky Holland at Bloomsbury for all of their patience and support and for their constant faith in the project. Special thanks to the production team, in particular Joseph Gautham at Deanta Global and Jophcy Kumar at Bloomsbury, for their huge support (and patience!) in the final stages of pulling this book together. Thanks also to Gurdeep Mattu at Rowman & Littlefield Publishing Group who championed the book from the beginning.

I would also like to thank the University of Sheffield and, in particular, the School of English; Headway and all at Headway East London, particularly Ben Platts-Mills for his insights into the complex intersection of functional/organic pathologies of brain injury; UKABIF; the Sheffield Community Brain Injury Rehabilitation Team at LTNC, Sheffield; Nicholas Royle and Nightjar Press; John Oakey Design; H&H Reeds Printers; Professor Jenny Kitzinger; and the Head Injury and Homelessness Research Group (HIHRG).

Many, many thanks to all members of *The Write Way* for sharing their stories and for their support for the project, for which I will always be incredibly grateful: Steph Grant, Caroline Waugh, Gwynfa Grant, Laurence Cox, Joel Wilde, David Stead, Lesley James, Heather Norton, Rachael Fox, Wilf Griffiths, Ste Jones and Jo Maricseonda.

I am extremely grateful to all of my friends and colleagues who have helped me along the way: Dr Steve Hollyman, Tom Carter, Antony and Kelly Buxton, Reanna Heath, Dr Hannah Merry, Dr Adam Smith, Dr Pete Walters, Dr Zelda Hannay, Dr Michael Flexer, Dr Sam Goodman, Matt McGuinness and his VAAST project (which has soundtracked the writing of this book) and Matt Jones. Special thanks to Paul Hare for giving me the push to embark on this research.

Above all, I am deeply grateful to my wife, Charlotte, for her endless encouragement; to Fred, for getting me out of the house on walks around the streets of Sheffield to help clear my mind and sharpen my focus; to Viv, Malc, Glyn and Janet; and to our new little addition, Flora, who has been the happiest, most mischievous of distractions during the final stages of writing. And of course, special thanks to mum and dad, for their constant support throughout this process and encouraging me to make the leap into this research.

Dad – I wish you were still here to see me see this through.
And so I dedicate this book to you.

Introduction

Towards the beginning of Quentin Tarantino's revenge thriller, *Kill Bill Vol 1*, we learn that the film's heroine, The Bride, while in a four-year coma, has endured years of sexual abuse and rape at the hands of a corrupt nurse who is in charge of her care. As the audience joins her in the hospital, she is bitten by a mosquito which triggers a sudden 'awakening'. Later, after taking revenge upon her abusers, she drags herself across the hospital and underground car-park, her muscles atrophied during her time in coma. Yet this physical consequence of her prolonged disorder of consciousness (PDoC, 'prolonged' being a diagnostic term relating to the fact that a patient has been 'unconscious for more than 4 weeks' (RCP 2020: 20)) is only temporary, as, lying on the flatbed of a commandeered van, she wills her 'limbs out of entropy' by repeating the mantra: 'Wiggle your big toe' (*Kill Bill Vol 1*, 2003).

This particular representation of coma within contemporary culture, it seems to me, is a good starting point for the discussions that will develop across this book. It does, after all, contain the visual language typical of so many fictional texts that portray this medical disorder: the idealized body of the coma-patient, beautifully groomed and often sexualized and/or fetishized; a sudden and immediate emergence from coma, cognition intact instantly, with no sign of long-term brain injury (BI). And while Tarantino does portray some of the effects of long-term vegetative states (muscle deterioration) this, again, is overcome through willpower and a linguistic imperative.

This image of an abused, comatose woman is similarly represented by the Spanish auteur Pedro Almodóvar in his 2002 film, *Hable con Ella* (*Talk To Her*). The film narrates parallel stories of two men who are supposedly in love with women who are in comas: one woman, Alicia, a former ballerina who lies in a vegetative state after being hit by a car; the other, Lydia, a female bullfighter who lies comatose after being gored by a bull in what seems to be a failed act of suicide. It is in the characterization of Alicia where the visual language of fairy tale is at its most extreme. Both Tarantino's representation of The Bride and Almodóvar's representation of Alicia are paradigms of what the neuroscientists Eelco and Coen Wijdicks term the '"Sleeping Beauty" phenomenon', a common trope that they discovered when analysing the representation of coma in 30 feature films released between 1970 and 2004. As they discuss, Alicia always appears on-screen perfectly groomed, serene, lips gently parted; as if merely asleep. Moreover, her body seems flawless and, as the Wijdicks further observe, there is no representation of the realities of the patient within a disorder of consciousness (DoC): bladder and bowel incontinence, muscle atrophy and decubital ulcers (bed sores) (2006: 3201). As Adrian Owen summarizes, 'In the Disney version of *Sleeping Beauty* . . . Aurora's condition resembles coma, akin to a bewitched slumber. In real life, the picture is far less romantic: disfiguring head injuries, contorted limbs, broken bones, and wasting illnesses are the norm' (2017: 4).

Throughout *Hable con Ella*, there is a prominent level of fetishization of the coma-body: the camera frequently lingers on the naked Alicia, peering at her through the half-open door of her hospital room or staring down at her from above, shots most often focalized through the perspective of the male protagonists. There are lengthy close-ups of the hands of Alicia's nurse, Benigno, as he massages her limbs in attempts to keep her muscles supple and her facial expression is constantly at rest and at peace; her lips softly rouged (Benigno, it is revealed, is both a medical professional and trained beautician), Alicia appears to await the kiss of some Prince Charming. The one muscle spasm she has occurs with an air of tranquillity, opening and closing one eye slowly, like the controlled, autonomic function of a child's doll.

The clinic in which Alicia is being treated is called El Bosque, or 'the forest': the contemporary setting in which the cursed or enchanted heroine resides, much like her fairy tale predecessors. As Adriana Novoa observes in her analysis of the film, '[C]oma is synonymous with the mysterious spells cast on beautiful, kind women in such stories as "Sleeping Beauty" and "Snow White"' (2005: 228). Alicia's 'protector' in the forest appears to be the nurse Benigno, but similarly to The Bride's guardian, Benigno turns out to be anything but *benign*. During a routine review at the clinic, hospital administrators notice that Alicia has missed several periods, although this is not immediately a cause of concern as this can be the case for patients within vegetative states. However, the explanation proves to be much more sinister as it is revealed that Alicia was raped by Benigno months before, again subverting the role of Prince Charming – or rather extrapolating the traditional heroic behaviour of the role to its most extreme, highlighting questions over the concept of sexual consent within fairy tale narratives. In the case of *Hable con Ella*, the 'kiss' of the Prince Charming, in the form of an extreme, sexual abuse of power, does conform to fairy tale ritual – it triggers an 'awakening' for Alicia, although through tragic circumstances: Alicia gives birth to a stillborn child which, in turn, breaks the 'curse'. Almodóvar, though, rather than depicting the actual moment of emergence from coma, instead focuses upon the aftermath, where it is revealed that Alicia, after her four-year coma (much like The Bride in Tarantino's film), has recovered with brain function intact, only requiring two sticks to help her walk.

Most recently, the violation of the comatose sleeping beauty appeared in David Lynch's *Twin Peaks: The Return*, the third instalment of his surreal horror-detective franchise. Within the series, it is revealed that Special Agent Dale Cooper's evil doppelgänger, shortly after emerging from the Red Room, visits the comatose Audrey Horne in hospital. It is only when we discover that the depraved antagonist Richard is her son do we begin to question what actually occurred within that hospital room the night of the doppelgänger's escape from the Red Room. It is a suspicion that is confirmed near the end of the series when the doppelgänger refers to Richard Horne as 'my son' (Ep.16, 'No Knock, No Doorbell', 2017). Lynch's co-writer, Mark Frost, further endorses this revelation in his literary series tie-in, *Twin Peaks: The Final Dossier*, with Special Agent Tammy Preston reiterating the fact that 'Cooper' was seen 'exiting the room in the ICU occupied by Audrey Horne' and that, 'Nine months later, almost to the day, Audrey Horne gave birth to her son Richard Horne. The birth certificate states the identity of the father as "unknown"' (2017: 21).

The representation of coma in these three media texts from contemporary culture not only reveals how writers and filmmakers perceive DoC but also the symbolism and language tropes with which they describe them. The sleep metaphor is one such example, with all three female protagonists emerging from prolonged coma with little or no long-term physical or neurological impairment (in Frost's *The Final Dossier*, Tammy Preston notes, 'Audrey awoke from the coma . . . after three and a half weeks. She apparently retained no memory of the event itself and at first seemed to be on her way to a complete recovery' (31)). This conflation of coma and sleep is not so surprising, the word coma, itself, derived from the Greek κῶμα (kōma) meaning 'deep sleep'. The confusion is compounded when looking at the Oxford English Dictionary's definition of coma: '"A state of unnatural, heavy, deep and prolonged sleep, with complete unconsciousness and slow, stertorous, often irregular, breathing", due to pressure on the brain, to the effect of certain poisons, or other causes, and frequently ending in death; stupor, lethargy.' This entry is conspicuous in that the first half borrows language from the *New Sydenham Society's Lexicon of Medicine and the Applied Sciences* in order to craft a definition of the 'sleep-like' state of coma – language to describe coma that itself first appears in 1882.

The prominent neuroscientist, Antonio Damasio, is quick to try and dispel the sleep mythology when he observes, 'It looks like sleep, it may sound like sleep, but it is not sleep' (2000: 236). So, if it is not a form of 'deep sleep' (as the name coma/kōma itself suggests), what is it? And how is it different from sleep? Baldly, a coma is a state of prolonged unconsciousness that can be caused by a range of problems: traumatic brain injury (TBI), stroke, brain tumour, drug or alcohol intoxication, alongside other pre-existing conditions, such as diabetes. Damasio discusses how when we sleep, we have the belief that we will wake up; that the concept and habit of sleep provokes no anxiety in the subject whatsoever. However, the comatose patient is quite different as, 'He cannot be awakened from the kind of sleep state he has been forced in, and the possibility of his recovering consciousness is not high' (2000: 237). Yet Damasio still can't seem to avoid those linguistic tics of 'awakened' and 'sleep state', despite warning against confusing coma with sleep. This use of the linguistic register of sleep when attempting to describe coma is common. The designation 'sleep-like' coma was used frequently throughout Fred Plum and Jerome B. Posner's seminal work on DoC, *The Diagnosis of Stupor and Coma* (1966), appearing in later editions up to and including the third edition of 1980. It is notable that the fourth edition, published in 2007, omits any reference to coma being 'sleep-like' and devotes more time to carefully drawing distinctions between sleep and coma. This edition clearly defines coma as, 'A state of unresponsiveness in which the patient lies with eyes closed and cannot be aroused to respond appropriately to stimuli even with vigorous stimulation' (Plum et al. 2007: 7). The patient may produce facial expressions in reaction to painful stimuli and limbs may withdraw from the stimulus itself but the patient does not exhibit defensive movements: movements that would reveal consciousness or comprehension. Coma is a DoC in which, 'A person is still alive but lacks any wakefulness or awareness' (Jarrett 2015: 273). Coma may also deepen, and as this occurs, responses to stimuli may dissipate or disappear altogether (Plum et al. 2007). Unlike sleep, there is no sleep/wake cycle in coma: patients do not experience REM (rapid eye movement) in which dreams occur and during which EEG readings appear to be similar to those of waking states.

The confusion caused by the slippage between language used to describe coma, though, doesn't start and end with the sleep metaphor. *Hable con Ella* introduces to us further confusions that are common in both fictional representations of coma but also in non-fictional reportage. Throughout the film, there are the constant references to so-called 'miracle awakenings' or recoveries (as represented, ultimately, by Alicia's own rehabilitation). There is also the slippage in language used to describe the PDoC that both Alicia and Lydia inhabit – Lydia is at once described as being in 'coma', while also having 'wakefulness', thereafter alternatively diagnosed as inhabiting a persistent vegetative state (PVS); and then there are numerous allusions to both Lydia and Alicia being 'brain-dead'. This is a diagnostic criterion (determining that a person has died if either their cardiovascular functioning has ceased or their brain has irreversibly stopped functioning (Jarret 2015: 278)) that would clearly negate their position as coma or PVS patients. Even though in the brain-death state patients lack all awareness and wakefulness, *as if in* coma, the diagnosis is different as 'their situation is irreversible and their lack of brain functioning is total – they are dead' (Jarret 2015: 279). While Lydia does indeed die later in the film, this is clearly not an accurate diagnosis for Alicia who later emerges from 'coma', with all brain functions immediately intact.

This interchangeability of language when describing very complex medical conditions seems to raise yet more questions: what exactly is the persistent vegetative state? And how is it different from coma? Returning to Damasio, he notes the possibility of what he terms 'deep coma' becoming 'lighter', eventually transitioning into a long-term state of unconsciousness: the persistent vegetative state (2000: 237). This term 'lightening' is a useful one, as it neatly sidesteps the linguistic trap of referring to a coma 'awakening'. It suggests a gradual emergence from coma with sleep/wake cycles appearing once more, as opposed to the hopeful possibility of a full and immediate recovery; as if merely stirring from sleep. However, this PDoC of PVS has a huge impact upon what I will discuss herein, exposing the phenomenon of the spectrum of consciousness upon which coma occupies but one position of many. For this reason, it is useful to look briefly at how the recognition of this complex spectrum of consciousness came about, before I examine the history of coma and its representation (alongside the language used to describe it) in more detail in Chapter 1.

In 1968, the Harvard Brain Death Committee made a ground-breaking decision that has shaped how we understand and define death and which has consequently helped to influence medico-legal policy: they developed a list of criteria that focused upon the diagnosis of death based upon the permanent failure of the brain to function. Prior to this, diagnosis of death was purely cardio-centric, based upon the irreversibility of cardio-respiratory functions. However, due to the increasingly inadequate and outmoded technologies (the basic empirical data gained, for example, from listening to the patient's heart through a stethoscope) and the rise in more advanced, life-supportive technologies (with machines that electro-mechanically provide and sustain cardio-respiratory functions), there was suddenly the need to move away from older cardio-centric diagnoses of death and towards a more satisfactory and ethically responsible one. There was also the development of MRI and CT scans, resulting in physicians being able to monitor the state of the brain, again allowing for more complex life-support mechanisms to be put in place. In 1971, a modification to diagnostic criteria of death was developed, known as the Minnesota criteria, which meant that, as Stephen Holland points out in his discussion of this landmark development in medicine and its impact upon bioethics, 'A patient is diagnosed as dead when their brain stem is dead' (2003: 71). As a consequence, there was a sudden rise of patients who were kept alive in near-death states, not least coma.

Then in 1972, a further complication arose. The two neurologists Fred Plum and Bryan Jennett identified what they called the 'persistent vegetative state', the PDoC in which patients who were previously in coma have 'progressed to a state of wakefulness without detectable awareness' (The Multi-Society Task Force on PVS 1994: 1499) and where 'sleeping and waking cycles return' (Plum and Posner 1980: 6).

This broadening of the divisions of DoC not only called into question the boundaries of consciousness itself, but also of the thresholds between life and death. Where exactly on the spectrum between consciousness and unconsciousness, life and death, does the coma patient sit? And what position on this spectrum does the patient in PVS occupy? This was to be complicated to an even greater degree when, in 2002, the 'minimally conscious state' (MCS) was diagnosed, defined as a 'condition of severely altered unconsciousness in which minimal but definite behavioural evidence or environmental awareness is demonstrated' (Fins, Schiff and Foley 2007: 305). Unlike PVS, the patient who reaches MCS has a good prognosis for significant recovery, although permanent disability is highly likely.

The recognition of these alternative PDoC has been significant both in aiding the developments of medical care for the coma, PV and MC patient and in simultaneously creating confusion and bafflement within the public arena, these conditions being often conflated or mythologized through popular representations – the conflation of PVS, coma and brain-death in *Hable con Ella*, for example. This is a repercussion that has also become common in media reportage that will often contain 'scientific inaccuracies, inconsistent diagnostic and descriptive terminology' alongside 'mismatches between the descriptions of [the patient's] state and the medical terms used to characterize it' and 'inaccurate prognoses' (Bernat 2008: 964).

One case in point that was much in the public eye concerning such confusions surrounding diagnostic reporting of coma and PDoC, arising out of the slippage of language to describe these conditions, is that of the Formula One driver Michael Schumacher. Since being brought out of his medically induced coma in January 2014 after suffering a severe BI during a skiing accident, media speculation over Schumacher's condition and the inconsistencies in language employed to voice these theories have been rife. An article from a January edition of *The Times* entitled 'Schumacher "is being brought out of coma"' (De Bruxelles 2014) included a photograph of the driver with the caption, 'Michael Schumacher: "can open his eyes and squeeze a hand"'. However, on reading the article, it transpires that this revelation was merely a speculation formulated by the French newspaper *L'Equipe* that was refuted by Schumacher's manager. The way this conjecture had been used by *The Times* as a pull-quote, however, imbued the article with a sense of hope and veracity to be later questioned by a report from *The Express* almost six months later. This article queried the 'level of progress' that Schumacher had actually made since coming out of coma, even writing of the 'fears that he could remain in a permanent vegetative state' (Hall 2014). *The Times*, around the same time as the report in *The Express*, ran the article, 'Michael Schumacher "an invalid for life" says coma specialist' (Charter 2014) and yet soon afterwards, *The Metro* ran a report in which the former Ferrari boss Jean Todt was quoted as saying that Schumacher could expect to lead a 'relatively normal life' (Mackay and Hall 2014) in the near future. Most recently, reports have been circulating that suggest that Schumacher is to undergo stem cell surgery, with one article from *The Guardian* noting that he 'is reported to have muscle atrophy and osteoporosis from being confined to bed for six years' (Richards 2020).

The professor of intensive care at Edinburgh University, Peter Andrews, reveals his deliberate decision to select carefully medico-linguistic terminology when talking about coma that is significant in this discussion. Quoted in an article concerning the Schumacher case in *The Guardian*, Andrews talks of how he avoids 'the term "awaken" because it could trigger too high expectations among relatives' (Oltermann 2014). This advocacy for the careful representation of DoC was likewise voiced by several doctors in an article that was openly concerned with the reportage of Schumacher's accident published in *The Telegraph* in June 2014. In this report, the former Formula One physician Dr Gary Hartstein described the overly optimistic recovery claims and the opacity and confusion of media reportage as 'a highly cynical use of language, using the truth to convey an impression that is almost certainly false' (Paterson 2014).

We can therefore see the precarious role that language plays within medico-cultural discussions. In truth, the prognosis for patients within long-term vegetative states is rarely positive. Plum and Posner assert how coma almost never lasts more than two to four weeks, after which the patient enters a chronically unresponsive state (1980: 3). This is a position reinforced by Dr David Bates who notes, in outlining an aetiology and sequelae of coma, that the longer a patient remains in coma the poorer his or her chance of recovery (Bates 2001: 21), a reality at odds with reportage of Schumacher's condition and the representations of coma in *Kill Bill* and *Hable con Ella*, whose heroines have both been in four-year "comas", and *Twin Peaks: The Return*, Audrey's coma lasting a little shy of four weeks.

In my discussions of the representations of coma thus far, I have been primarily focusing on one particular perspective; that is, the perspective of the coma patient in treatment, or the patient now out of coma: in 'recovery'. Whereas this constitutes what I would term 'exterior' coma literature where the focus is placed upon a third-person perspective of the patient still in coma, there is another category: 'interior' coma literature with a narrative focus upon the subjective experience of the coma victim. It therefore follows that if many of the external narratives treat the patient of coma as a sleeping subject, then the internal narratives represent the subjective coma experience using the language and imagery of dream, often creating complex, nightmarish worlds of the unconscious. BBC One's series *Life On Mars* (2006/7), for example, depicts an interior state of coma through representing and parodying the 1970s era, often drawing upon cultural icons from that period, not least the representation of the police force, metonymically embodied by the politically incorrect Gene Hunt, a parodic homage to such 'realist' police dramas as *The Sweeney*. The coma-protagonist

Sam Tyler, a noughties police officer trapped in coma after a near-fatal car accident, is drawn into solving crimes within this alternate reality. But even this reality is constantly threatening to break down, as clinicians in the outside world interact with his comatose body and attempt to trigger an emergence from coma. The television screen in his bedsit acts as a conduit between his comatose psyche and the outside world, with, for example, the little girl holding the toy clown in the old BBC test card and Open University professors with customary leather elbow-patches and helmet-strap beards offering advice to Tyler, attempting to force him into facing up to the reality of his coma.

The coma-as-dream device can similarly be seen in David Chase's series *The Sopranos*. In the final season, the central protagonist, Tony, spends several episodes within coma, this particular production exploiting the soft-focus 'white-tunnel' imagery of the near-death experience alongside, as in *Life On Mars*, representations of the interiorization of external stimuli. In one scene, Tony bangs on the wall of his hotel within the world of coma in order to silence the incessant chattering of his neighbour, language which enters his unconscious from the external world and becomes interiorized, assimilated and translated into his subjective experience of coma as a form of irritating white noise (*The Sopranos*, 'Mayham' 2006). The identity of the speaker in the world outside of coma is significant: the gangster and associate of Tony, Paulie Walnuts, with whom Tony has a volatile relationship. Despite not recognizing individual words being spoken, it is suggested that Tony, subconsciously in his coma, registers the identity of the speaker. All of Tony's frustrations and irritations that he associates with Paulie translate the distant flow of incomprehensible language into an overall impression and dream-symbol: the incessant, disruptive chatter coming through the wall of a neighbouring hotel room.

Kevin Bigley's *Comaville*, too, depicts the coma patient assimilating and translating external stimuli. At one point the protagonist Josh Husk, unaware he is in coma and navigating through an uncanny coma-dream stitched together from a kaleidoscope of memories, feels 'inky' raindrops 'spitting . . . down upon him'. When he looks around him, he finds that no one else in his immediate proximity is being rained upon (2019: 56). The following chapter, narrated from the external subject position of Josh's loved ones, reveals that Josh's partner is in fact crying over his comatose body, tears dripping onto his face, washing him in a 'salty rainfall' (57).

There are still many mysteries that surround what actually occurs within the subjective experience of coma patients. Damasio points out that patients who return to consciousness after being in coma often recall the descent into the 'nothingness' of the disorder, yet nothing is remembered of the period while in coma (2000: 95). What occurs within coma appears to be a blank in consciousness, but it also represents a blank in empirical knowledge. This, in turn, constitutes a blank canvas for writers of fiction, offering them a wealth of creative potential. Writers invariably draw upon classic dream imagery, tales of mythical quests and mythological symbolism and the language and ideas of depth and archetypal psychology in developing complex coma interiorities, often exploring coma as a psychological phenomenon. Yet survivors of long-term coma will most often sustain permanent, organic brain damage that not only wipes memory, but can also indelibly alter personality and identity, leading to ongoing trauma post-coma: what Catherine Malabou refers to as the 'shredded' psyche (2012: 48). However, the reality of BI is rarely depicted in fiction, writers seemingly less interested in the real-life consequences of DoC, resulting in the proliferation of what I term the 'soap opera paradigm' of BI. With this model, we see characters emerge from coma or sustain a BI after which they are 'changed' in some way, this change often manifesting as amnesia. It then only takes a second blow to the head for the protagonist to 'return' to his pre-injured self; to return from the 'abnormal' to the 'normal'. I will investigate examples of such 'soap opera' representations in more detail throughout this volume, but for illustrative purposes, I will revisit *Twin Peaks: The Return*. After Cooper escapes from the limbo (the 'dream-coma') of the Red Room, for the majority of the series he inhabits the life of insurance salesman Dougie Jones. But more than this: his emergence into the 'real' world has delivered a total stun to the senses and profound amnesia. In essence, Cooper has no idea of who or where he is, experiencing this new life for the first time – a man reborn. Living with this de facto BI, Cooper/Dougie gradually learns to function again as a 'whole' being, like a child developing within its environment. Yet all this changes when he is suddenly drawn to an electrical socket after hearing the name of his old boss, Gordon Cole, on the television. Cooper/Dougie pokes a fork into the socket and receives a massive electrical shock, sending him into coma (Ep.15, 'There's Some Fear In Letting Go', 2017). Later, on emerging from coma, he has returned to his self, all of Cooper's senses and memories and behaviours reinstated (Ep.16, 'No Knock, No Doorbell'). The electrical shock and second coma/limbo (after the coma/limbo of the Red Room) acts as the second blow to the head of the soap opera paradigm allowing Cooper to return. For Lynch, coma holds a particular fascination which maybe comes as no surprise given the director's interest in liminal states, transcendental meditation and dream, and the mysteries of coma that allow him to explore these ideas.

This elision of the permanence of BI on behalf of writers of fiction deploying the soap opera paradigm resonates with G. Thomas Couser's observation of a 'general rhetorical imperative' within first-person illness narratives that he terms 'the tyranny of the comic plot', that is, the 'strong preference in the literary marketplace for a positive "narrative arc", i.e., a happy ending' (2016: 4). Pertinent to this discussion of the translation of illness to narrative, Theodor Adorno, in his development of aesthetic theory, discusses authors' use of language to communicate suffering, referring to 'fantastic art in romanticism' with its 'presentation of the nonempirical as if it were empirical' (1997: 19). This perhaps provides a further explanation of what writers of coma fiction are doing: their depictions having no real origin in the empirical as in most cases, survivors of coma emerge with little or no memory of what occurs within the unconscious state. The historian and scholar of trauma studies, Dominick LaCapra, warns against 'fetishized and totalizing narratives', stories of trauma that are overly focused upon 'harmonizing events, and then recuperating the past in terms of uplifting messages or optimistic, self-serving scenarios' (2001: 78). In other words, he remains sceptical and critical of aestheticizing trauma and the rush towards the universal 'happy ending' for which Couser also holds suspicion. Returning briefly to *Hable con Ella*, we may deem it to be the classic soap opera paradigm of a fetishized and harmonized narrative where a full recovery is possible, despite the means of her metaphorical 'second blow to the head' – her stillborn child, itself a product of rape. Wijdicks and Wijdicks are similarly highly critical of such a comic plot, proposing that this 'may be a conscious decision to maximize entertainment but is a disservice to the viewer' (2006: 1301). Yet the American physician and medical ethicist Joseph J. Fins, known for his work on vegetative states and BI, in a rejoinder to Wijdicks and Wijdicks's commentary on coma and film, points out that while the portrayal of Alicia's recovery is fanciful, it is nevertheless 'metaphorically powerful', going on to assert that 'there can be little doubt about the accuracy of [Almodóvar's] portrayal of the personal and social isolation of severe brain injury' (2007: 79).

Throughout this book, I will discuss such complexities and controversies of interior and exterior representations of both coma and BI, across many works of literature, film and media, eliciting some of the creative and, occasionally, ethical challenges that arise in the field of illness and disability narratives. For this reason, I will draw on a range of both intertwining and competing theory: literary, cultural and narrative theory; trauma and disability studies; psychology and neurology. It is hoped that by doing this, I will succeed in developing nuanced analyses of texts from multiple perspectives that will help to fully interrogate society's fascination with coma and liminal states of consciousness.

Developing some of the central concerns set out here, Chapter 1 will discuss the medical condition of coma itself, alongside other DoC and BI. Taking the lead from Koehler and Wijdicks's informative yet concise historical overview of coma, I will expand this primarily from a linguistic perspective, exploring how the word 'coma' has shifted in meaning over time. Contextualizing this analysis within discussions of key historical events and scientific thinking, I will examine how such factors have helped shape our understanding (and misunderstanding) of coma. I will also look at how advances in neurology and the development of new technologies have allowed us to gain more knowledge of the workings of the brain (alongside insights into the sequelae of different forms of BI) but have simultaneously created confusion in the identification of multiple PDoC lying on a hierarchical spectrum, leading to a wide range of bioethical debates. Scientific advances have also given rise to confusion surrounding the BI survivor and his behaviours. Neuroscience and neuroscientific medicine recognizes the distinction between 'functional' and 'organic' sequelae of BI, that is, the distinction between 'mind' and 'brain'. This in turn has separated scientific and clinical disciplines, for example, psychology from neurology. This split is exemplified, as I will discuss, by debates surrounding the cause of shell shock that arose around and between the two World Wars, debates which are still raging today. Running parallel to this historio-linguistic/scientific analysis will be a literary and cultural study exploring the fascination with unconscious and semi-conscious states and BI, discussing, for example, the image of coma/rebirth in mythology alongside the popularity of somnambulism and the 'sleeping beauty' exhibit within Victorian-era 'freak shows' and how these fed into the coma-as-sleep paradigm, despite growing evidence to the contrary within the burgeoning field of neurology. Finally, taking Susan Sontag's *Illness As Metaphor* and *AIDS And Its Metaphors*, I will examine how current metaphors of coma often 'romanticize' the condition and how metaphors of BI 'demonize' and stigmatize the condition thereby building a theoretical bedrock upon which subsequent discussions of both fictional and non-fictional metaphors of coma and BI can be built.

Taking two contemporary novels (Irvine Welsh's *Marabou Stork Nightmares* and Alex Garland's *The Coma*) as a starting point, Chapter 2 will examine the use of memory and exile motifs within coma fiction, looking closely at how texts represent the comatose self in exile. I will look at how coma embodies the ultimate form of exile, with the 'self' wrenched out of society and plunged into 'the deep well of emptiness' (Owen 2017: 1). I will explicate my analysis by interrogating various theories of trauma and exile, paying specific attention to Edward Said's essay, 'Reflections on Exile'. As touched upon earlier, many works of interior coma fiction, in particular, equate the state of coma with dream narratives. It therefore follows that such works depict protagonists' descent into coma as a psychoanalytical confrontation with the repressed secrets of the unconscious which exacerbates the feeling of exile. For this reason, I will analyse the key texts in light of some core psychoanalytical theory of the twentieth century, most notably that developed by Freud and Jacques Lacan. In keeping with the theme of exile, I will also draw on Freud's work on traumatic departures, as well as Cathy Caruth's contemporary revision of Freudian trauma theory. In this way, I hope to redress the fact that, as Couser points out, 'Trauma studies has largely ignored disability as an area of trauma' (2016: 9).

Chapter 3 will focus on the resurrection/katabasis motifs in coma fiction, motifs also present within texts discussed in the previous chapter. Central to this analysis will be Stephen King's *The Dead Zone* (a mainstream exponent of popular fiction). I will look at how the image of biblical death (and resurrection) mirrors the idea of coma: a descent into a death-state whereby one is alienated from society; an 'awakening' (or resurrection) and subsequent 'transfiguration' in which the self may be altered inexorably. As part of my application and analysis of biblical motifs, I will look at Peter Redgrove's poem 'Lazarus and the Sea' and Sylvia Plath's 'Lady Lazarus', focusing on how these overt references to the famous bible story use the language and symbolism of the story of Lazarus to explore the coma-state. I will also look at how some coma texts adopt the language and imagery of the narratives of hellish 'descent' – tales of coma-katabasis that echo, for example, Greco-Roman mythologies. I will discuss such texts as Iain Banks's *The Bridge* and Liz Jensen's *The Ninth Life of Louis Drax*, drawing out and exploring images of the katabatic quest narrative. I will establish the context of my analysis by looking at traditional bible stories, most notably those of Lazarus, Jonah and Christ himself while drawing upon contemporary interpretations of these stories, not least Nikos Kazantzakis's controversial novel, *The Last Temptation*. I will similarly focus on katabatic imagery in Greek and Roman mythology, drawing links between coma texts and, among others, Homer's *Odyssey* and Virgil's the *Aeneid*. In addition, I will look at Freudian and Jungian theories of the mind, while examining the language of 'excavation' often used in the practice of depth psychology – the need to 'dig down' into the mind to locate a hidden trauma. This image of excavation is similarly pertinent to the notion of katabasis – of the descent into hell – and I will elicit how authors of coma fiction use the image of excavation for their protagonists who have to dig deeper into their interior state of coma in order to try and attain 'resurrection'.

Chapter 4 will herald the second section of the book, moving away from the focus on interior coma narratives and beginning to examine the other end of the spectrum: post-coma narratives that deal, specifically, with the trauma of emerging from coma and dealing with the effects of coma and BI. At the heart of this chapter will be Tom McCarthy's post-trauma novel *Remainder* which depicts an unnamed narrator, struggling to come to terms with his new identity post-coma and post-rehabilitation. I will examine the notion of authenticity of selfhood, and the ramifications of this post-traumatic BI, discussing the novel in light of Jean Baudrillard and Umberto Eco's theory of simulacra. The chapter will conclude with an examination of post-trauma simulacra in real-world scenarios, as detailed in the documentary film, *Marwencol*, which tells the story of Mark Hogancamp, a coma survivor and BI victim who now creates and photographs dramatic tableaux of dolls as a way of retelling the story of his traumatic attack that caused his coma and injuries. Throughout the chapter, I will interrogate Marco Roth's concept of the 'neuronovel' and, most recently, Stephen Burns's development of this concept, which examines how there has been a gradual shift from novels concerned with the mind towards novels concerned with the brain: from functional psychiatry to organic neurology, a boundary that is now commonly criticized 'for maintaining an artificial distinction between psychiatry and neurology' (Bell et al. 2020: 3).

Building on the discussion of stories of real-life coma survival, Chapter 5 will examine further the lived experience of coma survival and BI. Taking such texts as James Cracknell and Beverley Turner's *Touching Distance* alongside Catherine Malabou's philosophical analysis of trauma and BI, *The New Wounded*, I will discuss the experiences of coma and BI survivors and the language tropes used to describe both the coma itself, but also the lived experience of long-term neurological conditions. As part of this, I will discuss the patient narratives generated through a writing group I have been running for the past few years, drawing links between linguistic tropes within these narratives and other patient narratives in the public domain. I will explore how, rather than the coma-state being a form of complex dreamscape that much of fiction would have us believe, in most cases, patients remember nothing of coma.

Following on from the previous chapter, Chapter 6 will draw my discussions to a close, developing, in more detail, the disparity between the language used to describe coma in fiction and the language used by coma and BI survivors. Coming full circle, I will return to Sontag's theories of illness and metaphor but reappraising them in light of more recent theory, most notably Anne Hunsaker Hawkins's work on metaphorical tropes in autopathographies – first-person patient narratives. I will explicate this analysis by looking at the use of negative BI metaphors in the media, discussing the fascination with the figure of the 'neomort' (the 'new dead', residing within PDoC). Building on discussions here, I will examine how fictional representations impact upon our collective understanding of the condition of coma, often propagating mythologies of coma and overly hyped prospects of coma survival, thereby leading to what Nik Brown, among other academics, have termed the 'hope economy'. Analysing such texts as Robin Cook's *Coma* and Douglas Coupland's *Girlfriend in a Coma*, alongside numerous examples of media reportage (including famous right-to-die cases of patients within PDoC), I will examine in close detail the interface between metaphor and linguistic tropes of coma survival and this economy of hope.

George Canguilhem, in his brilliant treatise on concepts of health and disease and their relationship to institutional power and practices of normalization, observes that, 'It is the abnormal which arouses theoretical interest in the normal. Norms are recognized as such only when they are broken. Functions are revealed only when they fail' (1991: 209). What follows in this volume will be an interrogation of a range of texts that explore the 'abnormal' of coma and wider PDoC and yet which often erase this abnormality in favour of the normal – sleep; dream. Simultaneously, the 'abnormality' of BI is also most often erased in favour of the comic plot. In this way, many of the texts I will refer to employ what Mitchell and Snyder have termed 'narrative prosthesis', that is, 'disability as a narrative device' (2000: 51). The controlling theme of this book is what occurs when writers attempt to make 'comprehensible that which appears to be inherently unknowable' (Mitchell and Snyder 2000: 6) by using narrative prosthesis. In the process, I hope to illustrate how linguistic and literary analyses of a full range of texts can lead us to understanding our attitudes towards grave medical conditions, disability; even death.

For now, though, one final word regarding my use of the word 'coma'. Throughout this book, I will be referring to a multitude of texts which purport to represent the DoC, 'coma'. However, as touched upon in this introductory chapter, due to the protracted length of the period of unconsciousness that is often represented (a period that frequently exceeds four weeks), many of these texts, in reality, depict PDoC rather than coma – PVS or MCS, perhaps. And oftentimes, as seen in *Hable con Ella*, texts knowingly conflate these conditions. But more on that later.

1

Contextualizing coma and brain injury
A linguistic, cultural and medical history

Towards the end of his treatise on the psychology of dream processes in his seminal *The Interpretation of Dreams*, Sigmund Freud describes an anxiety dream he had as a child. He describes his mother 'with a curiously calm look on her face, as if she was asleep', being carried by a group of shadowy figures with birds' beaks who proceed to lay his mother upon a bed (2006: 598). In unpicking the symbolism of the dream, Freud writes, 'My mother's facial expression in the dream was copied from that of my grandfather, *whom I had seen in a coma*, snoring, a few days prior to his death' (2006: 599, emphasis added). Freud conflating coma with a form of deep sleep or stupor (describing his grandfather's 'snoring') is a telling insight, informing us of how the term 'coma' was applied well into the twentieth century.

So far, I have outlined some of the common confusions surrounding coma and BI, and some of the widespread cultural tropes employed to depict or interrogate these conditions (the coma-as-sleep metaphor being one key example and one used in Freud's moment of self-reflective psychoanalysis). This chapter will seek to explore exactly how and why these misunderstandings have proliferated over the centuries. What follows is a linguistic, scientific and cultural review of the development of the medical term coma (and its gradual shift in meaning and association), a term that appeared in the earliest medical texts by both Hippocrates and Galen. As Koehler and Wijdicks point out in their historical study of coma and its use in the arena of medicine, 'Over the centuries, several terms were used to describe the phenomena that were observed and to grade the level of (un)consciousness' (2008: 877). Over the course of this chapter, I will look at a range of these alternative terms, while simultaneously examining how developments in an understanding of the brain and consciousness (in both neurology and psychiatry) led to the streamlining of these terms as more precise and symptom-specific diagnostic labels. Not only has the understanding and treatment of coma, as a medical condition, undergone a gradual evolution over many centuries, so has the very meaning of the word itself, the current coma/sleep conflation, as we shall see, constituting a metaphorical and linguistic hangover of this evolutionary process.

1.1 The diagnosis of coma and brain injury: beginnings

The Greek term coma [kōma] ('deep sleep') appears numerously across the Hippocratic corpus, this early physician seemingly applying it to a wide range of diseases and medical case studies. Christos Yapijakis draws attention to the fact that it was Hippocrates (460–377 BCE) who not only established the basic praxis of clinical medicine still in use today (the system of examination; observation of symptoms; diagnosis; treatment) but that he was also responsible for introducing a range of descriptive terms for diseases still used in modern medicine; and 'coma', Yapijakis points out, was one of these terms (2009: 508). In describing the outbreak of 'causus', a febrile malady that appears to be an umbrella term for a number of common fevers in the Levant (typhoid being one example), Hippocrates observes that around the eleventh day of infection, especially in the case of children, 'The malady was associated with coma and these cases were the most rarely fatal of all' (1978: 96). The notion that protracted coma is equated with a good prognosis of recovery is a surprising one given the fact that survival rates decrease the longer the patient inhabits coma. Elsewhere, Hippocrates details the case study of a woman who 'was seized with a fever while in the third month of pregnancy'. He outlines her worsening condition up until her death, with her symptoms, on the sixth day, including 'coma, nausea, shivering and delirium' (1978: 111–12). This grants us the biggest clue as to how the denomination 'coma' was applied. The fact that what we now understand to be 'the deepest form of unconsciousness' (Mindell 1989: 74) in which 'patients are utterly unresponsive and unaware' (Jarrett 2015: 274) is paired with conscious, embodied actions of vomiting and shivering suggests that coma, in these early developments of medicine, was more closely associated with its original meaning, a deep sleep (or drifting consciousness associated with fever), rather than an unresponsive DoC.

This particular usage of the medical term is made clear in Hippocratic case studies whereby patients are described as slipping in and out of 'coma', moving between periods of lucidity, as in the case of a man suffering from 'heaviness of the head and right temporal pain'. Hippocrates observes that on the eighteenth day, he was 'not lucid, comatose' yet by the twentieth day the man 'slept, was fully lucid' (1978: 114–15). This is of particular value in examining the shifting meaning of 'coma' as medical diagnosis as Hippocrates makes the subtle implication that there is a difference between coma [kōma] and sleep [hypnos / ýpnos]. Similarly, in Book III of his *Epidemics*, Hippocrates, in writing of patients suffering from causus, observes that, 'They were also afflicted with a continuous coma but something that differed from sleep' (1978: 123). This lack of precision becomes even more apparent when examining the writings of another medical pioneer of the ancient world, and disciple of Hippocrates, the Greek physician, Galen of Persamon (AD 129–216).

Throughout his treatises on diseases and their symptoms (and in his continued development of the humoral theories of medicine proposed by Hippocrates) Galen discusses 'coma' as a symptom of many diseases while also discussing a range of other DoC which kaleidoscopically merge into one another, eluding precise definitions. In writing of what he terms the 'cold diseases', brought about through an imbalance (*dyscrasia*) of the four humours of phlegm, blood, yellow and black bile, Galen observes: 'Extreme constriction, for we certainly established this as the third cause of cold diseases, brings about unconsciousness (*karos*), coma (*koma*) and apoplexy' (2006: 165). Sitting alongside 'unconsciousness' and 'apoplexy', we may assume, again, that 'coma' was used to describe a kind of sleep-like state whereas apoplexy/*karos* may be assumed to be a deeper state of unconsciousness. The closest we get to a diagnostic definition and differentiation of *karos* and *koma* is in Galen's discussion of the differentiae of symptoms where he writes, 'There is something akin to paralysis, which is termed unconsciousness (*karos*) or catalepsy (*katalepsis*) . . . and something akin to a deficiency or weakness, as in comas (*koma*ta) and lethargies (*lethargia*)' (2006: 191). While this comes close to distinguishing between DoC (karos is equated with paralysis; koma with a certain 'weakness'), matters are further confused by the expansion of the spectrum of consciousness by introducing further terms that appear to elide with one another. Karos is comparable to katalepsis (itself a medical term in its own right, today defined as a nervous condition characterized by rigid muscles, fixed posture and heightened pain threshold) and koma is comparable to lethargia (defined, in today's medicine, as a pathological state of sleepiness or deep unresponsiveness and inactivity).

Buried within the works of Hippocrates and Galen we also discover passing comments relating to BI that reveal two polarized attitudes to the condition, its treatment and prognosis, attitudes that still abound today and which are often reflected, as we shall see, in fictional images of brain trauma. In Hippocrates's *Aphorisms*, there appears the following assertion: 'A lesion of the bladder, *brain*, heart, diaphragm, stomach, liver, or any of the small intestines, *proves fatal*' (1817: 129, emphasis added), thereby declaring a pessimistic prognosis for the BI survivor that was to become characteristic of the Hippocratic School of Medicine which viewed 'the treatment of brain injury as invariably futile' (Fins 2015: 32). However, in the marginalia of Galen's own copy of the *Aphorisms*, is a telling, hand-written refutation of this position by Galen himself: 'But I have seen a severely wounded brain healed', a surprising rejection of a central tenet of the Hippocratic school. Such is the significance of this boldly optimistic statement from Galen that the founder of the Montreal Neurological Institute (MNI, opened in 1934), the neurosurgeon and neuroscientist, Wilder Penfield, had these very words inscribed into the intricate ceiling of the building. This entrance to the MNI reflects, according to Adams and Fins, 'Galen and Penfield's shared faith in the brain's resilience to heal itself and in healers to heal the injured brain' (2017: 835). Galen's assertion was not merely born out of a theoretical or hypothetical fit of pique, though. Unlike the practice of Hippocrates, where there is very little evidence to suggest that there was any neuroanatomical research methodology developed, Galen did carry out public experiments and vivisections, even performing neuroanatomical surgery on live animals, thereby refining the Hippocratic technique through the addition of empirically testable experimental rigour to clinical medicine of the ancient world (Adams and Fins 2017: 855). In Galen's *On Anatomical Procedures*, we see such case studies of live experimentations (often on ungulates) which begin to reveal very early observations of how brain trauma can lead to DoC. Detailing his dissection of the brain of a live animal, Galen writes how compression of the 'two anterior ventricles' of the brain lead to a 'stupor . . . which is slight'. Compression of the 'middle ventricle' induces a 'heavier' stupor; 'And when pressing down upon that ventricle which is found in the part of the brain lying at the nape of the neck, then the animal falls into a very heavy and pronounced stupor' (1962: 19). These are hugely important findings, made more significant by the fact that Galen goes on to discuss how some animals, depending upon which parts of the brain (through incision) were traumatized (and how severely), could 'return to the normal condition'. We may assume, then, that these early neurological experiments led to Galen's own, anti-Hippocratic aphorism. Moreover, he also transposed such experiments to the human subject, drawing 'conclusions about prognosis and brain injury from his own clinical encounters with brain-injured humans who received trepanation'. Again, during this surgical procedure, Galen would apply pressure to both anterior ventricles to induce 'a slight stupor' (Adams and Fins 2017: 857). Adams and Fins further point out that, in distinguishing the different impact trauma has upon the anterior and posterior chambers of the brain in both ungulates and humans, 'Galen made one of the first attempts to localize cerebral function, establishing an early nosology' (837). It is also interesting to note in this particular translation of Galen's *On Anatomical Procedures* by W. L. H. Duckworth, that he uses the word 'stupor', from the original ΚάρΟς or *karos*, alternatively interpreted by Ian Johnston, in his translation of Galen's *On Diseases and Symptoms*, as 'unconsciousness'. Here again, we have confusion as to what, exactly, the PDoC being produced in these experiments (in terms of our current understanding) constitutes, yet at the same time providing valuable insight into and context surrounding earlier conceptions of states of unconsciousness and the language used to describe them.

1.2 The sleep/death metaphor in mythology and religion

Koehler and Wijdicks note that Galen recognized that DoC were associated with an increased tendency to sleep (878) and the medical terms adopted and attributed to a variety of levels of consciousness echo this position. Yet sleep, itself, within culture, religion and mythology was widely and metaphorically compared with death. This sleep/death metaphor has huge implications for our interpretation and understanding of the coma/sleep metaphor, leading to an increasingly complex phenomenon: the coma-as-sleep-and-death trope.

This elision between sleep, death and unconsciousness is particularly apparent within classical mythology and no more so than in the Greco-Roman tradition. In Greek mythology, for example, the god of death, Thanatos, and the god of sleep, Hypnos, are twin brothers – two sides of the same coin who dwell not on Mount Olympus, but in Hades, alongside the dead, disembodied inhabitants of the underworld. Morpheus, Hypnos's son and the god of dreams, also resides within Hades, and although he is primarily responsible for visiting (often in human shape) sleepers in the overworld, delivering to them dreams, he 'sometimes convey[s] messages from the dead' (Harris and Platzner 1995: 199). Hades, itself, is not just represented as a place in which the souls of the dead reside, or where they are punished with hellfire and torment, as in Christian beliefs. There is a special place within Hades reserved just for this purpose: Tartarus, 'An almost bottomless pit of anguish and despair, a divine torture chamber'

(Harris and Platzner 1995: 200). However, Tartarus is primarily reserved for punishing those who have sinned against the Olympian gods themselves; within Hades, more globally, the dead (or the 'shades') wander aimlessly, numbed and mindless, losing all connections to their past and what tied them to the land of the living. As Harris and Platzner note: 'While depriving the soul of substance, death simultaneously impairs memory, reason, and will', with Thanatos severing the most intimate bonds of 'kinship and affection' (194). This is a concept of death as a condition of stupor or apoplexy: as a sustained, numbing DoC. This stupefying nothingness of the Homeric underworld, Michael Shermer points out, was also the foundation upon which Jewish teachings built their concept of the post-death world of Sheol, an equivalent to Hades: 'Not the hell of Christianity, but rather simply *nothing*' (2018: 52); a place of absolute darkness. Shermer discusses how the author of Ecclesiastes reflects upon the notion that, 'The living know that they shall die: but the dead know not any thing, neither have they any more a reward; for the memory of them is forgotten' (Eccles. 9.5, in Shermer 2018: 52). This biblical language and imagery of the insensibility of death (or death being commutable with a DoC) has its equivalence in the concept of Lethe within Greek mythology. As originally conceived by Plato in the 'Myth of Er', Lethe was described as a plain within Hades through which, according to the philosopher, 'a river of unmindfulness' flows. Literally meaning 'oblivion', the name Lethe was later attributed to the river itself (Hades' fifth river) by Roman poets (Harris and Platzner 1995: 195), further contributing to the tradition of equating death and the underworld with psychological or neurological stupefaction.

In Christian teachings, throughout both the Old and New Testament the word 'sleep' is similarly used to signify 'death', once more emphasizing the symbiotic metaphor developed within the Greco-Roman tradition. In the book of Daniel, for example, written in the second-century BCE, there is the following reference to the future resurrection of the dead: 'And many of them that sleep in the dust of the earth shall awake, some to everlasting life, and some to shame and everlasting contempt' (Dan. 12.2). In the New Testament, there is the account of the raising of the daughter of Jairus where Christ says of the dead girl, '"Why make ye this ado, and weep? The damsel is not dead, but sleepeth"' (Mark 5.39). And in St. Paul's letters to the Corinthians, we find the following passage: 'Behold, I shew you a mystery; we shall not all sleep, but we shall all be changed | In a moment, in the twinkling of an eye, at the last trump: for the trumpet shall sound, and the dead shall be raised incorruptible, and we shall be changed' (1 Cor. 51–52). The resurrection from death, and subsequent transfiguration, is as simple as an arousal from sleep, a key image, as I will demonstrate in chapter three, for writers of katabatic coma fiction.

1.3 Towards a detailed understanding of the brain and (un)consciousness: scientific advancements in the nineteenth century

In the middle of the nineteenth century, there occurs an explosion of interest in the mysteries of the human brain and consciousness, as well as a fascination with disordered and altered states of consciousness. This leads to a proliferation of theories of mind and a further expansion of medical terms to describe, diagnose and form prognoses of a range of DoC.

Prior to this, the history of the word 'coma', alongside the use of wider terms to describe unconscious states, is a little patchy in detail. Koehler and Wijdicks observe that after Galen's prolific use of 'coma' as a medical term during the second century AD, the word is rarely used in the extant literature up to the middle of the seventeenth century. They also note how in this century, the terms coma, lethargy, apoplexy and carus are still being used in influential medical texts, most notably Thomas Willis's (1621–75) *De Anima Brutorum*. These are terms that resonate with Galen's lexicon though tellingly, Willis attempts to delineate between the terms, with lethargy defined as pathological sleep (which he localized in the outer cortex of the brain), coma (heavy sleeping), carus (a depravation of the senses) and apoplexy, 'into which carus could turn and which [Willis] localized in the white matter, . . . [this] sequence indicating increasingly deeper forms of unresponsiveness' (Koehler and Wijdicks 2008: 878). Willis therefore adopts the medically vague terms developed and applied by Galen to describe various DoC and attempts to formalize them into a diagnostical hierarchy or spectrum.

During the eighteenth century, this notion of DoC being associated with an 'increased tendency to sleep' (Koehler and Wijdicks 2008: 878) continues to be adopted, not least by the Dutch scientist Herman Boerhaave who wrote that coma 'is the perfect image of a very profound sleep' with there being 'little distinction unless by duration' (Koehler and Wijdicks 2008: 878, 882). This statement is evocative of Antonio Damasio's mantra, written over two-hundred and fifty years later, that coma 'may look like sleep, it may sound like sleep, but it is not sleep' (2000: 236). The coma-as-sleep trope, Koehler and Wijdicks discuss, continues to proliferate throughout the eighteenth century until the French physician Francois Boissier de Sauvages de Lacroix in 1763 identified his own spectrum of consciousness, defining 'comata' as 'diminution or total loss of the powers of voluntary motion, and perception, with somnolence' (882). We begin to see a definition, for the first time, that achieves some sense of parity with the contemporary definition and usage of the term: 'A state of unarousable psychologic unresponsiveness in which the subjects lie with eyes closed' (Plum and Posner 1980: 5).

Another key text of this period is the second book of William Cullen's *First Lines of the Practice of Physic* (1790) in which he includes a section devoted to DoC entitled, 'Of Comata, or the loss of Voluntary Motions', with sub-sections thereafter covering 'apoplexy' and 'palsy'. Proposing that this section of the book will discuss 'affections which have been commonly called the soporific diseases', Cullen goes on to make a key distinction between coma/apoplexy and, in effect, sleeping disorders: 'But they are most properly distinguished by their consisting in some interruption or suppression of the powers of sense and voluntary motion, or of what are called the animal functions' (1790: 303). Here, Cullen builds on Boissier's definition of the coma patient lacking voluntary motion with the omission of 'somnolence' as a symptom even noting how, 'Of all the diseases to be comprehended under our title, sleep, or even the appearance of it, is not constantly a symptom'. This is an important paradigm shift, a linguistic flashpoint in the history of medicine as the signifier 'coma' becomes detached from its signified, 'deep sleep'.

At the turn of the nineteenth century, the British physician John Cheyne published his book, *Cases of Apoplexy and Lethargy*, which incorporated an important subtitle: *With Observations Upon the Comatose Diseases* (1812). Like Cullen, though, Cheyne uses the word 'comatose' as an umbrella term that covers degrees of unconsciousness. Similar to his medical predecessors, Cheyne notes that, 'Apoplexy, to a common observer, often appears like profound sleep ... But the patient in apoplexy is not to be raised by shouting in his ear ... nor by shaking or pinching him' (1812: 11). While, like other early medical texts, it is difficult to discern exactly how this diagnosis of apoplexy relates to our current conception of coma, this reference to the use of pain stimulus (pinching) is important as it foreshadows one of the tests to determine the depth of coma that was to be included within the Glasgow Coma Scale (GCS), a diagnostic system I will discuss in more detail later in this chapter. Furthermore, Cheyne also makes another crucial observation of the 'comatose' patient that foreshadows one of the other tests of the GCS, pupil dilation, when he writes, 'But generally, as death approaches, the organs of sense entirely lose their faculty of receiving impressions: the pharynx is insensible, the pupil becomes dilated, the eye opake, the jaw falls, and the countenance is sunk: no kind of excitation affects the patient' (12–13). In these clinical remarks, Cheyne is beginning to diagnostically chart the levels of unconsciousness into which the patient is sinking, until brain death occurs.

Such advances by Cheyne in diagnostic and prognostic praxis increased over the course of the nineteenth century with the development of theories of the brain and consciousness, alongside surgical operations and experimentation on the brain. During the second half of the nineteenth century, experiments to actively explain 'observed phenomena in coma' were undertaken (Koehler and Wijdicks 2008: 884). The pioneering neurologist William Gowers, in his *A Manual of Diseases of the Nervous System* (1888) makes particular reference to some of these experiments on the brain in order to observe and chart the onset and symptoms of coma (or apoplexy, as he again refers to it). Writing of the certain 'loss of consciousness' that occurs when a brain haemorrhage causes 'an increase of the intracranial pressure', Gowers refers to animal experimentation: 'A dog becomes unconscious when there is a pressure on the surface of the brain equal to a column of mercury 130mm high' (1893: 102). These kinds of experiments being performed on animals in the late nineteenth century in order to define the causes of coma are a natural extrapolation from those performed by Galen upon ungulates. Gowers' first-hand clinical observation of DoC also provides another insight into the shifting attitudes towards and diagnosis of coma. In defining coma, he writes, 'Complete loss of consciousness, in which a patient cannot be roused, is termed "coma" if it is prolonged' (99). This is another very important moment in the history of the meaning of coma, and our current conception of it, as Gowers begins to try and establish diagnostic signifiers of coma, as distinct from wider PDoC. Furthermore, he goes on to outline the specific symptoms of coma that can be differentiated from other states of unconsciousness on the spectrum: 'In coma, the reflex action in the limbs may be preserved, but it is lessened or lost in the more severe degrees ... The pupils may be widely dilated or small: in stupor they act to light; but in deep coma they are motionless' (99). This is a hugely significant clinical description as not only does Gowers distinguish coma from stupor, he is also beginning to, like Cheyne, develop diagnostic tools to measure the depth of coma, even using the term 'deep coma', therefore recognizing gradations of severity.

The nineteenth century was marked by a profound fascination with, and research into, not only unconscious states, but also a wide spectrum of *altered* states of consciousness in an attempt to comprehend the human mind. It is this constant theorizing of identity and questioning of shifts or ruptures in identity that would give rise to psychoanalysis and psychiatry throughout the nineteenth century and beyond, alongside the burgeoning field of experimental and clinical neurology. In the 1820s, for example, the study of phrenology spread from continental Europe (primarily France and Germany) to England as part of the increasing obsession with new scientific-metaphysical movements (Kaplan 1974: 696). The key exponents of phrenology proposed a specific and rigid mapping of the human brain, including this pseudo-science's creator, German physician Franz Joseph Gall. We find that at the height of phrenology, key practitioners also played a key role in the proliferation of mesmerism, again a pseudo-science obsessed with brain function and liminal states of consciousness. Charles Dickens' close friend, John Elliotson, for example, was the single Englishman most responsible for the spread of mesmerism in England while also being the founder of the *London Phrenological Society* in 1824 (Kaplan 1974: 696). Yet the legitimacy of mesmerism would soon come under scrutiny and so practitioners, wishing to distance themselves from this increasingly debunked 'science', began to develop the practice of 'hypnotism' – a term coined by the erstwhile practitioner of mesmerism, and Scottish surgeon, James Braid in 1841. Braid's assertion in 1843 that the hypnotic trance was due to 'strong suggestibility between the mesmeric operator and his environment and subject' (Kaplan 1974: 702) rather than an organic 'magnetic fluid' was successful in legitimizing 'hypnosis' as a genuine scientific practice (Braid went on to coin hypnosis in the clinical setting as 'neurohypnology') that 'could play an important medical role as a curative agent' (Kaplan 1974: 702). And hypnosis was certainly used widely within the clinical setting, not least in the treatment of hysterics under Jean-Martin Charcot at the *Hôpital Universitaire Pitié-Salpêtrière* in Paris. Charcot's student, Pierre Janet, too, employed hypnotism to advance the psychoanalytical concept of the dissociative propensities of the human mind, seeing hypnotism as 'the momentary transformation of the mental side of an individual, artificially induced by a second person, and sufficing to bring about dissociation of personal memory' (Janet 1925: 291). This interest in hypnotism in the psychiatric setting reveals the growing interest in the brain and how the brain processes trauma and memory, alongside the need to try and regain access to 'dissociated' memories in order to reprocess them with a view to healing trauma. It was a pursuit present in the early work of Freud who studied hypnotism at the Paris school under Charcot and who was initially an enthusiastic supporter of hypnotherapy, employing it as a technique, like Janet, to help patients to recover (dissociated) memories. His early book of case studies, written with Joseph Breuer, *Studies On Hysteria* (1893), would prove to be a fascinating insight into the hypnotic states of patients. However, Freud would soon fall out of love with the practice, abandoning hypnosis in favour of psychoanalysis, emphasizing the interpretation of the unconscious (through his 'free association'), rather than relying on what he determined to be uneven results stemming from the use of hypnotic suggestion.

Hypnosis and mesmerism may have had a turbulent history throughout the nineteenth century but it underscores the fascination with the potential of humans to occupy liminal states in which they were not quite themselves, and in which they would often reveal the darkest, hitherto hidden sides to them. Public exhibitions and lectures, incorporating hypnosis of audience members, were tremendously popular throughout society. Robert Hanam Collyer, a student of Elliotson's and convert to mesmerism, even claimed to have used mesmerism (or what he termed 'phreno-magnetism', a portmanteau word incorporating phrenology and animal magnetism) to induce a 'comatose state in a child only twenty-two months, so that a fungus, involving the globe of the eye' might be surgically removed (Collyer 1871: v). This recollection of the powers of mesmerism includes a useful reference to the state of coma, here being more akin to an anaesthetic stupor than a DoC. Collyer would frequently mesmerize party-goers across American polite society, writing of one occasion when, acting on the request of a certain lady to 'magnetize' her, within 'less than five minutes the voluntary muscles were all paralyzed, and the most profound coma supervened' (Collyer 1871: 49). Collyer once more uses the term coma to describe a kind of sleep or trance-like state and this reveals how this fascination with the hypnotized subject and the ability to alter behaviour and personhood through suggestion gave rise to a further obsession with another altered, liminal state of consciousness: somnambulism. Collyer writes of the case of a seven-year old girl who, 'During a state of somnambulism would with her lips imitate the violin and the piano' and enact other strange behaviours after which she 'did not appear to have any recollection of what had occurred in her sleep', despite demonstrating acuity of skills which, in her waking life, she seemed to lack. As Collyer observes: 'She was, when awake, a dull, awkward girl' (61–2). Janet was also interested in the mechanisms of somnambulism, undertaking, in 1899, a systematic study of the case records of 388 hysterical patients displaying physical symptoms of paralysis (both in waking states and states of somnambulism) in order to ascertain whether there was any observable relationship between the side of their body afflicted with paralysis and other sorts of ailments (Harrington 1985: 624). In this regard, Janet was combining his psychoanalytical training with neurological techniques, trying to localize the causes of external, physical symptoms in specific areas of the brain. As he had predicted, 'There was a significant tendency for language-related disorders to occur in conjunction with right-sided hysteria' but, and particularly germane to our present discussion, 'Somnambulism, fugue and attacks of pathological sleep were found to be significantly more frequent with left hysteria', thereby giving credence to the fact that the left hemisphere of the brain was more concerned and in control of motor functioning than the right (Harrington 1985: 624–5).

There are other key examples of this fascination with the liminal state of somnambulism throughout the nineteenth and twentieth centuries. Tom Norman, the longest persistent travelling showman, and the last 'exhibitor' of John Merrick in 1884, included in his show a long-running act entitled 'Man In A Trance' which he toured right into the early twentieth century. Robert Wiene's German-expressionist film of

1920, *The Cabinet of Dr Caligari*, even plays on the intersection between mesmerism and somnambulism, and the fear of the hidden, sinister and violent faculties of the psyche that can be summoned to the fore within the hypnotic, somnambulist state. In the film, Caligari, a mesmerist and performer in a circus sideshow, controls the somnambulist Cesare (Figure 1.1), willing him to sleep and awake whenever he chooses – and also to commit murder on demand.

Alongside this preoccupation with somnambulism, from the late nineteenth century until the middle of the twentieth century we begin to see a fascination with the antithesis of the somnambulist shows: the 'sleeping beauty' exhibit. Hoffman notes that, 'Strollers through European fairgrounds were liable to chance upon pretty young women, dressed in white satin, reclining on silk-draped beds. Some lay in state in glass coffins, resembling, at first glance, improbably displaced relics' (2006: 139). In *Caligari*, too, Cesare, when not reanimated by the mesmerist, lies inert in a coffin-like box. This tradition of the performance of death-like, unconscious states can be traced back to a certain Colonel Townsend who, according to Collyer, could, '*(To all external appearances)* die whenever he chose, and after having lain for a considerable period in that state, could resuscitate himself by a voluntary struggle' (63, original emphasis). This demonstrates the widespread appeal of what Hoffman refers to as the 'various imaginaries of death and somnolence that developed across the decades and formed part of fairground entertainments: from nineteenth century mesmerism and magnetism displays to magnetic evangelism, table-turning, catalepsy, anaesthesia,

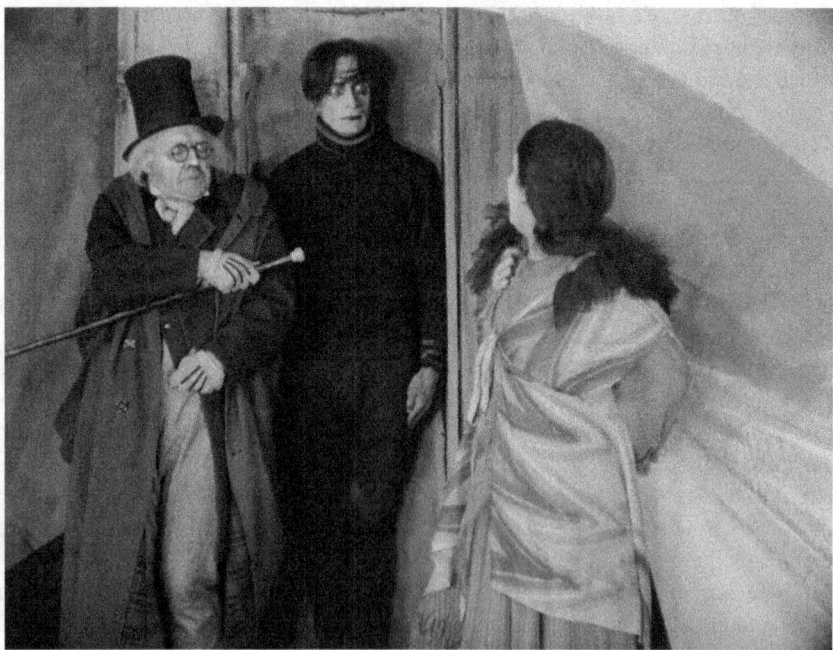

Figure 1.1 Still from *The Cabinet of Dr Caligari*, dir. Robert Wiene. Copyright © 1920. Courtesy Friedrich-Wilhelm-Murnau-Stiftung, Wiesbaden, Germany.

coma, somnambulism, ambulatory and then hypnotism' (50). Hoffman, in her whistle-stop yet insightful overview of the variety of sensational (and sensationalized) acts within this period interlinks 'death' with 'sleep', thereafter listing 'coma' as one such imaginary of these states – an embodiment of the multi-faceted coma-as-sleep/death metaphor. Hoffman goes on to discuss how this tradition extended deep into the twentieth century, as embodied by Price's 'Sleeping Beauty' (Figure 1.2). Taken around the 1950s, it 'shows a live young woman in a spangled suit, draped in white fabric, lying in a brightly lit glass coffin. A sign above her warns: 'Do not touch glass"' (Hoffman 2006: 152).

The writer and artist John Collier wrote about such exhibits in his mid-twentieth century short story, 'Sleeping Beauty'. The story follows a repressed, controlling and moderately wealthy young man who falls in love with and purchases a sleeping beauty exhibit from a disreputable carnie who has been exploiting her by clandestinely selling her for sexual favours to unscrupulous carnival-goers, an ancestor of the abusers of comatose 'sleeping beauties' in *Hable con Ella*, *Kill Bill* and *Twin Peaks*. Once the young man has transported her back to his English country house, he spends all his money trying to rouse her, eventually paying hard cash for a potion that will allow her to be awake for a certain portion of each day (subject to him administering the drug at the exact same time each day). But to his dismay, the Beauty shows nothing but utter contempt for him, seeing him immediately as a 'son of a bitch who'd take advantage' of her (2003: 321) – another sexually corrupt Prince Charming. After he has blown all of his money, and after she rejects him for the final time by embarking upon an affair with his neighbour, he ceases giving her the potion that sustains her wakefulness, regaining his fortune by exhibiting her as a sleeping beauty within his own carnival...

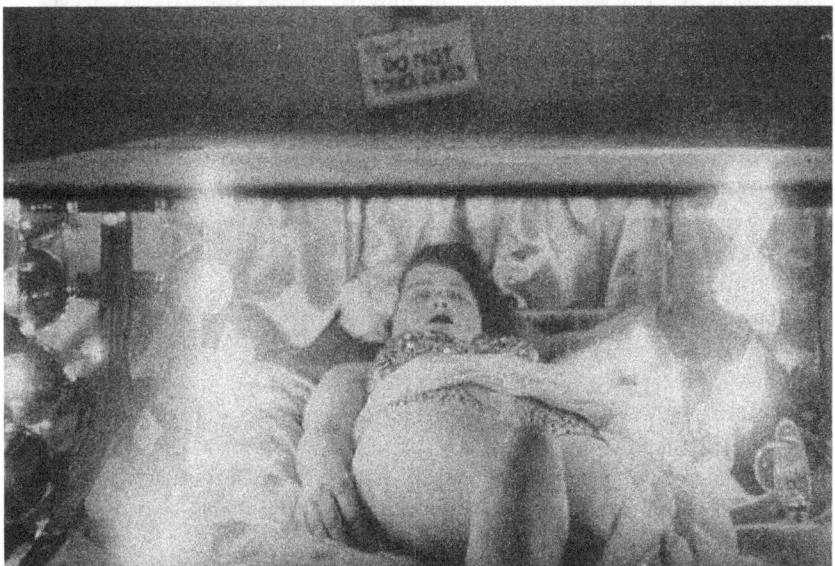

Figure 1.2 Photograph of Price's 'Sleeping Beauty', c.1950s. Source unknown.

and by, it is implied, charging visitors money to have sex with her. Adapted for film by James B. Harris in 1973, *Some Call It Loving* follows the source material relatively closely with the key exception that the sleeping beauty of the film, Jennifer, like the original fairy tale, is passive and deferential (emphasised by the virginal white gown she wears) and falls in love almost immediately with the protagonist, Troy. Troy, himself, wishes to fall in love with Jennifer in order to feel genuine emotion, rather than the manipulated feelings of desire he experiences through his life of voyeuristic sexual role-play that takes place within a cloistered mansion belonging to Scarlet, his partner in these sex games. Yet by bringing Jennifer into this mansion, he cannot simply start again with a 'perfect' relationship. Instead, Jennifer is brought into these games, gradually revealing to Troy that he is, in James B. Harris's words, 'masochistic [. . .] stimulated by his own betrayal' as well as by his original voyeuristic encounter with Jennifer, 'watching guys come up and kiss her'. In the end, he accepts that his relationship cannot be pure, cannot rescue him from his own manipulative desires, and so he drugs Jennifer back into her comatose sleep and establishes his own sleeping beauty exhibit, an inversion of the role of Prince Charming in the fable and similarly represented in Collier's story. Within the film, there is one particularly disturbing scene in which Jennifer describes her experience of her deep, coma-like sleep. She talks about the multiple abuses of the men at the carnival, kissing and touching her and 'doing other things', yet she says how she did not want this to stop as it was preferable to the nothingness of consciousness that would stretch intolerably between the moments of violation.

Now while these disturbing tales and depictions of unconscious disorders and somnambulism reveal a fascination with altered and liminal states of consciousness throughout the twentieth century, empirically testable neurological and psychological investigations into the brain and injury also begin to gather apace, and it was the advent of two world wars that contributed significantly to this new wealth of knowledge.

1.4 Shell shock and brain injury in the two world wars: the organic / functional conundrum

With the development of advanced ballistic technology and engineering and the use of this in modern warfare, there came an increase in brain injuries being sustained on the battlefield and most notably in the two world wars, a sharp rise in battlefield brain trauma that has continued into the modern era. As Shively and Perl note, 'The increased use of improvised explosive devices, rocket-propelled grenades, land mines, and other high explosives, traumatic brain injury (TBI) has become the "signature injury" of current warfare' (2012: 234). Yet during the First World War, clinicians were only just beginning to be confronted by the aetiology and impact of such injuries so while new advances in warfare gave rise to brutal trauma and injury, it also allowed for a development of neurological (organic) and psychological (functional) approaches to understanding and treating BI and trauma.

It is important to note that what we term "shell shock", now primarily associated with the psychological trauma of war and post-traumatic stress disorder (PTSD), was initially identified and diagnosed as an organic, neurological trauma. The first clinician to publish findings using the colloquial term "shell shock", and the person credited with coining the term, was the psychiatrist and war doctor, Charles Myers (Fueshko 2016: 41). Throughout his articles on the subject, Myers offered his suspicion that the syndrome was more psychological than physical (Fueshko 2016: 40). This was in contrast to the generally accepted thinking at that time, with doctors looking for 'physical disturbances to the nervous system rather than psychological explanations in their patients' (40). In Myers's 1915 article for *The Lancet* entitled 'A Contribution to the Study of Shell Shock', he discussed several symptoms including amnesia, 'total anosmia', loss of 'sense of taste' and loss of eyesight with one patient, in particular, 'unable to see letters until they were quite near' (1915: 316–17). In his conclusions, however (and partially based upon the successful use of hypnosis to retrieve amnesic memories), Myers stated that ,'The close relation of these cases to those of "hysteria" appears fairly certain' (320), even despite several of the patients having long-term physical disabilities, including sustained problems with eyesight which would suggest some kind of organic damage also. Nevertheless, Myers's clinical publication was influential in shell shock becoming synonymous with a psychological disorder.

It was the work of another doctor, working with shell shock patients within the Maudsley hospital, a research psychiatric hospital outside of London, that helped to define the neurological manifestation of shell shock and pinpoint the long-term effects of organic brain trauma. Major Frederick Mott was trained in both neurology and pathology and served as medical director at Maudsley. Mott proposed that sclerosis of the brain could be responsible for the effects of organic shell shock. Mott went on to discover that a patient found dead forty-eight hours after a severe case of shell shock was found, post-mortem, to have multiple brain haemorrhages. He concluded that this would have resulted in 'areas of sclerosis, possibly sufficiently severe to occasion definite symptoms' (Fueshko 2016: 45). Mott began to look at the potential permanent impact organic (neurological) brain damage could have upon behaviour and personhood. He went on to perform a number of post-mortem examinations of patients who had suffered shell shock and who had since died, publishing his findings in two articles for *The Lancet* in 1916, a year after Myers's article which had drawn a link between shell shock and psychological hysteria. Mott reported neuropathological findings in two soldiers, in particular, who had died soon after 'exposure to an explosive blast' while serving during the First World War and, 'In neither of these cases was there physical evidence of external trauma to the head'. However, post-mortem examination of their brains 'revealed multiple . . . haemorrhages' (Shively and Perl 2012: 235). Mott therefore was instrumental in proving that shell shock within modern warfare could cause closed head trauma: that BI, as will be discussed in detail later in this book, can be an invisible disability.

Soon after the publication of Mott's findings, Myers published his follow-up study on shell shock patients which saw some improvement in all cases 'with case four going back to duty, suggesting shell shock was curable' (Fueshko 2016: 44). This led to two polar interpretations of shell shock: the neurological model, viewing it as, 'A poorly understood organic disorder' versus the psychiatric model, viewing it as a 'functional disorder, a "psychoneurosis", related to insidious emotional turmoils' (Shively and Perl

2012: 235–6). Fueshko cogently evaluates this battle for the definition of diagnosis of shell shock during the First World War between the fields of neurology and psychology, highlighting the fact that it is 'an issue still debated today: when do neurological (physical) issues become mental issues, and vice versa?' (2016: 47). In the end, though, Mott's work on determining a physical aetiology of shell shock (alongside the work of others who supported this diagnosis) was ignored and a British governmental commission designed to investigate the cause of shell shock concluded that it was a 'convenient evasion of duty, if not disguised malingering' (Shively and Perl 2012: 236). The term 'shell shock' was abandoned and, as Shively and Perl highlight, 'Any idea that exposure to an explosive blast might produce lasting pathology in the brain was no longer considered worthy of investigation. The field of psychiatry had won the dispute over shell shock'.

By the beginning of the Second World War, the term shell shock remained banned by British authorities for the purpose of avoiding 'another epidemic of shell shock' (Jones, Fear and Wessely 2007: 1643). Instead, the term 'posttrauma concussion state', coined by W. F. Schaller in 1939, came into common usage, thereby replacing the more violent and emotive term 'shell shock', and by 1941, the term 'postconcussion syndrome' became popularized. As in the First World War, scientists and clinicians were split over whether this was a psychological or pathological condition, with Sir John F. Fulton, in a paper of 1942, sensitively concluding that, 'The problem of distinguishing such cases from organic concussion resulting from blast is delicate and often difficult' (Fulton 1942: 8). Jones, Fear and Wessely point towards two further, separate studies in 1942 from Lewis and Guttman that 'underlined similarities in the presentation of head-injured and non-head injured soldiers seen in many psychiatric units' (2007: 1643), highlighting the frequent difficulty of diagnosing behaviours as the product of functional or organic brain damage, despite the fact that the separation defines the two distinct fields of neurology and psychology. But perhaps by far the most in-depth study of organic shell shock that arose within this period was led by the Russian neuro-psychologist, A. R. Luria. With a strong belief that, 'Psychology should develop in a manner that was consistent with, but not entirely dependent on, the neurosciences' (Cole and Levitin *in* Luria, Cole and Levitin 2010: 8), Luria is considered to be one of the founding fathers of neuropsychology who recognized, for the first time, that behaviours of the brain injured or impaired patient may not necessarily be explained by either functional or organic factors, but a combination of the two. As Anne Hunsaker Hawkins explicates, in his 'clinical biographies' (a term coined by the contemporary neurologist Oliver Sacks), Luria's 'explicit aim [was] to understand a particular clinical feature in relation to the whole configuration of the individual's personality' (1986: 5).

Working with brain-injured patients, Luria's aim was to, in his own words, 'Develop psychological methods for the diagnosis of local brain lesions' (2010: 131). His work with brain-injured soldiers during the Second World War (and beyond) was therefore a natural extension of this pursuit and his most groundbreaking work in this area was that conducted with Russian soldier Zasetsky. As detailed in Luria's book *The Man with a Shattered World*, Zasetsky, while advancing on a German battalion on the Russian front, was shot in the head and went into 'a prolonged coma' (Luria 1975: 31). After emerging from coma, and seemingly 'recovering' with the 'wound appear[ing] to have healed' (27), it transpired that Zasetsky had severe, permanent organic brain damage that affected him both physically and mentally. In his observations, Luria notes how, 'On the surface his [Zasetsky's] life may appear no different, but it has changed radically; owing to an injury to a small part of his brain, his world has become an endless series of mazes' (1975: 40). Short-term memory loss, failure of speech comprehension and severely impaired vision impacted upon Zasetsky profoundly and Luria worked for many years with his patient in order to both aid his rehabilitation but also to learn about the localization of BI and the effects of injuries within different parts of the brain. One illustrative example of this was how Luria was quick to point out that, 'Patients with frontal lobe lesions show no gross disturbances of the structure of neural operations ... Their articulation of words and their auditory recognition are not affected' (2010: 149). Yet while such patients 'return the content of their thought ... their difficulties are in the dynamics of their thinking' (151). In short, Luria observed shifts in behaviour, emotion control and disinhibition that arise from frontal-lobe damage. In his book *Traumatic Aphasia* he describes his findings based on diagnostic tests and therapy with more than 700 victims of head wounds inflicted by the bullets and shrapnel of the Second World War (1970). Luria noted that, 'Paradoxically, this period of disaster [the Second World War] provided an important opportunity for advancing our understanding of the brain and of psychological processes' (Luria 2010: 140). Luria's work with Zasetsky also illustrates the use of rehabilitation in order to achieve a 'radical reconstruction of the entire functional system of articulation so that it is carried out by completely different mechanisms' (Luria 2010: 146). What is remarkable about *The Man with the Shattered World* is that while it does include Luria's clinical observations of his patient, the book is primarily comprised of Zasetsky's memoir of his lived experience of injury and rehabilitation – the earliest example of first-person testimony of TBI. Hawkins notes that in doing this, Luria 'create[s] a picture of a human being, not an explanation of a disease – a "real image" that is not reducible to mechanistic principles but retains the richness and the mystery of the living reality' (1986: 13). Luria's clinical biography springs from the intersection of functional and organic approaches to BI, rejecting what Couser refers to as the medical establishment's typical response 'to the paradigm, not the patient – the syndrome, not the subject' (1997: 31).

Both Zasetsky and Luria outline the incredible struggle of the young soldier, initially being only able to read 'printed material letter by letter' (Luria 1975: 66), an affliction reflected in one of Myers's research subjects from the First World War, referred to earlier, whose vision was so badly impaired that he could only see individual letters in a document – yet who was diagnosed with psychological shell shock. In the case of Zasetsky, his sight disability manifested two-fold as the part of his brain responsible for language recognition and optical impulses was so badly damaged. At the same time, his BI was so severe that, while reading, moving onto the next letter in a word, he would forget the previous letter it had pained him so much to recognize initially. In the end, Zasetsky embarked upon a determined process of 'morbid writing' (Luria 1975: 77) in order to record his life story, a process that involved a series of both physically and psychologically exhausting 'rote' tasks of letter/word associations and recitals of the alphabet to himself, until he found the letter (and association) which he required in order to piece together the word he was trying to form: 'I began to make some progress', he writes, 'By finding words that would work as memory props. But sometimes I could only remember these for a minute or two before they'd slip my mind completely' (65). Again, Luria used this work with Zasetsky to fine-tune his research into traumatic aphasia and brain localization, observing that by reciting the alphabet out loud, Zasetsky was 'using a long-established oral-motor skill instead of trying to visualise each letter'. He also noted that this required a faculty of the brain that had not been damaged by his war injury, concluding that, 'Only the part of the cortex responsible for gauging visual spatial relationships had been affected, not the verbal-motor functions' (65). Clearly, Luria was highly influential in developing a neuropsychological methodology of rehabilitation, using and exercising other areas of the brain to compensate for damaged ones, a method still in use today. As Luria reflects, the Second World War 'had greatly increased our understanding of the role played by separate areas of the brain' (2010: 157).

1.5 Towards a further understanding of coma and the spectrum of consciousness

Despite advances in knowledge regarding BI, the use of coma as a medical term still continued to be inconsistent during this period, with wide-ranging interchangeable terms in use. Coma and apoplexy were still popular (and barely distinguishable from each other), in a sense moving away from the attempt to streamline terms to describe DoC (alongside their diagnosis and aetiology) made by Gowers towards the turn of the twentieth century. Nevertheless, by the middle of the twentieth century, and in line with the growing understanding of the relationship between coma, ICP (intra-cranial pressure) and ensuing BI, the term 'coma' itself starts to become more defined and consistently used. Koehler and Wijdicks note that several books published throughout the 1940s and 1950s begin to have stand-alone chapters on coma: Biemond's *Brain Diseases* (1946) being one example which describes the 'systematic examination of the 'comatose' patient' (Koehler and Wijdicks 2008: 887). DeJong's *The Neurological Examination* (1950) even included a separate chapter describing the level of 'coma', referring to a condition 'semi-coma', a 'nebulous' term, according to Koehler and Wijdicks, described by DeJong as a 'state of partial or relative loss of response to the environment in which the patient's consciousness may be impaired in varying degrees' (887). While this might be nebulous or vague, again we see a recognition of a spectrum of consciousness and degrees of severity alongside an attempt to distinguish the DoC coma from longer-term PDoC. But it was the work of Fisher, Plum and Posner in the latter half of the twentieth century that was to have a profound impact upon defining coma as we understand it today and outlining a detailed diagnostic and prognostic framework, moving towards a more neurological definition of brain disorder.

In 1969, C. M. Fisher published a pioneering, yet often ignored and neglected, fifty-six-page paper on the examination of the comatose patient. This paper was the 'first full clinical description of the comatose patient, the first classification based on CSF [Cerebrospinal Fluid] results, the first serious questioning of the clinicopathological correlation with brain herniation, and the first major emphasis of relevant eye findings in coma' (Wijdicks 2017). Another forerunner to the Glasgow Coma Scale, Fisher also used pain, voice and eye stimuli to try to gauge severity of coma. However, advances in coma diagnosis and clinical care of the comatose patient really started to be noticed with the first publication of Plum and Posner's *The Diagnosis of Stupor and Coma* in 1966, arriving three years before Fisher could publish his research. At once a historical review of neurophysiology and overview of the aetiology and sequelae of a range of DoC, *The Diagnosis* detailed diagnostic tools, prognostic indicators of the comatose state and a practical approach to the comatose patient. It also provided a clear definition of coma: 'A state of unarousable psychologic unresponsiveness in which the subject lies with eyes closed. Subjects in coma show no psychologically understandable response to external stimuli or inner need' (1980: 5).

During the 1970s, Fred Plum and Bryan Jennett contributed to two watershed moments in defining and delineating both coma and PDoC, while also moving towards more testable frameworks of clinical diagnosis. In 1972, the term 'persistent vegetative state' was coined by Jennet and Plum to describe the condition of patients with severe brain damage in whom coma has progressed to a state of wakefulness without detectable awareness. Unlike coma patients, it was observed that such patients have sleep-wake cycles but no ascertainable cerebral cortical function (The Multi-Society Task Force on the Persistent Vegetative State 1994(1): 1499). The subtitle of Jennett and Plum's paper on the vegetative state referred to a 'syndrome without a name', but their research stemmed from observations of patients who are awake but whose 'eyes are unaware and undiscerning' (Fins 2015: 35). This condition, and the ability to examine and clinically diagnose the condition, was, as Fins summarizes, an 'emerging diagnostic category brought about by medical technologies like the ventilator, which now could keep patients alive who decades earlier would have died' (2015: 35). Reflecting later, in 2002, upon these early in-roads into defining and diagnosing PVS, Jennett rightly points out that such physical signs of mental awareness alongside the 'wide range of reflex responsiveness in some vegetative patients ... can give rise to suspicion of meaningful mental activity' (2002: 355). However, Jennett goes on to discuss how data from the analysis of 754 published acute cases of PVS patients (research led by The Multi-Society Task Force on the Persistent Vegetative State and published in 1994) found that, 'Of those vegetative at one month 43% had regained consciousness, by one year, 34% were dead and only 23% were still vegetative. The longer the vegetative state had lasted, the fewer recovered – after six months, only 13% regained consciousness' (2002: 356). The Task Force reports upon how, 'For patients in a vegetative state as a result of traumatic brain injury, the prognosis for recovery remains unfavourable' (1994(2): 1572). Dr David Bates discusses the unfavourable prognosis of DoC in relation to coma patients, pointing out that, 'The longer a patient remains in a coma the poorer his or her chance of recovery', stating that, 'By the third day [of coma] the chance of making a good recovery is reduced to only 7%, and by the 14th day is as low as 2%'. By the end of the first week, he continues, almost half of those patients who have not regained consciousness are in a vegetative state (2001: 21).

This development of an understanding of and diagnostic/prognostic framework for both coma and vegetative states is important when considering the language and imagery of fictional representations, particularly in those texts that, as I will demonstrate, portray coma as lasting anywhere between three and five years. In reality, such texts are not really portraying coma as such, but the PVS – or, more accurately, what might be termed 'permanent vegetative state', a further sub-category of unconsciousness defined, by Niall Cartlidge, as the point at which 'there can be a high degree of certainty of irreversibility' (2001: 19). The Task Force, as Fins points out, is more specific in defining 'permanence', concluding that, 'When a vegetative state continues beyond thirty days it is described as persistent and that permanence sets in three months (six months in the UK) after anoxic injury (severe oxygen deprivation) and 12 months after the insult resulted from trauma' (Fins 2015: 69). It follows that, beyond the grim prognosis of recovery, patients who do emerge from PVS will, in all likelihood, have severe and permanent physical and cognitive disabilities.

Despite defining PVS in 1972, it was actually eleven years later, in 1983, when the President's Commission for the Study of Ethical Problems in Medicine and Biomedical and Behavioural Research accepted Plum and Jennett's definition, while defining unconsciousness as the inability to 'experience the environment' (The Multi-Task Force 1994(1): 1499). Yet prior to this ratification of the medical term and diagnosis, Jennett, together with Teasdale (and a mere four years after the recognition of PVS), contributed further to the study and diagnosis of coma and vegetative states by creating and defining what would become the Glasgow Coma Scale (GCS), a system that aimed to define 'in mathematical terms the probability of various outcomes [of coma] derived from the different combinations of predictive features shown by individual patients' (Jennett and Teasdale 1976: 1031). In short, Jennett and Teasdale developed an objective system that could test the 'depth' of a patient's coma or unconscious state by measuring the degree of three physical responses: eye (pupillary dilation), verbal and motor (response to pain stimuli). Published in *The Lancet* in 1976 (though conspicuous in its failure to acknowledge Fisher's work in this area, eventually published in 1969), Jennett and Teasdale's GCS was a numerical system measuring the severity of coma based upon the patient's response to these three stimuli, each response scored on a 1–5 scale (Figure 1.3). Clinicians would arrive at a total numerical figure designed to diagnose level of consciousness and

Eye Response	4 = Eyes open spontaneously
	3 = Eye opening to verbal command
	2 = Eye opening to pain
	1 = No eye opening
Motor Response	6 = Obeys commands
	5 = Localizing pain
	4 = Withdrawal from pain
	3 = Flexion response to pain
	2 = Extension response to pain
	1 = No motor response
Verbal Response	5 = Oriented
	4 = Confused
	3 = Inappropriate words
	2 = Incomprehensible sounds
	1 = No verbal response

Figure 1.3 The Glasgow Coma Scale.

potential prognostic outcome. The lowest possible score, 3, indicates deep coma; the highest (for a fully conscious person) is 15. As Middleton observes, 'Prior to this, most descriptions of altered levels of consciousness revolved around very subjective portrayals such as "comatose", "drowsy", "obtunded", and "stuporose"' (2012: 176) – emphasizing the vague terms that had the linguistic register of somnolence which obfuscated a precise diagnosis. In this way, the GCS led to the possibility of 'a summary overview of injury severity' within and between series of patients (Teasdale et al. 2014: 13).

This intricate spectrum of consciousness was to become even more complex in the twenty-first century when the minimally conscious state (MCS) was recognized and defined. First described in 2002, it was diagnosed as a 'condition of severely altered consciousness in which minimal but definite behavioural evidence of self or environmental awareness is demonstrated'. The key distinction between MCS and PVS lies in the fact that, 'Cognitively mediated behaviour occurs inconsistently, but is reproducible or sustained long enough to be differentiated from reflexive behaviour' (Giacino et al. 2002: 350–1).

This further delineation on the spectrum of consciousness has had a huge ethical impact. Fins, Schiff and Foley point towards the fact that, 'Cases of patients who began to recover long after injury are now sporadically making headlines and causing confusion because media reports and public comments often make no distinction between VS and MCS' (2007: 305). Aside from this misreporting and conflation of PDoC, there has arisen deeper ethical considerations, specifically, the existential positioning of the patient within a PDoC and the implications for clinical care and end-of-life decision making. The development of definitions and diagnostic criteria of coma and VS has given rise to a number of high-profile right-to-die cases brought to court, both in the United States and the United Kingdom, leading to a marked increase in the ethical debates surrounding these difficult decisions. As Stephen Holland queries in his bioethical approach to 'ambiguous' cases of living beings, 'How can a PVS patient who spontaneously respires and perspires, responds to temperature change, digests food, and so on, be dead?' (2003: 73). Derick Wade, professor in neurorehabilitation, further explores such ethical questions when he reflects that, "The vegetative state is simply one end of a spectrum of awareness, and there is no obvious cut-off between the vegetative state and the low awareness state [MCS]", leading him to philosophically ask, 'In the absence of any test, can we accept that any human being is unaware?' (2001: 353). These were concerns held by both Jennett and Plum immediately after defining PVS, commenting, even before the publication of their paper, that the growth in cases of PVS, due largely to advances in life-support technology, is 'provoking comment both in the health professions and in the community at large [of] ethical, moral, and social issues' (Fins 2015: 36).

Such volatile ethical and moral questions and dilemmas have been complicated further in recent years. In 2011, Bruno et al broadened the category of MCS even further by proposing to 'subcategorize MCS patients based on the complexity of their behaviour'. They suggested two sub-divisions: MCS Minus (MCS-), describing patients with 'minimal level of behavioural interactions without command following'; and MCS Plus (MCS+) where patients 'show higher level behavioural responses such as command following' (2011: 1088). 'Such diagnostic fine-tuning', Nettleton et al argue, can lead to what they term a 'diagnostic illusory'; that is, 'the imperative for diagnostic conviction could generate as many anomalies as it seeks to resolve', thereby exacerbating 'existential doubt' (2014: 134). In 2010, Laureys et al proposed to replace the term 'vegetative state' (an 'outdated' term (3) with a 'negative connotation' (1)) with 'unresponsive wakefulness syndrome (UWS)' in order to avoid 'inadvertently risking comparisons between patients and vegetables and implying persistency from the moment of diagnosis' (4). Since then, VS and UWS have been used interchangeably. And in 2018, the term *'permanent* vegetative state' was called into question by Giacino et al, asserting that *'chronic'* would be a suitable replacement, noting that permanent 'implies irreversibility, which is not supported by the current research' (2018: 455-6). The research team proposed that the term 'chronic VS' should be used, 'accompanied by a description of the current duration of the VS/MCS' (456). Yet the Royal College of Physicians (RCP) maintained the term 'permanent' in their 2020 PDoC guidelines, reserving 'chronic' for VS/MCS- if it has persisted for three months (non-traumatic BI) or one year (traumatic BI) and MCS+ if it has persisted for nine months (non-traumatic BI) or eighteen months (traumatic BI) (2020: 37). It should also be noted that because of the confusion that often arose with the acronym PVS which described both 'persistent' and 'permanent' vegetative states, 'The UK National Clinical Guidelines for PDoC therefore replaced the term 'persistent' with 'continuing', both for VS and MCS' (RCP 2020: 36). Here again, we see the importance (and precarity) of language in diagnostic criteria and in the moral and ethical debates that surround the existential state of patients within PDoC, alongside the medico-legal decisions that have to be made.

1.6 A return to metaphor

The latter half of the last century saw the gradual drift of the term 'coma' from its original meaning of 'deep sleep' as the drive towards a more organic/neurological, 'hard' science diagnosis and definition of both DoC and BI gained pace. As Bell et al. note, 'The mid-20th century birth of cognitive psychiatry and computational approaches to the mind saw a conceptual shift. 'Functional' was associated with software and the mind, and 'organic' with hardware and the brain' (Bell et al. 2020: 4). This shift culminated with President George H. W. Bush designating the nineties as 'The Decade of the Brain', a declaration coming directly out of this deep interest in the brain and neural phenomena, alongside huge progress being made, as we have seen, in developing diagnostic criteria and imaging technologies throughout the 1970s and 1980s. The decade of the brain continued to build on these new advancements, seeing significant accomplishments in, for example, the discovery of neural plasticity and development of functional Magnetic Resonance Imaging (fMRI). Yet despite coma now having a set of neurological aetiology ascribed to it, distancing it from its connotations of sleep and dream, in linguistic and metaphorical terms, this has proven to be a difficult tradition to slough off. It is useful therefore to also look at Susan Sontag's theory of illness and metaphor to help explicate both how and why metaphors of coma and BI have developed and become embedded within culture and public consciousness.

In her seminal work *Illness as Metaphor*, Sontag traces the use of the metaphors of tuberculosis and cancer throughout the history of literary and socio-political language. She examines how, traditionally, TB was often romanticized, with the dying victim 'pictured as made more beautiful and more soulful', whereas the victim of cancer was often 'portrayed as robbed of all capacities of self-transcendence, humiliated by fear and agony' (1991: 17). She exemplifies this theory by looking at how the metaphors are manifested: the 'spiritualizing of consciousness' of TB juxtaposed with the 'obliterating of consciousness' of cancer (68). The literary and medico-social language of these two diseases contribute to a sense of metaphorical polarity: TB described in terms of a certain 'vigour' or vitality (32) which it instils in the patient; cancer in terms of invasions of the 'Other', of 'alien' or 'mutant' cells stronger than normal cells' (69), sinister and potentially stigmatizing imagery that is immediately evocative of the invasion of parasitic alien bodies depicted typically within the science fiction genre. Similarly, Sontag refers to metaphors of warfare in relation to 'attacking' or 'invading' cancer cells. Couser highlights some of the ethical dilemmas arising from this kind of figurative language to describe disease, remarking, 'Such metaphors conscript patients into wars fought over, on, and in their bodies; among other things, such tropes may encourage the use of "heroic" measures of questionable effectiveness that may cause unnecessary suffering' (1997: 45). However, despite this 'privileging' of one disease over the other, the real-world gravity of both is undermined because of the metaphorical implications. There is a similar paradigm in the cases of what I term the C-Met (coma metaphor) and the B-Met (brain injury metaphor) and their uses in contemporary society and literature. Coma is frequently described as an ethereal, transient dreamscape and a place where transcendent enlightenment and revelatory knowledge of the self and society can be found; BI, on the other hand, is often ignored altogether or accumulates the linguistic register of an insult, becoming synonymous with a lack of intelligence, or with a sense of existential or creative lack. During an interview given in 2011 for the BBC documentary *Faulks on Fiction*, for example, the author Martin Amis deployed a typical manifestation of the B-Met. While discussing whether he would ever consider writing a children's book, he commented, 'People ask me if I ever thought of writing a children's book. I say, 'If I had a serious brain injury I might well write a children's book' [. . .] I would never write about someone that forced me to write at a lower register than what I write'. What is most startling about Amis's insult against BI survivors is that much of the backlash came from those who were offended by a perceived slur against children's fiction and its authors. Indeed, the sub-heading to an article in *The Guardian* reporting on this incident illustrates this rather misdirected outrage: 'Children's authors have expressed anger over 'insult' to their work on BBC programme' (Page 2011). This same article also cites the children's author Lucy Coats who sees Amis's faux pas as an 'implicit insult to those of us who do write children's books', yet she fails to mention how this is an explicit insult against those living with BI.

The use of the equally misleading C-Met is no less prevalent, not least in the sociopolitical arena. On accepting the Democratic Party's nomination for Vice President in 1988, Senator Lloyd Bentsen, recalling the Reagan administration, declared that, 'America has just passed through . . . an eight-year coma' (Sayer 1989: 207). Over a century prior to Bentsen's speech, in another era of contentious political debate, the suffragist Sarah Emily Davies, during a paper delivered at the annual meeting of the National Association for the Promotion of Social Sciences in 1868, proposed that, 'We have persuaded ourselves that Englishmen of the present day are such a nervously excitable race, that the only chance for their descendants is to keep the mothers in a state of coma' (1910: 104). These examples, set 120 years apart, illustrate how long the coma metaphor has been employed in political rhetoric. In both, the word 'coma' is synonymous with a state of sleep or stupor (harking back to its original meaning) from which the public need to be 'awakened' and greet a new world order. The C-Met is still frequently used in political writing and debate. Stephen Bush, the political editor of *New Statesman*, for example, in critiquing the proposed plan by opposition parties in the UK to prevent a no-deal Brexit by forming a 'government of national unity', writes, 'From time to time, a political story emerges that is so silly that I begin to worry if I am in fact not covering politics at all, but have actually been hit by a large object and fallen into a deep coma, or perhaps have accidentally ingested a great quantity of mind-altering drugs' (2019: 17). Deep coma, here, is a hallucinatory experience, a political nightmare that warps reality.

The C-Met similarly emerges within the literary arena, beyond extended representations of the condition itself. In his poem 'And Others, Vaguer Presences', John Ashbery, in typically minimalist style, muses upon the dislocation of the self within a brutalist architectural landscape, describing this sense of alienation as like emerging from 'a coma that is a white, interesting country' (1978: 48). Ashbery's reference to coma is evocative of the so-called 'white tunnel' phenomenon of the near-death experience (NDE), seen also in David Chase's *The Sopranos*; a transition through a liminal state towards a form of transfiguratory afterlife, suggesting a certain simplicity and 'ease' of movement between extreme states of consciousness. And in Chuck Palahniuk's *Diary*, while an actual coma is depicted (and in trademark, visceral style, protagonist Misty Wilmot's husband described as a 'brain-dead vegetable' with 'a tube up [his] ass' (2003: 38); a 'withered skeleton' (40)), the author also uses the C-Met throughout the novel to satirize the widespread use of the metaphor within an affectless, modern society. As she gazes upon her husband, 'hooked to a zillion very expensive gadgets' to keep him alive (38), Misty muses, 'Everyone's in their own personal coma' (39).

Sontag writes of the 'predilection for psychological explanations of disease' and that such an understanding 'undermines the 'reality' of a disease' (56). This dynamic similarly arises out of the production of the C-Met, depicting coma as a purely psychological disturbance, thus causing it to become detached from reality. As we shall see, recovery from coma is most often depicted as being quick and immediate, with the survivor's cognition being immediately intact.

From a literary perspective, the critic and poet John Hollander discusses how these metaphors of consciousness are created. He examines how even the process of writing about altered states of consciousness becomes 'immensely complicated by the impulses to use language to represent them'. He notes that, 'The rhetoric of such representations will liken a direct experience of such a state, or an imagined one, to that of another such condition' (2001: 589). This 'likening' of one state of consciousness to this unconscious state within the literary arena can be examined further through Sontag's notion that such psychologizing and figuring of illness leads to 'the promise of a triumph over illness', therefore creating a feeling of hope of full and immediate recovery.

This privileging of coma over BI, and the consequences this has for the utility of each metaphor, is exacerbated by representations within popular culture. Danny

Boyle's 2013 film *Trance* depicts how someone with amnesia arising from a TBI (caused by the stereotypical blow to the head, another "soap opera" paradigm of TBI amnesia) undergoes hypnotherapy to recover his memories. Consequently, Boyle's film, through its characterization and narrative development, serves to propagate an archetypal medical mythology: that the 'cure' for BI can be found exclusively by locating traumatically suppressed memories in the injured brain.

The role of the coma metaphor as narrative device is likewise seen in another of Boyle's films, *28 Days Later*. In the opening minutes of the film, the central protagonist, Jim (Cillian Murphy) emerges from a month-long coma, both with cognition fully and immediately intact, but also with unimpaired motor functions. In almost a mirror-image of this initiating dramatic event, in the first book of Robert Kirkman and Tony Moore's zombie-apocalypse comic-book series *The Walking Dead*, the central protagonist Rick Grimes similarly emerges from a month-long coma with cognition intact. In this text, though, slightly more attention is paid to the degradation of muscle strength and motor functioning. A full-page panel depicts Rick 'gasping' as he exits coma suddenly. Immediately after, we have a regular, 9-panel page, depicting Rick getting out of bed; struggling to walk; holding onto his IV stand for support; stumbling to the ground, his legs and body clearly weakened from muscle atrophy while in coma. Yet the last three frames are interesting: frame one, Rick sits on the floor, legs stretched out, leaning against his hospital bed, head hung in dejection; frame two, his head is now raised, his attention drawn to something; frame three, he is now standing, opening a drawer to get his belongings (2013: 10–11). Given that the frame size is identical and, more importantly, the white space between frames is also identical, implying an even, regular passage of time occurring between the action depicted in the frames themselves, Rick's weakness and physical atrophy is very short-lived, disappearing almost as quickly as it lasted – much like Jim in *28 Days Later*.

In both *28 Days Later* and *The Walking Dead: Days Gone Bye*, the coma is used as a narrative device which allows the writers to collapse time and quickly move beyond the narrative timeframe during which the rage virus spreads (*28 Days Later*) and the dead start to reanimate (*The Walking Dead*). The second text is most effective in the use of the coma device and an immediate "awakening", depicting Rick being shot within the first six frames of the comic, and then having him emerge from coma in the seventh frame. In Boyle's film, there is a version of a 'pre-credit' sequence during which the audience sees the moment of break-out of the virus, an expository device that is absent in *The Walking Dead* comic and first episode of Frank Darabont's TV adaptation (2010). In this use of the coma metaphor in *The Walking Dead*, Rick is also metaphorically represented as 'awakening' from 'death' only to encounter those who have similarly 'awoken', only in a much more literal sense: the living dead. This immediacy of coma 'awakening' allows the audience to be also awoken in the midst of this apocalyptic scenario.

A recent counterpoint to such representations in popular media is Todd Phillip's DC comics reboot, *Joker*, in which we find a fascinating portrayal of BI. In alluding to Arthur Fleck's functional/psychological trauma (yet without explicitly identifying a specific condition) while simultaneously referring to a neurological/organic BI he sustained as a child, Phillip's film represents the overlap that may occur between functional/organic sequelae of BI. In this way, he subtly dismantles the 'misleading, dualistic distinction between mindless matter and matterless mind' (Zeman 2014: 142). In short, in depicting Fleck's hallucinations, delusions, even the pseudobulbar affect that causes Joker's trademark, uncontrollable laugh, Phillips blurs this artificial divide between psychiatry and neurology.

For a neurological disability like BI that lacks the aura of mystery and ethereality of coma, it has inevitably acquired darker and more pejorative connotations. Amis's use of the B-Met certainly isn't an isolated example, its use as a cultural slur apparent later in 2011 when, during an edition of BBC2's *The Review Show*, the writer and critic A. L. Kennedy suggested that the writer of the Channel 4 fantasy-drama *Camelot* must have had a 'brain injury' as an explanation for why it was so badly written. And during the 2014 World Cup qualifying match between Portugal and the United States televised on BBC One, football commentator Mark Lawrenson, by way of explaining the erratic ability of the Portuguese player Nani, commented: 'A great description of Nani – promising career ruined by a niggling brain injury'. While Lawrenson's use of the metaphor has the same register and effect as Amis and Kennedy's usage (referring to BI as a means of describing a perceived creative 'flaw'), it has even more stigmatizing implications. The fact that Lawrenson refers to a 'niggling' BI grossly undermines the gravity of this neurological disability on several levels. It at once describes BI as persistent yet simultaneously reduces its severity to a 'nagging' or even 'petty' complaint, something that, while persistent, may be intermittent, negating its permanence. Yet this particular B-Met, Lawrenson maintains, is a 'great' description.

Writing about the punitive notions of disease inherent in the cancer metaphor, Sontag explicates this development of the negative medical metaphor. She discusses how traditionally in debates about cancer, the illness itself is seen as the enemy, but that conversely, 'It is also the cancer patient who is made culpable.' Moreover, the onus of responsibility both for becoming ill and for getting well falls upon the cancer patient, thus the illness is imbued with a moralistic meaning (59). As Couser explains, 'Sontag has brilliantly illustrated how cancer discourse has tended to stigmatize and marginalize the ill, condemning them in two senses – simultaneously censuring and sentencing them' (1997: 45). Sontag also lucidly describes the process an illness has to go through in making its transition into metaphor. The first stage, she explains, invokes the identification with the disease of negative associations, 'subjects of deepest dread'. It is at this point that the disease has become a metaphor, but in order for it to be sustainable, it has to enter the secondary 'adjectival' stage, during which the disease and all of its horrific associations are imposed upon other targets as we have seen in the case of the B-Met. As Sontag concludes, 'Something is said to be disease-like, meaning that it is disgusting or ugly' (60).

I will return to Sontag in the final chapter, reappraising her thesis on illness and metaphor in light of new and emergent theory while also examining the influence and impact of C-Met and B-Met within public fora. For the time being, what follows is an examination of key examples of C-Met within a range of fiction and non-fiction, interrogating how authors use figurative depictions of coma (and BI) and what they reveal about our belief systems with regard to these conditions, and how coma, as narrative device, functions as a springboard from which writers can reveal wider existential questions, fears and dilemmas.

2

Coma, trauma and the exilic self

Anne Hunsaker Hawkins, in her analysis of mythologies used by writers of what she terms 'pathography' (an 'autobiographical or biographical narrative about an experience of illness' (1999: 229, n.1)), highlights one trope which is particularly instructive to my ongoing analysis of coma metaphor in fiction: the 'journey' mythology. This mythology, Hawkins notes, takes several forms: the 'familiar quest motif', for example, 'where the hero journeys into distant lands, undergoes various ordeals and trials, and returns with some gift or trophy' (78–9). I will return to this sub-set of the journey myth and its connections to metaphors of rebirth and hellish descent in the next chapter, but for now, I wish to explore another 'variant of the journey myth' which Hawkins highlights: 'the theme of exile' (79). As Hawkins observes, 'Unlike the quest, exile is involuntary and evokes feelings of estrangement, alienation and separation. The exile is condemned to wander in strange and foreign territories' (79). This is a particularly prevalent motif in coma fiction, with the coma itself represented as a form of neuro-psychological exilic outland, the victim banished from the homeland of the outside world and trapped within strange, nightmarish territories. In using this particular C-Met, writers of fiction represent a profound exile from the self and within the self.

2.1 Coma, exile, trauma: an overview

This image of exile within the body or mind is prolific across many works of coma literature: physical and neurological representations of the exilic coma patient offering an imagined subjective experience of being trapped within oneself. Ma Jian's novel *Beijing Coma* depicts protagonist Dai Wei's exile in coma, his DoC triggered after being shot in the head at the Tiananmen Square protest that occurred ten years earlier. As is the case with many works of coma fiction, the coma itself is portrayed as being exceptionally protracted despite the fact that, as discussed, coma soon progresses to the PVS (or continuing VS). Dai Wei is described, though, in the blurb of the novel, as a 'prisoner in his own body', evoking the trope of exile within the comatose body. Throughout the novel, he is also a prisoner to his own memories with irruptions of an italicized, second-person interior voice reminding the comatose Dai Wei of his medical exile: '*A portion of your brain is still alive. You wander back and forth through the space between your flesh and your memories*' (2009: 5). In essence, Dai Wei is in an exilic limbo, trapped within the corporeal place of exile and by the oppressive flood of memories from which he cannot escape, alongside the clear awareness of his exilic status as comatose patient.

A similar conceit is at play in Kevin Bigley's *Comaville* which follows protagonist Josh Husk (an aptronymous surname, perhaps, given Josh's entrapment within his own body) who lies in coma after a road-traffic accident while riding his bike. Like Dai Wei in Jian's novel, Josh is engulfed by memories of his past but unlike his counterpart in *Beijing Coma*, these memories are amalgams of remembrances from different times of his thirty-six years of life. Despite awakening 'in a bed that had once belonged to him' (2019: 1), wandering around the house in which he awakens, he realizes that each room, each feature is taken from various houses that he has lived in throughout his life: 'a Frankensteined home of memory' (4). Despite the fact that his individual memories are so precise and vivid, Josh begins to feel a profound sense of alienation and exile due to the fact that the combination of memories is inaccurate – a collage of memory which he soon finds emotionally draining: 'While the buildings and familiar faces fomented feelings of warmth and comfort, he could not help but feel exhausted by the amount of familiarity and its impetuous stitching' (51). Significantly, however, one gap in memory which he does possess is that of his parents. When trying to conjure an image of them, 'Their faces, shapes, and voices were absent from even the furthest reaches of his brain' (3). In short, those memory traces that immediately connect him to the world beyond coma, the familial aspect of the homeland, have been severed, thereby underscoring his sense of exile.

In contrast to *Beijing Coma* and *Comaville*, Mike McCormack's *Notes On A Coma* sees the medical condition as a means to escape (self-exile), rather than a condition from which a return from exile is desired. The novel is centred around the young protagonist, J. J. O'Malley, the adopted son of Irish farmer Anthony O'Malley who rescued J. J. from one of the infamous Romanian orphanages and raised him in a quiet rural community in West Mayo. Yet J. J., despite this new life, is incapable of finding happiness, cursed with an immense intellect that causes him to spiral into nihilistic philosophical debates – his 'mindrot meditations' (2005: 42). After the tragedy of his best friend dying, an event for which J. J. blames himself, he suffers a crippling nervous breakdown, eventually deciding to enrol for a trial for a new penal system that involves placing prisoners into induced comas on a repurposed cargo ship off the West coast of Ireland. McCormack depicts an entire landscape of exile, with the coma itself one manifestation of this: a self-imposed exile both from the central protagonist's own self and from his community. The prison ship itself is renamed the *Somnos*, embodying that common conflation of coma and sleep, yet McCormack is particularly interested in the fusion of flesh and machine: the 'pipes draining and feeding' J. J. (15), alongside the physical consequences of DoC, noting, at one point, that, 'Coma patients need their bodies to sustain them. Muscle atrophy is an inevitable effect of long-term coma' (109) in a rebuke to the sleeping beauty motif. But he also addresses questions that DoC raise in relation to the existential positioning of the comatose patient: the 'neither-here-nor-there ontologies' (27) that I will discuss further in the closing of this investigation. Indeed, McCormack refers to J. J. as 'inhabiting the realm of the undead' (42), another popular trope of coma fiction that I will address in the following chapter.

McCormack goes on to craft a delicate satire on the nature of reality television, as J. J., alongside his fellow volunteers, become 'celebrities', viewers glued to their broadcast EEG readings and live-feeds. In fact, McCormack drily suggests that the broadcast of the live coma patient is the ultimate form of reality-TV, the high-drama and tantrums of previous shows now 'flatlined to a series of minimal cues and responses, decipherable only to a specialist audience' (193). J. J., therefore, in an attempt to exile himself from the world by inhabiting coma actually only succeeds in embedding himself further into that world as a cultural icon on a global scale.

The language and imagery of corporeal exile is similarly exploited in what I would term pseudo-coma texts; that is, those texts that depict the interiority of exile of consciousness, trapped within the body. Dennis Potter's futuristic play *Cold Lazarus*, for example, depicts the cryogenically-frozen head of writer Daniel Feeld, and the experiments of scientists, employed by an American media tycoon. Their goal is to chemically induce Feeld's memories to broadcast to the world, reaching, as Professor Emma Porlock, the head scientist in charge of extracting Feeld's memories reflects, 'Into the actual memory, the actual mind, of a human being who died three hundred and seventy-four years ago' (1996). Similar to *Notes On A Coma*, Potter's pseudo-coma sees his protagonist's condition become a hot media property, breaching ethical boundaries, particularly when it is revealed that Feeld's cryogenic brain is still conscious but trapped, exiled, at the hands of the corrupt media conglomerate – his head also physically exiled from his body.

Dalton Trumbo's *Johnny Got His Gun* may, too, be seen as a work of pseudo-coma fiction, maybe even proto-coma fiction, and a very early representation of consciousness trapped and exiled within the body. Written in the 1930s detailing the horrors of the First World War, Trumbo depicts an American soldier in a war hospital who suddenly becomes aware that he has 'no legs and no arms and no eyes and no ears and no nose and no mouth and no tongue' (2009: 64): he is trapped within the 'outland' of his own body. What follows is a frantic kaleidoscope of memories of the past, horrors of the present and terrifying hallucinations that plague Joe Bonham's exiled consciousness. While clearly not a work of coma fiction per se, what is fascinating about Trumbo's novel is its use of linguistic and semiotic tropes that would go on to be similarly adopted by writers of coma fiction. At one point, Trumbo writes, 'He was trapped in his own brain tangled in the tissues and brain-matter kicking and gouging and screaming to get out' (189), a description that evokes the plight of many comatose protagonists, as we shall see. Like *Notes On A Coma* (and alongside wider texts to be discussed in Chapter 3), there are multiple allusions to the underworld and resurrection, at one point Joe musing that, 'Never before in the world had the dead spoken never since Lazarus and Lazarus didn't say anything' (224). Trumbo, aside from the image of death, also conjures the image of birth, alluding to Joe being 'in this womb forever and ever and ever' (83), a mythology of rebirth, as Hawkins explicates, that is often used in pathography (1999: 33). And towards the end of the novel, Trumbo even writes that, 'It seemed to him that he was lying in some kind of dream coma' (241), drawing a connecting line between his protagonist's own corporeal exile through physical trauma and the neurological exile of coma.

This depiction of consciousness exiled within a corporeal outland through a catastrophic medical condition or injury is similarly portrayed in Jean-Dominique

Bauby in his autobiographical bestseller, *The Diving Bell and the Butterfly*, later adapted for the screen by Julian Schnabel (2007). Bauby went into coma after suffering a massive stroke, yet his memoir depicts a different exile of consciousness: that of locked-in syndrome, 'A state in which selective supranuclear motor differentiation produces paralysis of all four extremities and the lower cranial nerves without interfering with consciousness' (Plum and Posner 1980: 9). In short, consciousness becomes trapped within a body that has no motor functions, with Bauby dictating his memoir through an excruciating sequence of blinks, a struggle represented, by Schnabel, through blurred, restricted and obscured point-of-view shots that mimic Bauby's subjective experience of the world, only being able to observe (and communicate with) his one working left eye. Once more, Bauby depicts the body as a place of exile, his 'cocoon' that is 'oppressive', in contrast to the 'butterfly' of his mind (2204: 13), echoing the limbless, paralysed cocoon of Joe Bonham's body.

Yet it is perhaps Duncan Jones' 2011 film, *Source Code*, that most comprehensively draws together the linguistic and semiotic tropes established by Trumbo's novel of corporeal exile. Itself a work of coma fiction, the film tells the story of an American air force pilot, Captain Colter Stevens, who is repeatedly inserted into an eight-minute 'source code' that constitutes the last moments of memory retrieved from a victim of a terrorist bombing on a train. Stevens must keep repeating this eight-minute sequence, inhabiting the character and mind of the victim, in order to uncover the identity of the bomber so as to prevent a subsequent, larger-scale attack taking place.

However, it is gradually revealed that Stevens is actually in coma and the scientists who communicate with him do so through direct contact with his brain synapses – Stevens' visualization of his communication with his superior officers is merely an invention of his vegetative brain. In reality, his spoken words appear as written text – brain impulses translated into written language. Even the simulation-chamber of the source code in which we see Stevens communicate and from where he is inserted into the source code is an invention of his comatose mind (what one of his superiors refers to as a 'manifestation' of his brain); a way of coping with the trauma and reality of his coma-exile. In the end, when the audience comes face-to-face with the 'real' Stevens, his body is revealed to be akin to Joe Bonham's – his lower-half blown off, a corporeal 'cocoon' in which his comatose mind is exiled and which, like Dennis Potter's pseudo-coma protagonist, Daniel Feeld, is at the mercy of unscrupulous scientists.

What all of these examples demonstrate is coma-exile as a site of profound trauma, sometimes physical, sometimes psychological; oftentimes both. In several of the texts, we also find that the exilic condition is perpetuated often by the memory of the place from which one was exiled: the 'homeland'. The persistence of this memory and the yearning to return to the homeland has its equivalence with traumatic memory. Memory will not allow the exile to become fully contented and at peace in his present surroundings and will not allow him to move forward and beyond the feeling of exile. Just as the traumatic memory entraps the survivor of trauma within a ruptured temporality of existence in which the traumatic episode of the past is repeated and relived, so the memory of the homeland for the exile entraps him in a constant yearning for the past, haunted by the traumatic associations of displacement and upheaval that it evokes. Edward Said, in his influential essay on exile, refers to this predicament as 'the loss of something left behind forever', a loss which is embodied by the 'unhealable rift forced between [. . .] the self and its true home' (2000: 173). Said's language resonates with the traumatic condition, the 'unhealable rift' of exile mirroring the 'wound' of the traumatized subject that is constantly reopened through reoccurring encounters with the traumatizing event. The word trauma itself (from the Greek τραῦμα) translates as 'wound'; today often interpreted as a psychological wound that may remain unhealed if not confronted or 'worked through'. For Cathy Caruth, in her reflections upon Freud's theories on trauma, the traumatizing event 'is not fully perceived as it occurs' (1995: 8), a phenomenon that is applicable both to the exiled subject and the victim of coma. Developing Freud's work on traumatic neuroses, Caruth discusses the 'haunting' nature of trauma, postulating that, 'To be traumatized is precisely to be possessed by an image or event' (1995: 4-5). Within Freud's language on the subject of trauma there are frequent references to this notion of 'haunting', with the mind's compulsion to repeat embodying a form of psychological possession. His core example of Tancred from Tasso's romantic epic *Gerusalemme liberata*, cited in *Beyond the Pleasure Principle*, describes the spectral nature of trauma and it is significant that Caruth uses this as a foundation for her own theory of what Anne Whitehead terms the 'possessive influence' (2004: 5). After unwittingly killing his lover, Clorinda, Tancred enters a charmed and frightful forest, where he attacks one particular tree with his sword, at which point 'blood gushes from the wound, and the voice of Clorinda, whose spirit magically entered into that very tree, accuses him of yet again doing harm to his beloved' (Freud 2003: 61). In this, Freud introduces the notion of the repetitive, inwards-turning nature of trauma and the compulsion to repeat the traumatic event of the past, an event that 'perpetually escapes or eludes our understanding' (Whitehead 2004: 13). Through repetition, the victim of trauma hopes to reassimilate the rupture of temporality and of identity, thereby mastering or coming to terms with the traumatizing event. But this example also emphasizes the ghostly form of trauma; its haunting quality. The voice of Clorinda manifests itself as a ghost, and cries out to Tancred against his will. Just as he unwittingly killed her the first time, he unwittingly kills her the second time and this traumatic repetition takes the form of a ghostly voice, a spectral re-run of the traumatic event. Freud proposes that this poetic repetition is akin to the dreams of those 'possessed' by traumatic neuroses, the survivors of the First World War, for example, who were at the forefront of his mind at the time of writing *Beyond the Pleasure Principle*. Thus, as Whitehead concludes in her appraisal of the development of trauma theory, for Freud, 'Trauma is inextricable . . . from the ghostly or spectral, and it testifies to the profoundly unresolved nature of the past' (2004: 13).

In coma literature, the traumatizing event, often caused by a violent action enacted upon or within the physical self (road-traffic accident/brain tumour) is likewise often not perceived as it occurs. In such texts, the plight of the coma victim is centred upon the attempt to face up to the event that has caused such a catastrophic 'break in the mind's experience of time' (Caruth 1996: 61) but which has also caused such a rupture within the victim's sense of selfhood. What is most interesting is that in interior coma narratives this attempt to 'reunify' the self through a rediscovering of the haunting, past event occurs within the world of the unconscious. Once the victim of coma has confronted the traumatic event, then the process of their survival has only just begun. In many of these narratives, it is the confrontation with the traumatizing event that catalyses the victim's emergence from coma, the texts concluding at the point of 'awakening' or, in the case of *Source Code*, the hero's realization and acceptance that he is exiled within coma and his only escape is death.

Whitehead, in discussing the traumatizing event reinterpreted by Caruth in her development of the Freudian structure of trauma, asserts that it is 'not available in the usual way to memory and interpretation'. While Whitehead goes onto discuss how the traumatic event 'cannot be possessed in the forms of memory or narrative', nevertheless the 'haunting quality' of trauma continues to 'possess the subject with its insistent repetition and returns' (2004: 12), once more evoking the language of the supernatural and uncanny.

It seems to me that there is a clear parallel between the language of such trauma theory and of the theory of exile. Said's notion of the 'loss of something left behind forever' conveys a sense of death, or of a ghost, with the lost object (in this case the homeland) repeatedly haunting and possessing the memory of the traumatized exile. As Catherine Reuben succinctly posits in her reflections upon the interplay between exile and identity, 'There is a strong link between exile and memory. Without memory, one would not know that one was in exile' (2003: 202). This is a sentiment supported by Said in his suggestion that, 'Almost by definition exile and memory go together' (2000: xxxv). Said proposes that in order to attempt to move beyond this traumatizing memory of exile, the victim must refuse to 'sit on the sidelines nursing a wound' (2000: 184), again evoking a notable parallel with the language of trauma theory. According to Said the only way one can cope with the trauma of exile is to cease the reopening of the wound of the traumatizing incident – the initiating moment of exile.

This complex nexus between trauma, memory and exile can also be extended to the medical state of coma and the plight of the coma victim. For the individual who survives coma but has sustained brain damage, they not only return from the exile of coma but return to a 'homeland' in which they still feel exiled due to the indelible changes in personhood. Even if the survivor has no memory of who they used to be, these memories will still be held by proxy by friends and loved ones and shared with them, perpetuating not only a sense of exile within the homeland (the world outside of coma) but also a sense of exile from their former self. It follows that memory, whether disrupted or obliterated completely through the impact of coma and BI, has the ability to sustain the exilic state. The homeland, therefore, can never be the same again; the feeling of exile will always persist and be perpetuated by the memory of loss. Said also addresses this concept of the exile's 'unreachable' homeland to which a return can never be made, suggesting instead that, 'The pathos of exile is in the loss of contact with the solidity and the satisfaction of earth: homecoming is out of the question' (2000: 179). This statement can be considered as a powerful metaphor for the plight of the 'coma-exile' who loses contact with the solidity and familiarity of the homeland while within the 'outland' of coma and who then returns from exile only to find that the homeland can never be the same again. Baldly, even if the exile does eventually return, a true 'homecoming' is impossible because the homeland is now loaded indelibly with the traumatic memory of exile and loss.

Coma fiction frequently depicts this triumvirate of trauma/coma/exile. Marc Levy's novel *If Only It Were True* is at once a fascinating example of the fetishization of the coma-body (and the use of the 'sleeping beauty' trope) and an examination of key concepts arising out of the theories of trauma and exile, most notably the idea of traumatic hauntings. The novel tells the story of Lauren, a young doctor who 'dies' in a car crash, only to be brought back to life moments later. Trapped in coma, an astral projection of her 'self' inhabits her apartment, now being sub-let by a new tenant, Arthur. He is the only one who sees her and he soon falls in love with her, becoming increasingly desperate to save her before her life-support machine is switched off. An exponent of romantic fiction, Levy's novel recycles the stories of Snow White and Sleeping Beauty to create a modern fairy tale, complete with 'sleeping' Princess and dashing Prince Charming. Rather than the cursed apple or spindle, though, it is a car crash that precipitates the heroine's descent into the deep 'sleep'.

In the description of the crash itself, Levy uses the figure of the coma patient that further exemplifies the glorification of the traumatized body. Lauren is described, post-accident, as being 'peaceful, at rest' with 'calm' features and 'slow and even' breathing. Levy writes how, 'There might even have been a small smile on her slightly parted lips', and how, 'She seemed to be sleeping'; her 'long hair framed her face' (2000: 11). This description exudes a sense of serenity that is at odds with the violence of the traumatizing incident: the car crash that sees Lauren flung through a shop window. The lingering upon the physical aspects of Lauren's body is sexualized, romanticizing the coma in much the same way as other texts discussed earlier, most notably Almodovar's *Hable con Ella*. Again, the coma is portrayed as a tranquil state of deep sleep, the sibilant reference to the 'small smile' implying that this is a blissful liminal state in the aftermath of the violence of the crash.

However, this fetishized coma aesthetic becomes more complex as Levy gradually integrates factual medical detail seen, most prominently, at the point at which Arthur and the astrally-projected Lauren visits the corporeal Lauren who still lies in her hospital bed: 'The motionless woman was paler than her double, and thinner. Her hands had begun to turn inward in the seizing up that occurs in long-term coma patients, and she looked frail, but the resemblance was striking' (2000: 44). The romantic notion of the sleeping beauty intersects with the degradation of the body occurring within actual cases of long-term coma victims. Later, images of the 'IV drip to irrigate her' and the 'catheter to carry away her waste' (2000: 45) are once more at odds with this modern-day fairy tale narrative and serve to deconstruct the earlier, sexualized depiction of Lauren post-accident. Levy portrays the sleeping beauty figure as a physically flawed heroine, who nevertheless captures (and maintains, despite these flaws) the romantic attention and commitment of the Prince Charming.

In Lauren, there is also the manifestation of the haunting nature of trauma and exile, the protagonist literally becoming the ghost of her trauma, constituted by a violent accident of which she has no memory. We see the connection between the 'haunting' of traumatic memory and the 'haunting' of the post-coma, post-traumatic memories of the coma survivor. We also see a representation of another key strand of trauma theory and one of Freud's foundational theories of traumatic neurosis: the phenomenon of latency (*nachträglichkeit*, or deferred action), a concept that can likewise be applied to the exilic condition. In *Moses and Monotheism*, Freud writes of a hypothetical situation in which a man walks away from a train wreck 'apparently unharmed'. It is only after a delayed period of time that he begins to develop, 'A series of grave psychical and motor symptoms, which one can ascribe only to his shock or whatever else happened at the time of the accident' (1939: 109). In a similar example to that of Tancred cited in *Beyond the Pleasure Principle*, the traumatic condition only takes hold after a certain delay in time: after a traumatic *departure*. As Caruth explicates in her development of Freudian thought, 'So trauma is not locatable in the simple violent or original event in an individual's past, but rather in the way that its very unassimilated nature – the way it was precisely *not known* in the first instance – returns to haunt the survivor later on' (1996: 4). In the cases of both the trauma survivor and coma survivor, the traumatic event is not confronted or understood as it occurs and only makes its impact belatedly, often in the form of traumatic repetitions and psychological 'hauntings'. The psychoanalyst Jean Laplanche translated Freud's *nachträglichkeit* to describe this belatedness of traumatic memory as 'afterwardsness', a concept that he describes as 'contain[ing] great richness and a certain ambiguity, combining a retrogressive and a progressive direction' (1999: 265). It is a term that, as Roger Luckhurst points out in his discussions of Laplanche's redevelopment of Freudian theory, '[F]oregrounds the odd temporality of an event not understood as traumatic until its return' (2008: 9) – the spectre of trauma.

Within the pages of Levy's novel, this 'afterwardsness' of Freud's hypothetical train wreck survivor is re-imagined through the depiction of Lauren's car-wreck trauma that is not comprehended as it occurs. Instead it is repeated and confronted as she continues to exist (through her astrally-projected self) after leaving the scene of the accident. Lauren is both haunted by this traumatic event but also actively *haunts*, forcing Arthur to become the witness to her trauma in all of its forms: the trauma of the accident; the trauma of her coma; and the potential future trauma of her death as the decision to switch off her life-support machine draws ever closer. The figure of Lauren becomes an embodiment of the multi-faceted traumatic experience of coma, both in the trauma of her lost past, and in her struggle to work through this and to survive. Lauren therefore represents the 'traumatic memory [that] persists in a half-life, rather like a ghost, a haunting absent presence of another time in our time' (Luckhurst 2008: 81). The coma is emblematic of this half-life that sustains and preserves Lauren's existence but which prevents her from fully living. She is trapped in spiritual form within her old apartment and so is both absent and present, a ghost of the trauma that is etched upon and within her physical body. This paradox of trauma is heightened in the novel's denouement when Lauren, emerging from coma, has no memory of who Arthur is or what her relationship is to this strange man who holds vigil at her bedside. Levy by no means paints a wholly romanticized depiction of coma survival. Ultimately, Lauren has only survived the first stage of her traumatic ordeal: the emergence from coma. The next stage of her traumatic experience and survival awaits: her rediscovery and rebuilding of selfhood, albeit a trauma that is somewhat romantically buffered by Arthur's faithful, optimistic role of Prince Charming. Peculiarly, the paratextual tagline of the novel, 'Fall in love again', does not relate to the storyline contained within the pages of the novel but pertains to the future lives of Arthur and Lauren that exist in the world beyond the ending of the story. The romantic repetition implied in this tagline is indicative of the traumatic ordeal (we can only imagine that this process of falling in love 'again' for the protagonists will not be straightforward, as testified to by Lauren's lack of recognition of Arthur) and so the very act of falling in love also becomes traumatic set against this backdrop of coma and survival. The unease that this example of romantic coma fiction engenders is highlighted by the Hollywood film adaptation, *Just Like Heaven* (2005). The film departs from Levy's treatment of the most common medical consequences of coma – the void of the post-coma consciousness – by adapting the genre fully into 'romcom', focusing upon comic 'meet-cute' scenes between David (Arthur, in the novel) and Elizabeth (Lauren). In this adaptation, Elizabeth is unaware that she is in coma, unlike the novel, thereby exploiting the boy-meets-girl conceit at the heart of the romcom genre but also heightening the sense that she might be a ghost (there is even a scene of a comedy exorcism) as the last we see of her before a smash-cut to black is her car crashing into an oncoming truck. When she eventually does confront her comatose self lying in the hospital bed, David exclaims, 'It's way better than being dead – you don't have any scars, you look pretty!', a comment at odds with the representation of the degradation of the body in Levy's source material and underscoring the sleeping beauty trope. And at the end of the novel, Elizabeth's status as sleeping beauty is ratified as she is finally 'awoken' by a kiss from David although, true to the novel, she does not remember him. Having said this, the film's coda is a sequence in which Elizabeth learns to rediscover her feelings and astral experiences she had with him while in coma – the 'fall in love' again tagline of Levy's novel played out on screen.

While Levy's novel paints a complex picture of the relationship between coma and the haunting nature of trauma, it simultaneously draws a link between these conditions and the exilic state. There is a multi-faceted representation of exile: the traumatic event of the car accident exiles Lauren from the world through her ensuing coma; yet Lauren is also exiled *from* her own body, the corporal and psychological elements of her identity separated from one another. However, Lauren's astral projection does return to a certain manifestation of her homeland, her apartment, but this in itself is alienating, a reminder of her exilic condition. To return to Said, Lauren (literally), has lost all contact with 'the solidity and satisfaction of earth' making 'homecoming' impossible.

2.2 The role of memory and language in coma-exile

While much of Said's discussion of exile focuses upon the physical and geographical dislocation of an individual *from* his homeland, David Bevan, in his introduction to a collection of essays analysing the relationship between literature and exile, proposes a model of exile that occurs *within* the homeland. He writes, 'Exile within a place is often still more poignant than exile from a place or exile to a place. Exile, viscerally, is difference, otherness' (1990: 3). Much of coma fiction inhabits this idea by portraying the interiority of coma, and the feeling of exile the patients experience; exile from both the world outside of coma (exile *from* a place) and also exile felt *within* a place: the homeland of the mind and body. The coma victim exemplifies this concept of exile within a place, still physically inhabiting the homeland and yet, through the distinct otherness of coma, exiled from it, reflecting Magda Stroińska's assertion that it is possible to 'feel exiled in one's own country' (2003: 97); in this context, the homeland of the mind or body.

The Coma by Alex Garland and *Marabou Stork Nightmares* by Irvine Welsh explore this 'internal' exile of coma and how memory and language impacts upon and often perpetuates the exilic self. In his analysis of the work of another prominent literary exile, W. G. Sebald, Philip Schlesinger highlights a common connection between violence and exile: 'Typically, violence – actual or threatened – propels people into exile, although we cannot exclude the inner compulsion to depart' (2004: 46). In the case of Carl in *The Coma*, it is certainly a violent initiating event that heralds his exilic departure from the homeland: a vicious attack on a tube train. For Welsh's protagonist, Roy, his departure is an altogether more complex manifestation of departure, triggered by an act of self-violence: a botched suicide attempt. The two novelists, however, present the characters' respective comas in two sharply contrasting ways. For Carl, it is an exile from which he is desperate to escape; for Roy, self-imposed and self-sustained exile becomes a safe haven in which he can attempt to hide from the realities of his homeland, realities that led him to suicide in the first place. Despite this difference, both novelists explore how traumatic memory (and the distortion of memories) plays a key role in sustaining these fictional comas. Said notes, 'For an exile, habits of life, expression or identity in the new environment inevitably occur against the memory of these things in another environment' (2000: 186). This description of the 'doubling' of exile (geographical, physical detachment from the homeland and the habitual behaviours of the homeland enacted within the outland) again suggests that it is the memory of the homeland that makes it impossible for the exile to live comfortably; that he can only compensate for the real sense of loss by 'creating a new world to rule' (2000: 181), rather than trying to recreate the old world in a new place. Thus, the exile will attempt to create a new conception of selfhood in order to learn to accept and overcome the feeling of exile and assent to a future self that can live comfortably within a new land. However, as Said suggests, the memories of exile cannot be completely put out of mind and so this attempt to develop control over how one perceives and accepts a new life and a new land will be inevitably superimposed over those distant memories of the homeland. Like Josh Husk in *Comaville*, both Carl and Roy, while in their respective comas, are trapped within traumatic psychological projections of geographical landscapes, new worlds over which they try to rule despite the memories of the homeland impinging on this. For Husk, these memories are 'profoundly exhausting' (51) and 'anxiety-inducing' (52), his 'new world' full of familiar faces which he struggles to recognise and work out where they sit 'in the timeline of his life' before they are 'replaced by another acquaintance', disallowing a chance to 'connect with them' (52).

At the start of *The Coma*, Carl narrates the details of his attack and his emergence from coma, describing a nightmarish homeland to which he has returned. However, it soon transpires that this entire 'memory' of survival and rehabilitation is a falsification, a 'new world to rule' that was formed while still within his coma. Considering Said's theory of exile, Carl's existence within this fake re-imagining of his homeland occurs against the backdrop of memories of his real homeland, again in a similar vein to Josh Husk. Unlike most of Husk's memories, though, Carl's lack definition and are maddeningly intangible and so this new world, to once more refer to Said, becomes 'unnatural and its unreality resembles fiction' (2000: 181). Said acknowledges the inevitable consequence of the attempt of the exile to 'build' a new world upon memories of the homeland. Such an existential palimpsest can only have one result: the alienation from the new world as memories of the homeland irrupt, leading to an overall and persistent traumatic memory of exile. These haunting feelings of displacement, alongside the memories of the homeland that leak through the cracks of consciousness, are represented in Garland's novel, creating an unnerving sense of disorientation and dislocation within Carl's comatose mind. His attempts to reside within a 'fictionalized' version of his homeland continually remind him of the place from which he was exiled and so it is only a matter of time before the façade breaks down to reveal the truth: he is still trapped in coma.

Throughout the novel, Garland represents a highly complex relationship between memory and coma-exile. Even before Carl realizes his initial memories of awakening are false, the reliability of his memory as a whole is brought into question as he describes his attack as an outer-body experience, seeing himself *'hovering between the external glass and the subway walls'* and *'walking backwards through the carriage'*, concluding that, *'From my position outside the carriage, I watched as the young men kicked me into unconsciousness'* (2004: [4],[1] original emphasis). Immediately, the reliability of Carl's memory comes under scrutiny. Carl positively affirms that as the incident took place, he stood as an external witness to his own trauma. However, this suggests that he has a somewhat distorted memory or that his consciousness is creating Freudian 'screen memories', a psychological mechanism, Freud postulates, that assists the subject in concealing the 'memory of a more significant or painful event than that which is superficially remembered' (2000: 109). Carl witnessing his attack from an objective subject position creates a sense of separation between him and the trauma of the violence which constituted his point of departure into the exilic state of coma. It is as though the attack were happening to someone else and the flat, apathetic tone of the narrative voice represents the self-preservative function of the screen memory, distancing the subject from the trauma. Yet the fact that Carl's memory of his attack takes this objective form calls into question the very reliability of his memory itself. As Freud explicates in his discussion of the phenomenon of seeing oneself from an objective subject-position within certain memories, 'Wherever one appears in a memory in this way, as an object among other objects, this confrontation of the acting self with the recollecting self can be taken as proof that the original impression has been edited' (2003: 20). Freud also refers to this phenomenon in his discussions of how one perceives one's own death, proposing that, 'Our own death is indeed unimaginable, and however often we try to imagine it, we realize that we are actually still present as onlookers' (2005: 183). In Carl's memory 'edit', he describes only what he imagines the attack (a death-encounter) would have looked like from the point of view of an external witness. Garland's use of italics adds weight to this sense of unreality, creating a certain distance between the recollected memory of the attack and Carl's attempts to move on with his life. The experimentation with form constitutes one technique commonly utilized by writers of trauma literature as observed by Roger Luckhurst in his critical review of the traumatic memoir 'boom', noting that in such texts, 'Disjunct strands of self, typographically separated on the page' often represent the eruptions of traumatic memory that have not yet been confronted or assimilated – in this case, a disjunct strand of Carl's traumatized psyche, trapped and exiled in coma. Carl's attack is not fully perceived 'as it occurs', resulting in the Freudian memory edit in which he detaches part of his identity from the violent event in an attempt to disassociate himself from the attack and to initiate a screen memory of survival and awakening from coma, thus repressing both the physical and psychological traumatic reality of his situation. In essence, this function of memory represents a splitting of the self – a 'cloning or twinning', as Michael Seidel discusses in his work on narrative representations of exile (1986: 20) – in which part of the self is left within the external world (his corporeal self) while the other part of him (his unconscious) is trapped within the interior world of his coma. This fragmentation of self is often symptomatic of the condition of trauma in which part of the self and the traumatic experience may be repressed, only to come resurfacing in the form of traumatic echoes or episodes. But it is also symptomatic of the exilic condition whereby the subject stands astride two worlds, trying to reside here but inevitably residing elsewhere and so generating, as Schlesinger explains, a 'hybrid . . . sense of identity' (2004: 46). Carl cannot remember how long he has been in his coma, a gap in memory that embodies the 'incubation period' which Freud discusses: the limbo in which the memories of the traumatic incident begin to coalesce to form an overall traumatic neurosis (1939: 109). Between the end of the attack and the first memories Carl experiences within the coma, the exilic, traumatic condition takes hold, leading to a 'hybrid identity' and moreover, a hybrid, fictionalized world within which he temporarily resides, thereby causing a fragmentation of selfhood which Carl must attempt to reunite if he ever wishes to escape from his coma.

The first stage of this reunification is to confront the fact that his 'memory' of leaving the coma and embarking upon rehabilitation is false, constituting a distorted reality: a coma 'dream'. In his discussion of the exile's use of coping strategies, Seidel suggests that, 'Another imaginative solution to the exile's anguish is to export just enough of the homeland to the outland to metonymically purify it' (1986: 10). This approach to dealing with the traumatic nature of exile is adopted by Carl who transposes certain memories and relationships extant within the homeland to his false narrative in order to 'purify' the exilic, alien landscape to which he has been banished. However, in doing this, his consciousness creates a doubling of exile, a traumatic echo that he has to live through twice: facing up to the trauma of his coma within his fake narrative of 'awakening' before confronting the fact that he is still in the exilic state of coma, heralding the end of this false experience of return and the illusion of recovery.

The function of Carl's memory within his exilic state, therefore, becomes even more complex and paradoxical. As with Husk (who also 'awakens' within his coma into a new, uncanny world), Carl's false memories of awakening from coma both protect him from confronting the psychological trauma of his exile, but at the same time prevent him from commencing his return to the homeland. Garland's depiction of dream-like narratives and memories to convey a form of coma consciousness consistently highlights Carl's fractured sense of self, both preventing his unconscious from revealing the reality of his situation while conversely encouraging him to accept the new rules and conditions of his exilic territory. His early encounter with his 'friends'

Anthony and Mary exposes this tension between memory and exile. Throughout this episode, Carl is confronted with 'uncanny' occurrences which reflect 'the helplessness we experience in certain dream-states' (Freud 2003: 144). In the first instance, he has no memory of how he arrives at their house, a confusion he expresses when he says to Anthony: 'One moment I was lying in the bath, the next I was ringing your doorbell' (2004: [24]). He also mentions how there was 'nothing in between', like the dizzying jump-cuts that occur in dream narratives or the 'detached shreds of the scenes we have really experienced' to which the sociologist Maurice Halbwachs refers in his extensive analysis of the appearance of deceptive memory-scenes within dream-states (1992: 42). It is also soon revealed that Anthony did not come to collect Carl from the hospital, with Anthony himself confessing that, 'A real friend should have been there' (2004: [23]). When Anthony hands over a cup of coffee to Carl, Carl says: 'I felt mildly irritated that Anthony had given me the mug in the first place, because, considering our friendship, I thought my dislike of coffee was the sort of thing he ought to know' (2004: [27]). Significantly, while with Anthony and Mary, Carl feels 'a sudden and terrific feeling of despair' (2004: [29]), which is akin to those feelings he experienced as a child when he had 'very powerful fever dreams'. What he experiences is the ultimate 'fever dream' of his coma. Thus, Anthony's comment that 'a real friend should have been there' becomes an unconscious signpost that points to the fact that he isn't a 'real friend' after all. Instead, as is revealed, Anthony is a cypher, a character created within Carl's coma consciousness and based upon the patriarchal frontman of a 'bland family' (2004: [145]) at the centre of an advertising campaign in Carl's homeland. One of Carl's last memories before he is attacked on the train is seeing 'Anthony' on a poster within the tube station. His constant meetings with this cypher within his fake coma 'dream' is a traumatic echo of his last, fractured memory before slipping into unconsciousness.

This representation of linguistic and symbolic signposts within the coma consciousness that attempt to guide the protagonist out of coma similarly appear in an altogether different kind of text: Ubisoft's 2011 high-octane driving simulation game, *Driver: San Francisco*.[2] The sixth instalment of the Driver video game franchise, *Driver: San Francisco* kept the first-person, sandbox format of its predecessors, but what marked its key departure was the narrative twist. Within the first segment of the game, its central protagonist, Tanner, a cop for the SFPD, is involved in a violent car-crash while in pursuit of his criminal nemesis. From this point on, the rest of the gameplay unfolds within the coma unconscious of Tanner, the narrative plotting allowing a new gameplay dynamic: the 'shift'. This 'shifting' allows the player to astral project across the city and 'possess' the driver of any car he chooses. In terms of narrative, much like Sam Tyler in the BBC series *Life On Mars*, Tanner must solve crimes within his coma, in order to come closer to comprehending his true state of consciousness and emerge from coma. Embedded within the world of the game are generic motifs inherent within works of coma fiction. Throughout, Tanner is confronted with road-signs that contain subliminal messages concerning his condition, signposts that try to guide him out of coma: 'Wake Up', one sign subliminally orders him. As in Garland's novel, the interior world of coma works to remind the protagonist of its unreality and the need to escape from it: the process of the unconscious that creates these exilic worlds works against itself in order to allow a return to the homeland.

Said's exegesis of exile can again help to illuminate the processes of both Carl and Tanner's coma-state when he proposes that, in extreme cases, 'The exile can make a fetish of exile, a practice that distances himself from all connections and commitments' (2000: 146). This resonates with Carl's false reality created by his coma-dream. The comfort provided by his unreal friend, Anthony, no matter how traumatic, initially outweighs the need to face up to the reality of his medical dilemma. Said's notion of exilic 'fetish' is personified by Anthony and Mary, themselves creations spun from a paradigm of cultural fetishization: advertising. In Said's warning against the fetishization of exile, we see a fascinating mirroring of Dominick LaCapra's similar misgivings in regard to the fetishization of trauma within writing, discussed at the beginning of this book. Although LaCapra specifically looks at 'totalizing narratives' in trauma writing while Said proposes a model of fetishization that can occur within the lived experience of the exile, there is a clear parallel between how both critics interpret the role of fetish within the two scenarios they describe. The fetishization of trauma in writing and of exile in the *living* of it, they argue, serves to undercut and draw a veil over the gravity of the situation, acting as a form of defence mechanism that, as LaCapra posits, recuperates 'the past in terms of uplifting messages' or, as Said posits in the case of the exile, prevents him from possessing the 'moral courage' to challenge the injustice of exile, instead living a shallow existence 'as if everything around [him] were temporary . . . and trivial' (2000: 146). It becomes inevitable that Carl, following the encounter with Anthony and Mary, feels a sense of 'powerlessness in [his] adopted land', to refer to Lucy Wilson's analysis of the exile's relationship to the outland (1990: 78), the shallow fetish of his coma eventually ceding the power it holds over Carl to a confrontation with reality. He is led to his own hospital room where he comes face-to-face with a vision of the corporeal self within which he is still medically exiled. This proves to be the first step towards accepting the severity of his circumstances (at the point of confronting his body, he says, 'Not for the first time in this dream, I woke up' (2004: [56])) and the catalyst for his quest to reunite his fragmented identity. In other words, returning to Said's theory of the fetish of exile, Carl finally makes the 'connections and commitments' that are required to accept the truth of his exilic state, enabling him to 'cultivate a scrupulous . . . subjectivity' (2000: 147).

But the complex and paradoxical nature of Carl's initially fetishized exile and his screen memory of awakening can also be cogently elucidated through an adaptation of Jacques Lacan's psychoanalytic theory. Throughout the novel, Garland attempts to render a model of consciousness manifested within the coma-state that resonates with much of Lacan's work on the formation and processes of the unconscious. Carl's confrontation with a psychological projection of his physical self, still locked in coma, echoes the Lacanian mirror stage, that point at which the child's Subject is formed, allowing the child to move towards having a unified image of itself. In many examples of coma literature, we discover that the coma is viewed as a form of birth or, more accurately, rebirth. In describing her son's coma and subsequent TBI, for example, the academic and writer Ruthann Knechel Johansen repeatedly uses the language of (re)birth in outlining her son's rehabilitation process, referring to his emergence from coma as his 'second "birth"' (2002: 16). And in Steve Hollyman's novel *Lairies*, there is a similar comparison of the emergence from coma with birth, as the author, in describing one character's coma 'surfacing', writes: 'This is how it felt to be born. Unwombed and taking the first breath, back when I was nameless' (2021: 11). This concept of a second, traumatic birth (the rebirth from coma) evokes another theory of development as proposed by Lacan: the inherent trauma and loss, as he saw, experienced by the child as it is born. In revisiting Freud's concept of *das ding*/the Thing (the object of yearning or desire for the Subject, lost from the moment of birth; a primordial, subconscious 'lack'), Lacan equated the Thing with the mother; not necessarily the 'real' mother, but the mother-who-is-lost or the absence of mother (Bailly 2009: 137). As Lacan postulated, 'The Thing is characterised by the fact that it is impossible for us to imagine it' (1992: 125). Lionel Bailly, in his reappraisal of the Lacanian Thing, proposes that, due to the inherently unsymbolized and unsymbolizable nature of the Thing, 'The Thing is what is lost at the point of birth: the environment *in utero*'. The fact the child once occupied this perfect state of being, this other existence in which 'all of its needs were being met by the functioning of the mother' (Bailly 2010: 137) – the Ideal-mother, if you will – creates a huge sense of loss: both the loss of this perfect other life, but also of the perfect (m)Other. Bailly concludes that the Thing only manifests itself as a concept after the event of its loss, and this is a 'representation of an unrepresented object – a representation of pure loss' (2010: 138). This intersection between the loss of this Ideal-existence, and the fact that, for Lacan, in children there is, 'A veritable *specific prematurity of birth*' (Lacan 2006: 78) – that is, 'the child is born unfinished' (Sarup 1992: 64) – creates a perfect storm for the feeling of lack and the desire to recapture the unsymbolizable Thing: a nexus between an awareness that one is not complete once one is born and the knowledge that one once occupied a perfect state of being where all one's needs were met. I would suggest, also, that the Lacanian Thing resonates with the notion of the Freudian traumatic 'departure' – the trauma that is not experienced as it occurs, and yet leaves the subject with a traumatic, spectral haunting or echo that keeps on returning. Through the lens of Lacanian psychoanalytical theory, birth becomes essentially an exilic process – exile from the Ideal-mother, and ideal state of being. It is the mirror stage that is crucial in drawing the child away from the potential psychosis of this traumatic 'pure loss' by allowing it to, as Sarup argues, 'seek and foster the imaginary wholeness of an "ideal ego"' (65).

Through this Lacanian perspective, the comparison of the post-coma condition to a form of birth becomes even more complex. Due to the fact that often, in cases of serious coma, memories and even whole identities may be lost in the void created by brain injury, there nevertheless remains an awareness, a knowledge, that something has been lost, yet it cannot be symbolized because of the ruling condition of the BI: that the previous self is lost forever to this new self that has been (re)born. The victims of coma may therefore emerge as a completely different person – the (re)birth of a new self that, often, may have to learn (or, more accurately, *re*-learn) everything it once knew. While Garland doesn't concern himself with this post-traumatic, post-coma condition, what he does do is imagine this secondary mirror-stage occurring *within* coma, evoking the 'transformation that takes place in the subject when he assumes an image' (Lacan 2006: 76). In Garland's novel, Carl's self-image is lost to himself. At the point at which Carl sees himself lying in the hospital bed, a manifestation of the Lacanian recognition of self occurs. Just as the baby recognizes itself for the first time 'as a unitary being'

(Bailly 2009: 29), Carl is finally able to resolve the elements of the disturbing, uncanny 'otherness' of his exile and confused sense of self he has encountered up until this moment: 'One moment I was opening the door to the ward room and seeing myself lying on the bed [. . .] The next moment, I was lying on the bed. *I* was lying on the bed' ([55]). Metaphorically, Carl, through this secondary mirror stage, is able to unify all of his fragmentary actions and conceptions of himself into this one revelation of selfhood, just as the baby is able to reconcile all of its fragmented actions and functions into one unified body and self-image, with 'a flutter of jubilant activity' (Lacan 2006: 76) within the mirror. However, as Lacan further proposes, despite this moment of unification, this mirror stage is still an alienating, exilic and misleading experience constituting simultaneously a 'splitting' of the self, a necessary rift separating the Subject from the Object-self which is responsible for the creation of the ego. For Lacan, this split allows the Subject to enter what he terms the Symbolic realm, heralding the acquisition of complex language signification which is vital for the creation of the Subject and the elaboration of the Object: the ego or 'Ideal-I'. The mirror stage, therefore, is an intellectual action in which the child begins to recognize the function of metaphor. The building of the ego 'comes with the gradual acquisition of language', as language attaches ideas to the objectified idea of self, first acknowledged in the mirror (Bailly 2009: 34). Essentially, this pivotal moment in a child's development marks the entry point into the Imaginary realm of consciousness where it creates an 'imaginary' vision of a unitary self: an 'alienated relationship of the self to its own image' (Sarup 1996: 66). It is also where it begins to understand metaphor: *that what I see in the mirror is not really me, yet I will still regard it as though it is me*. This imaginary sense of self acts as 'a kind of bridge' (Bailly 2009: 95) to the Symbolic realm, a realm constituted by the language, laws and social structures of the world. Returning to Hollyman's *Lairies* and the comparison of coma with birth, the allusion to Shaun being both 'unwombed' and 'nameless' embodies this idea of the comatose protagonist/foetus inhabiting a state of limbo before they are (re)born into the language system of the Symbolic realm. For Lacan, the Symbolic is where the unconscious resides and where the Subject is created; structured like language, it holds all the rules and hypotheses that organize and regulate human society and thought, comprised of repressed signifiers. The fact that, as Bailly explicates, the image held in the mirror '*is* oneself and simultaneously *not* oneself' establishes both a pleasurable but also traumatic rift between and interdependence upon the Subject and the Object, a splitting and separating of self *within* the self emblematic of a kind of psychodynamic exile. As Bailly summarizes, 'The foundation stone of the human Subject or identity is an intellectual, schismatic act of narcissism' (2009: 31).

As a novel of psychology rather than neurology, *The Coma* is preoccupied with such psychoanalytical concepts. As Carl re-experiences this Lacanian act of 'schismatic narcissism', gazing upon his mirror-image in the form of the Object/ego of selfhood lying in the hospital bed, he re-enters language, or rather, the schema of language and metaphor that he had developed up until his attack. Carl once more acquires the ability to comprehend metaphor, allowing him to interpret his false screen memory of awakening and thereby confronting the truth of his exilic state, allowing him to attempt a return to the homeland. Looking once more at the interchange between

Anthony and Mary, every action and utterance they perform constitute repressed signifiers that signpost his true exilic state within coma, 'blurted' by his unconscious Subject. The true meaning of these Carl has repressed into his unconscious, in much the same way as a child will repress negative or hurtful signifiers into its unconscious in order to preserve the embellishment and perceived 'perfection' of its Object-ego – its Ideal-I – in a process of wishful thinking that denies reality. The child, then, will create 'master signifiers', linguistic 'tics' that will sometimes emerge from the unconscious Subject in the form of blurts, denegations, language slips and dream-images. The master signifiers 'usually mask their opposites' (Bailly 2009: 63), working to preserve the Ideal-I in re-orientating signifying chains to support the ego. Carl's guidance out of exile relies upon the interpretation of master signifiers. Anthony's failure to pick up Carl from hospital; his unawareness of Carl's dislike of coffee; Mary's insistence upon him going to hospital (an insistence that leads Carl towards the moment of his secondary mirror stage); Anthony's 'language-slip' that a 'real friend should have been there' all constitute a preservation of the ego – in this case an 'ideal' scenario in which Carl has emerged from coma and is engaged in a process of successful rehabilitation with the (albeit questionable) support of his friends. The notion and repetition of 'friendship' is the master signifier which masks and re-orientates the reality that within his coma, Carl has no friends and that he is isolated in his medical exile.

However, even after this revelation following his secondary 'mirror stage', this process of following the signifying chains is further complicated for Carl due to the fact that the chains themselves contain gaps or are shattered completely. Throughout the novel, in an attempt to trigger an "awakening", Carl must follow various signifying chains in an attempt to piece his life together and move out of exile. However, these chains frequently come to an abrupt end, or fail to go anywhere at all due to the disruptions in traumatic memory, thus exacerbating and sustaining the exilic state. This suggests that exile is also a condition that is embedded in language: that it is the understanding of language, metaphor and signifying schemes that allows the state of exile to be perpetuated. The exile experiences this sense of permanent, personal loss because the homeland comes to represent a fundamental part of the individual's identity, with the place of habitation often becoming personified and the relationship with it being deeply personal: a relationship that one understands through the grasp of metaphor and language signification. Magda Stroińska, in discussing the role of language in the re-construction of identity in exile, asserts that, 'Language, or languages with which we grow up are factors in identity construction', going on to explore how, 'Language is so closely intertwined with all aspects of our identity that it may at times seem inseparable from it' (2003: 95, 97). For the exile, there is always the possibility of 'the loss of one's language' leading to 'a loss of identity' (97). Certainly, this seems to be the situation in Carl's case – a splitting or 'twinning' of identity, with the shadow-Carl continuing to 'live' a parallel life of coma recovery within the coma-psyche of the real-Carl. This echoes Norman Manea's examination of the role of language and translation in the development of the exile's identity, when he observes that, 'The exile often swings, for a long time, if not forever between the past and the present. Between formation – deformation – reformation, between different possible egos until, gradually, *the double* appears to represent him on the new social stage' (2012: 266).

Carl does precisely this, oscillating between the deformation/reformation of identity, moving further away from a clear sense and grasp of selfhood the closer he gets to it. Stroińska also notes that, 'It is possible to feel exiled in one's own country [...] where the same national language is spoken' (97). Applying this to Garland's representation of the inner exile of coma and Lacan's concept of the unconscious self, structured like language, we might conclude that Carl's exile within his own mind is sustained by the breakdown in understanding of language and metaphor.

2.3 Coma-exile and traumatic compulsion

This operation of language and memory functioning within the exile of coma is also of paramount concern to Irvine Welsh in *Marabou Stork Nightmares* yet unlike *The Coma*, the circumstances surrounding the event of traumatic 'exilic departure' for its protagonist, Roy Strang, is withheld from the reader for much of the novel. Roy consistently comes close to revealing the cause of his coma-exile, but always shies away from revealing the truth. These constant narrative sidesteps represent Roy's reluctance to confront the cause of his coma: his guilt over his involvement in the violent rape of a young woman. It is gradually revealed that this has led to his unsuccessful suicide attempt and subsequent condition, exemplifying Schlesinger's notion of the exile who possesses (and is possessed by) an 'inner compulsion to depart', a compulsion similarly felt by J. J. O'Malley in Mike McCormack's *Notes On A Coma*. In Roy's outland of coma, instead of obliterating all memories of the atrocity he has committed, he repeatedly and traumatically re-enacts them in the form of his 'Marabou Stork nightmares'. However, we might also consider another of Schlesinger's ideas that is germane to our current discussion: that 'suicide is one response to exile' (2004: 52). Roy's self-induced exile of suicide unintentionally leads to his coma-exile, but Schlesinger is speculating about the possibility of suicide as a *response* to exile, not necessarily as a point of departure *into* it. Roy's quest to discover his true self is revealed through the tripartite narrative of his coma: a 'surface' narration that is triggered by the constant threats of 'awakening' and which registers the comings and goings of nurses and loved ones in the homeland outside of coma; his autobiographical narration (reflecting upon the events of his distant and most recent past); and his twisted, fantastical coma nightmares on the hunt for the Marabou Stork. Through this structure, an unending cycle of exile is gradually uncovered. Roy implies that, from birth, he was exiled from his family and homeland (an example of Bevan's exile *within* a place), referring to his immediate kin as a 'genetic disaster' (1996: 19) and the housing 'scheme' in which he was brought up as 'a concentration camp for the poor' (22). In this metaphor, Welsh uses another example of an exilic people, the Jews (whose multiple histories of exile are most often predicated upon violence) to create a connection with Roy's early feelings of exile. Welsh also criticizes Scotland's post-war housing redevelopment and rehousing schemes that saw old communities demolished and the inhabitants relocated to either the new developments or to other areas entirely. As Clandfield and Lloyd note, in likening the scheme to 'a concentration camp for the poor', Welsh uses a 'hyperbolic metaphor that appears to speak to the social dysfunctionality of rehousing schemes, which removed communities from their histories and thus effectively denied them the chance to grow organically' (2007: 126); rehousing and redevelopment schemes that mirror the condition of exile. Elsewhere, genetics continues to play a key role in his childhood alienation as he is bullied because of his physical features inherited from his cruel and violent father, not least his large ears giving fuel to the nickname 'Dumbo Strang', again serving to exile him from the collective group. In the attribution of this epithet, Roy is dehumanized and deemed cartoonish; his ears become a symbol of stupidity, his Disney counterpart christened with this name by his cruel peers who interpret his over-sized ears as a mark of freakish idiocy. Yet we might also consider the original meaning of the word 'dumb': to be 'destitute of the faculty of speech' *(OED)*. The Disney Dumbo is precisely this: he lacks language, exacerbating the magnitude of isolation and exile he feels within the pack. And while Roy in Welsh's novel is in possession of the faculty of speech, he does not have access, as we shall see, to the language that would enable him to vocalize the trauma that he experienced as a child, or the trauma to which he subjects his rape-victim as an adult. Instead, these exist as signifiers repressed into the Symbolic realm of his unconscious and played out as nightmares within his coma. Like Dai Wei in *Beijing Coma*, Roy is trapped and exiled both within his own body and by the oppressive flood of memories that battle for supremacy within his comatose consciousness.

Roy only seems to find peace when his family decides to emigrate to South Africa, yet Welsh cleverly uses the oppressive ideology of apartheid to create an unyielding feeling of exile, much like the function of Mike McCormack's multiple incarnations of exile within *Notes On A Coma*. Again like McCormack, Welsh is interested in the idea of self-imposed exile, depicting Roy's father's masochistic hatred of Scotland and his desire to leave his own homeland behind. But this is not an act of emigration; it is one of self-exile, another manifestation of Schlesinger's 'inner compulsion to depart'. Despite Roy's relative 'contentment' in this environment, because of Welsh's multi-faceted, heteroglossic unreliable narrator, we have to dig much deeper to find the final reason for Roy's exile of coma. In his 'autobiographical' narrative recollecting his childhood, despite projecting a sense of belonging and new-found contentment in South Africa, he reluctantly reveals that he had to suffer sexual abuse at the hands of his Uncle Gordon. Within the coma, however, Roy persists in creating screen memories to conceal the horrors of what was actually done to him so that, to return to Freud's exegesis, 'Instead of the memory image that was justified by the original experience, we are presented with another, which is to some extent associatively *displaced* from it' (2000: 7). This process of 'displacement' (in which the unconscious shifts the emphasis of important elements to unimportant elements) occurs within Roy's coma 'dreams' in which he is back in South Africa with his fictitious friend, Sandy, on the hunt for the Marabou Stork. The stork is a displacement of attribution where Roy displaces his own undesirable characteristics and behaviours onto the image of the stork – an act of psychological projection. This particular displacement is so loaded with multiple traumatic associations that it gradually develops into an example of 'condensation', whereby a single image becomes symbolic of many other associations or ideas. The stork is a symbol that represents all of the horrors Roy has experienced and, ultimately, the immoral 'monster' that Roy had become prior to his suicide attempt. During the quest for this stork, Roy's pre-coma memories are assimilated into screen memories, prolonging the cycle of repression. The character of Dawson, for example, with his corrupt sexual proclivities and white supremacist beliefs becomes a projection of Uncle Gordon, despite the fact that the latter was 'a thin, spindly man' (19) whereas Dawson is an obese 'desperate old queen' who appears 'to be covered in a strange, translucent oil', an uncanny manifestation of a sexual predator which symbolizes the disgust Roy felt for Gordon at the time of his abuse. Despite these physical differences, they are both described as having breath that is 'sweet and rancid' (41), a transference of negative memories that brings to mind Paul Tabori's definition of the exile: 'someone who inhabits one place and remembers or projects the reality of another' (1990: 68). Roy attempts to evoke and inhabit the positive memories of his past place of habitation, South Africa, yet also projects the negative memories of the sexual abuse that occurred there and which served to exile his child-self further in this outland to which his father brought him. Thus, this new place in which he tries to reside, in which he tries to sustain his self-imposed coma-exile, is constantly turning against him, causing him, as an adult, to perceive an affinity between Scottish 'schemies' and black South Africans, derogatorily referred to as 'Kaffirs' (80). Gavin Miller describes this as a 'contentious comparison between Scottish class structures and South African apartheid' (2007: 90) yet similar to Welsh's reference to the schemes as 'concentration camps', this image of apartheid serves to develop the ongoing saturation of the theme of exile throughout the novel. It also, as Miller explicates, elicits the fact that Roy is 'morally suspect because he is seeking to deny his individual guilt as a rapist and to present his working-class origins as a moral counterweight to the privileged status he enjoyed in South Africa' (97). Again, screen memory is deployed so that Roy can avoid facing up to his moral culpability for his actions in the outland of coma.

Roy's processes of screen memory, displacement, condensation and projection are not just employed in his coma quest-fantasies: they are also utilized in his seemingly 'factual' autobiographical narration. Whenever Roy is in danger of nearing a painful truth in his life, he shifts into his fantasy narrative, creating a rupture in memory and narrative cohesion in order to repress both the severity of his sexual abuse and the degree of his involvement in the rape. He reflects upon how, 'It didn't really feel like abuse at the time', how he found it 'mildly funny and amusing watching Gordon making a drooling tit of himself'. Critically, exile allowed him to 'find' himself, and a new place to rule.

In these early autobiographical narrations, Roy describes the abuse as non-traumatic events of masturbatory titillation that cedes to him 'power [and] attractiveness' (72) by permitting Gordon access to his body in exchange for gifts and favours. In the dream-like outland of coma, this perversion is transferred to Dawson who is frequently portrayed as masturbating and defecating in public: a carnivalesque, derisory figure – though not necessarily a figure to be feared. Towards the end of the novel, however, as the division between fantasy and reality increasingly threaten to corrode completely, Roy enters into what Luckhurst refers to as the 'emergency phase', a common feature of trauma fiction characterized by the 'intrusion of occluded memories into an identity built on an excised version of the past' (2008: 105). In Welsh's novel, Roy's narrative voice explodes into a confessional, capitalized stream of violent language: 'GORDON WITHDRAWING HIS BLOOD-STAINED COCK FROM A FRIGHTENED YOUNG BOY BENT OVER A WORKBENCH' (1996: 255). In a similar way to Carl in Garland's novel, Roy sees the traumatic event from an external position, disassociating his current self from the impersonal 'boy' of the confession, but the most significant implication of this is that he was never in control; that the abuse he suffered was total, brutal and unrelenting. Both the fantasy and the autobiography are screen memories and distortions, created in childhood and held onto throughout adulthood in order to protect the ego (the Ideal-I): attempts not to face up to the full extent of the abuse that are now challenged and broken apart by Roy as he delves deeper into the Symbolic realm within his exile of coma. This is often a consequence of traumatic experience as Kalí Tal proposes in her extensive work on the trauma of sexual abuse when she observes that, 'The dislocation of trauma, which removed meaning from the world, is gradually replaced by new stories about the past that can support a rewritten personal myth' (1996: 125). For Tal, this 'myth-making' is an essential element of the process of trauma survival. It allows the traumatized subject to speak of and testify to their past, to render this traumatic history into language, in order to retell their trauma and attempt to make it seem more 'real' so that future communities can bear witness to and learn from this past. However, for Roy, this 'myth-making' becomes a way of creating a screen between himself and the trauma so that he does not have to face the real gravity of his past, a form of deceptive self-protection and preservation. Even at the end of the novel, Roy still insists that his involvement in the gang-rape was merely as a bystander, dragged into the horrific act by his psychotic friend Lexo. It is only when, in his collapsing fantasy in the Symbolic realm of his hunt for the Marabou Stork, Sandy turns against Roy by pointing his shotgun at him, that he begins to see through the screen memories and face up to the fact that far from being a bystander, he was the actual instigator of the rape. The actions he fervently attributes to Lexo throughout the novel are revealed to be his own as Roy finally realizes that, 'Lexo isnae the stork' (258): the stork is Roy.

In Welsh's representation of the repression and recovery of traumatic memories through a confrontation, in coma, with the screen memories which have concealed the trauma, one of Freud's central concepts of his model of psychology may again be applied: repetition compulsion. Through his sexual violence, Roy, seen through the lens of Freudian theory, 'Does not remember anything of what he has forgotten and repressed, but acts it out . . . he repeats it not as a memory but as an action' (1958: 150). It therefore follows that the repetitious nature of his coma-dreams and his transference of traumatic memories, not least his creation of the symbolic Marabou Stork, become Roy's way of 'repeating and working through'. Roy follows his own 'dream' narrative towards the origin of his neurosis, Welsh's psycho-narration of the interiority of coma reflecting how (un)consciousness might cope with both physical and psychological trauma. Dorrit Cohn's work on narrative modes for representing consciousness, in particular the function of the self-narrated monologue (a technique at play in *Marabou Stork Nightmares*) is particularly instructive in understanding Welsh's narrative construction. Cohn suggests that, 'Unable to cast a retrospective light on past experience, [the narrator] can only relive his dark confusions, perhaps in the hope of ridding himself of them' (1978: 168). Cohn's concept of 'dark confusions' is embodied by Roy's quest for the Marabou Stork, a quest which is hampered by narrative non-sequiturs and interruptions due to the fact that the stork, itself, represents the evil of Roy's crime, which he is not yet ready to face. The linguistic revelation, at the end of the novel, that Roy's physical affliction was not large ears but a large nose ('*Beaky* Strang', not 'Dumbo') substantiates this idea that the Stork is Roy: the moral corruption that needs to be, as Roy repeatedly insists, 'eradicated'. Yet this linguistic slippage continues to hold significance: at the point at which the signifier 'Dumbo' is erased, Roy ceases to be voiceless, or rather, the voice with which he has been speaking, replete with lies, half-truths and fantasies (a fetishized voice portraying an idealized version of himself) is replaced with a voice of painful and traumatic veracity.

The ways the protagonists of both novels use memory in their exilic states of coma are starkly contrasting. Carl is desperate to eliminate false memories; Roy is desperate to preserve false memories. In this sense, like J. J. O'Malley in *Notes On A Coma*, Roy sees the exile of coma as a means of escape from the pressures of the homeland. Despite this divergence, the structural models of memory *in* coma that both Garland and Welsh portray are similar, representing levels of consciousness lying in vertical relation to each other: the deeper the level, the more repressed the memory. Yet in this, we also see what Nicola King describes as Freud's 'two contrasting models of memory' (2000: 11) – a puzzling aporia lying at the heart of psychoanalytical theory. The 'archaeological analogy' in Freud's writings, that is, the topological, vertical model of mind in which the subject can dig deep to locate the source of the repressed, traumatic memory is, as King observes, at odds with the concept of *nachträglichkeit* or 'afterwardsness' which 'unsettles the belief that we can recover the past as it was and unproblematically reunite our past and present selves' (12). In both *The Coma* and *Marabou Stork Nightmares*, we see this aporia of trauma theory appear in the depiction of coma-exile. In splitting *Marabou Stork Nightmares* into three narrative identities, Welsh develops voices which are again in a vertical configuration, with the voice of the narrative present being at the surface, the autobiographical memory being at the intermediary level, and the fantasy-quest (the source of Roy's trauma) lying at the deepest point of coma, akin to Freud's primal, instinctive Id. It is also where initially (and until the fantasies begin to break down and Roy begins to decipher the linguistic and symbolic signifiers) refuge and protection is provided for Roy: it is the place to which he goes when the truth of his traumatic departure into coma-exile comes knocking at his door, commanding his coma self to go:

DEEPER
DEEPER
(181, and throughout)

Yet the magnetic pull of the homeland constantly threatens an 'awakening', Welsh consistently manipulating *mise-en-page* to physically represent this tension within the coma consciousness:

      up
    up
  up
up
(181, and throughout)

When an uncomfortable memory threatens his exile, he uses the linguistic signifier 'DEEPER' to find shelter from it within his fantasies. However, the closer he gets to the truth, the more the command loses its potency. The layers of consciousness and narrative identity move closer together and become a coherent narrative that unifies the fractured elements of Roy's psyche, therefore revealing the truth of his self-imposed exile. Welsh emphasizes this reunification of selfhood through his use of language and dialect. Initially, as Roy embarks upon his quest for the Marabou Stork, his story is narrated in the RP style of a *Boy's Own* adventure story, with frequent exclamations in the vein of, 'Gosh Sandy, you're a Hungry Horace today' (7) and, 'Let's do the blighter!' (13). The closer the layers of memory and consciousness move together, the closer Roy gets to his Scottish identity, as conveyed, for example, when Roy processes, while in coma, a comment made by his nurse, Patricia Devine: 'Your Girlfriend looked nice'. This acts as a trigger for Roy to leave behind the polite, middle-class, measured language of his coma fantasy and slip back into the vernacular of his native Scottish tongue: 'What girlfriend? Surely that fat hoor wisnae back. Some mistake surely. She'll be getting fucked by somebody else long ago and good riddance'. As this voice returns to Roy, so does the violence and misogyny of his language, to the point whereby yet another voice breaks through, a voice of emergency that challenges and berates the brutal unpredictability of Roy's Id-like psyche: 'No don't talk about her that way don't talk about Dorie' (38). It is a heteroglossic, traumatic conflict that consistently threatens the haven of Roy's coma-exile.

Duncan Petrie notes how the use of dialect is also an important feature of contemporary Scottish fiction, hugely influenced, in particular, by the work of James Kelman. By using dialect consistently throughout his work, Welsh 'reaffirms both the validity and necessity of vernacular to convey both first-person subjectivity and third-person narration as a means of challenging the hegemony of Standard English – the language of a political and cultural establishment from which its characters are estranged' (2004: 90). This allusion to 'estrangement' is pertinent to this discussion of exile. Marina Mackay, for example, further discusses how the use of standard English in the *Boy's Own* adventure pastiche of Roy's fantasy narrative 'glorify the British imperialist adventure', the novel thereby illustrating 'a British Scotland impossibly implicated in political repressions, global and domestic' (2003: 280). Welsh strategically deploys vernacular and dialect as a way of depicting the complexity of alienation and the feelings of exile of a comatose anti-hero trapped between Scottishness and a British identity, an 'exploration between Scotland's imperial legacy and damaged masculinity' (Petrie 2004: 94). In addition to the language he uses, Mackay also discusses how, 'Welsh's graphic disruptions are used as a way of showing all the novel's seams, of illustrating its patchwork construction and, by extension, the patchwork identity of a Scottish self that is divided by tradition and by multiple linguistic identities' (279). In this way, *Marabou Stork Nightmares* is representative of what Cairns Craig refers to as 'schizophrenic texts' (1999: 113) that capture the dilemma of 'a nation which is not an independent state and [which] is uncertain whether its nationality is British or Scottish' (14). Welsh's novel is firmly aligned with what David Goldie describes as 'the long-standing Scottish preoccupation with themes of division and the divided self' (2015: 55), this denomination of the 'divided self', as Craig highlights, adopted as the title for R. D. Laing's seminal psychoanalytical work on schizophrenia (Laing, himself, being another famous son of Scotland). Craig further posits that, 'The divided self is a self which refuses to acknowledge its dependence on the other, whereas a healthy 'self', a 'person', is always an interaction with the Other' (112). In Roy's attempts to repress the Other into his coma unconsciousness (the half of his divided self that he wishes to rewrite or ignore altogether), he maintains a sense of exile both from the outside world but also between his two senses of self. Roy therefore constantly refuses to engage with the 'inner dialectic' which, Craig asserts, is 'essential to selfhood' and which, if refused, 'destroys the self' (112). Yet his divided self, while in coma, keeps threatening a dialectical interchange to force Roy into confronting his demons (the unconscious mind, as with Garland's protagonist, constantly working against itself). It is at these points that he issues the command 'DEEPER' in order to journey further into the exile of coma and to deny a reunification of his divided self, inhabiting, instead, fantasy, heroic manifestations of selfhood. In portraying these competing selves within one entity, Welsh writes in the Scottish tradition of Caledonian anti-syzygy, 'a yoking together of opposites in which both aspects remain distinct' (Tim Middleton 1999: 6). The exile of coma becomes a site of battle between the 'double or buried self' (Middleton 1999: 7) and the 'surface' self and so at the point at which the dialectical relationship is restored (rather than the divided self existing separately), Roy's emergence from coma is triggered.

In Garland's novel, the vertical structure of memory is emphasized when Carl says: 'Waking is rising, and dreaming is sinking. You wake up, you fall asleep' (Garland 2004: [109]). This comment also emphasizes Garland's approximation of the state of coma to the states of sleep and dream. Unlike his counterpart in Welsh's novel, Carl is desperate for a 'rising', as one would 'rise' from sleep – or even 'rise' from the dead (a metaphor in coma literature I will elaborate upon in the following chapter). However, before this 'rising' can occur, Carl begins to develop, first, a certain amount of control over his coma – like Roy, he is able to move between the levels of consciousness by simply willing it, proposing that once he realized he 'was dreaming', he could then get 'a sense of place', allowing him to 'shift' from 'one location to another' ([68]). This trope of the astral projection, similarly utilized in Levy's *If Only It Were True*, is again visually present in *Driver: San Francisco*. At one point Tanner, while in coma, utters, 'Maybe if I could hop a whole building . . . or a whole block', comprehending his ability to shift between locations. He no longer has to use the physical 'shift-stick' of his car but can 'shift' psychically, possessing the minds of other drivers scattered across the cityscape of his coma. The linguistic tone here is markedly similar to that used by Garland: this ability in the game is allocated, by the game designers, the designation 'shift', echoing the language Carl uses to describe his own ability to shift between locations within his coma. This moment of realization, the tentative yet confident understanding that the ability to 'shift' can be illimitable, is present in both of these texts with the coma seen as an alternative reality that allows the protagonist boundless possibilities and over which he can develop a certain sense of control. Carl creates these transitions, these shifts, between memory scenes in a moment of empowerment, thereby negating the fear and panic he felt, earlier, when discussing his disjointed memory with Anthony. He begins to use this method of moving between the layers of his consciousness to try and locate memory triggers (the signifiers within particular chains) that will put an end to his exile. However, the scraps of memory and the blank spaces in between only serve to bring him so far to the surface of his coma before, at their worst, sending him spiralling back into a black void of his unconscious (the deepest level in the vertical model) where the only trace of his identity is a disembodied voice that gibbers, 'Random words, strung together. Strings of words. Simple and unhinged. Without pattern, no looping, no meaningful repetitions' ([116]).

This nadir of his exilic existence is initiated by following the trail of a certain signifying chain which he feels is sure to trigger a unification of his fragmented self: it is a trail that leads to a house he lived in as a child. Just as he appears close to breaking through 'the boundary of full consciousness' ([104]), he realizes that the two figures he thought were his parents are again empty cyphers: blank, featureless silhouettes, an overwhelmingly traumatic gap in memory akin to that experienced by Josh Husk in Bigley's *Comaville*. For Carl, this schism in such an existentially significant, familial signifying chain initiates a descent into a coma void, the darkest depths of the Subject, smashing any connections with the Ideal-I. Any Object-identification is made impossible by the fact that all he becomes is a 'consciousness' in a black void, losing 'track of any understanding of physicality at all' ([112]). At this deepest level of coma, not only does Carl lose sense of all physicality but this also leads to him losing language altogether, until eventually the 'strings of words' come back to him: 'BENT UNION TRACK OVER FINE CUBA ORE UNDER RED SORT ETHER INK TOKE INTRO SATURN NILE OR TRAP' ([116]). Garland creates an idea of the Subject trying to reform signifying chains (almost like a 're-booting' of the brain) emphasizing the importance of language in order for Carl to unify his fragmented, exilic self. Even in these 'simple and unhinged' babblings, the signifying chains can be detected, reconfiguring themselves into an overall discourse of Carl's unconscious. For example, the words 'UNDER', 'ETHER' and 'TRAP' signify the state of exile and alienation within his coma. As Lacan proposes, language, even at phoneme level, is essential for the individual to listen to and comprehend the utterances that frequently emerge from his unconscious Subject. Magda Stroińska observes, for the exile, 'Language is part of the process of gaining or maintaining power and access to power is often determined by language skills' (2003: 106). At this point of *The Coma*, this language chain, no matter how fragmented, helps Carl to access and begin to reunify his identity, regaining the power he needs to re-embark upon his journey out of exile.

2.4 Recovery/return: coma-exile, psychoanalysis and abreaction

The models of memory that both authors use adhere to the model of repression in Freudian psychology whereby, 'What is repressed is pushed downwards, into the unconscious. The subject no longer has access to it' (Van Der Kolk and Van Der Hart 1995: 168). This lack of access to the unconscious is akin to Lacan's redevelopment of Freud's concept: that direct access to the Subject is impossible. However, Lacan is not interested in a process of repression occurring within a vertical model of consciousness. Instead, he is much more concerned with horizontal models of repressed language signifiers that need to be traced in order to reach their signified meaning, a concept that is also explored in these novels. In psychoanalysis, of course, one way to access these repressed memories can be through dream-work, hypnosis or, more specifically, through hypnoanalysis in which hypnosis is employed in order to seek out the root cause of the problem, often stored deep within the unconscious. As previously discussed, Freud famously abandoned the practice of hypnosis, opting, instead, for psychoanalysis and free association (his so-called 'talking cure'), emphasizing the interpretation of the unconscious, rather than the power of hypnotic suggestion. The coma, as described in these novels, is a model of the unconscious state within which both protagonists can tap into the unconscious, accessing, rejecting and ultimately accepting the memories and fragments of experience that are at the root of their respective traumas: their exile within coma. The coma, in these novels of psychology, is equated to a hypnotic trance or psychoanalytical 'session' of free association, occurring within the unconscious interiority of coma, in which the victims can attempt to recapture or reinterpret repressed memories through an abreactive process during which the repressed emotions are released by 'acting out' (through language, behaviour and the imagination) the memory-trace that is causing the traumatic conflict. The divided or split self in both novels sees the characters become their own psychoanalysts, if you will, their own guides to lead the way out of their exilic landscapes, regardless of whether this exodus is desired or not.

There are several instances of abreactive interchanges in *The Coma*. Prior to the recognition and acknowledgement of the fact that he is in a coma, Carl interacts with characters within his coma-dreams that play the role of psychoanalytic guides to help lead him out of exile. Chief among these is the taxi driver who transports Carl between potential memory triggers. All of the conversations that Carl has with 'the Cabbie' are mediated through the taxi's rear-view mirror, or delivered to his profile as he drives the cab. In both situations, his face 'looks familiar', although Carl can never quite 'place it' ([43]). It follows that all of these characters are conjurations from Carl's unconscious. But they are also, inherently, manifestations of Carl himself and of various aspects of his fractured identity. Even the coma-version of Catherine, his girlfriend, is not really Catherine but rather a vessel that Carl can inhabit and speak through, appropriating a familiar face in order to create a trustworthy, inner psychoanalyst with whom he can cathartically discuss ideas and plans for a potential escape from exile. She also becomes a figure of the Lacanian Other, someone who represents the outside world with all of its mores and functions and habits. This Other/Catherine figure helps to generate a discourse of the unconscious which has the potential to guide Carl out of exile; it is Catherine who often suggests areas of memory which could possibly trigger an awakening for Carl. The Cabbie, too, is a manifestation of part of Carl's unconscious self and so the two-way conversation in the rear-view mirror becomes ever more significant, embodying the first mirror-gaze that occurs between a mother and child; an interchange in which the latter first becomes aware of itself. This primal connection is key as it is the Cabbie who guides Carl to the hospital. At this point, Carl realizes why he recognizes the Cabbie – he is also the hospital Nurse who then leads him to the vision of himself in the hospital bed, in much the same way that the mother might lead the child to the mirror. As Sarup posits, for the mirror stage to function successfully in child development and for it to adopt 'the tendency that leads him or her throughout life to seek and foster the imaginary wholeness of an 'ideal ego'" (1992: 66), the child 'must be able to turn around and see someone else *as* someone else. That is, it must be able to sense its discrete separation from an Other' (64). At the point of this secondary mirror stage, when Carl recognizes himself as an Other among other Others, he describes 'awakening' for a second time, in the company of Catherine. Despite the fact that 'her face was blank' ([61]), it is this creation of another Other, arising from this secondary mirror stage, that helps to guide him out of the exile of coma and that is a reminder of the homeland and, eventually, of the role and identity he once occupied.

In *Marabou Stork Nightmares*, Roy, too, has multiple guides out of coma, embodying abreactive episodes. Unlike Carl, however, he doesn't always want to follow where they lead. Constantly, the voices of his guides are appropriated by the apparitions of his past in a desperate attempt to make him confront the truth at the heart of his coma. When meeting Dawson for the first time, for example, Roy's heroic sidekick and alter-ego, Sandy, begins 'rocking in his chair and letting out a low sound. – Mmmmm' (1996: 53). Elsewhere, in the autobiographical narration, it is revealed that Elgin, Roy's autistic brother, exhibited similar behaviour when confronted with stressful situations. Sandy's terror is an unconscious formulation of condensation (as would occur in a dream) to force Roy into accepting the true nature of the abuse to which his Uncle (in the guise of Dawson in these stork fantasies) subjected him. But the Dawson figure is far more complex than being simply a screen memory for a traumatic childhood. He is also the character who charges Roy with the task to eradicate the Marabou Stork. In essence, Dawson is an unconscious creation in the Symbolic realm that simultaneously represents Roy's childhood abuse but which also guides Roy towards the quest that will force him into hunting himself down and re-entering the dialectic with his divided self. In Lacanian terms, the protagonist (or analysand) of each novel eventually reaches the point whereby he will 'reveal him to himself' (Bailly 2009: 191).

The exilic state of coma and the manipulative power of memory are not just communicated by the authors through narrative technique. As mentioned, Welsh plays with *mise-en-page* to represent visually the exile of the coma and the fine line between reality and fantasy. But it also, as previously discussed, captures the crisis of Scottish identity, the 'use of narrative fragmentation, interior monologue, and typographic experiment hav[ing] a socio-political purpose in creating a fictional form adequate to a complex representation of Scottish working-class life' (Goldie: 54) which, to Welsh, is alienating and exilic in itself. It is important to note that Garland, too, uses unconventional presentational techniques to achieve a similar outcome. The lack of pagination, for example, which Philip Tew sees as parodying 'the expectations of trauma culture' (2007: 192)[3], denotes a lack of specificity so that just as Carl is alienated by the collapsing, kaleidoscopic patterns of his exilic coma-dreams, the reader is alienated by and lost within the fluidity of the unnumbered pages of the novel itself. Most interesting, though, is the use of monochrome, abstract illustrations, woodcuts created by the author's father, Nicholas Garland. These clearly make visual the nature of Carl's exile, while highlighting the rupture in memory that has occurred

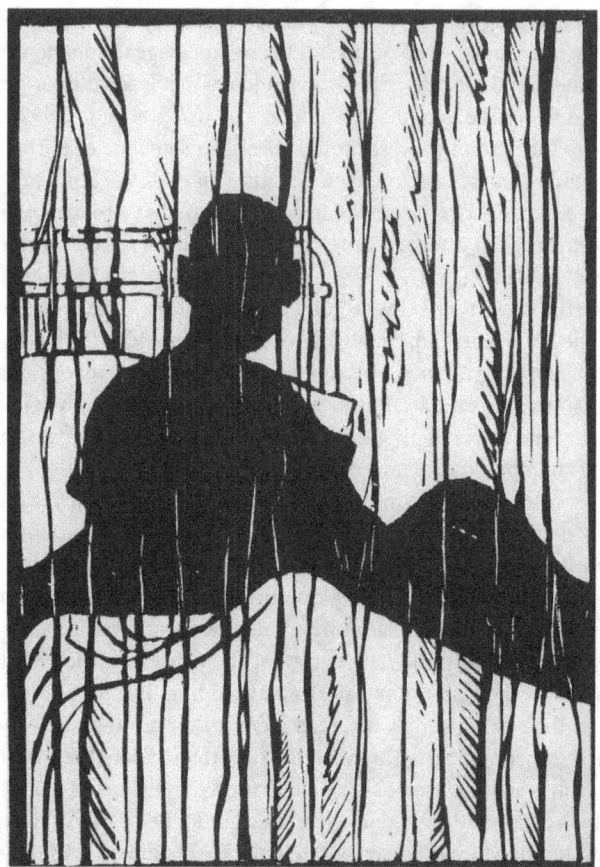

Figure 2.1 Facsimile of woodcut illustration from Alex Garland's *The Coma*. Illustrations by Nicholas Garland, copyright © 2004 by Nicholas Garland; from THE COMA by Alex Garland, illustrated by Nicholas Garland. Used by permission of Riverhead, an imprint of Penguin Publishing Group, a division of Penguin Random House LLC. All rights reserved / Copyright © 2004 by Nicholas Garland; from THE COMA by Alex Garland. Courtesy of Faber and Faber.

within the exilic state (Figure 2.1). The images depict silhouettes of specific episodes of the coma-dreams, yet the images are conspicuous in their absolute lack of specificity: facial features blacked out in cameo-style woodcuts, representing the rupture in Carl's identity and his traumatized memory; landscapes and cityscapes depicted from skewed angles that are evocative of German-expressionist films, or points of view that obscure scenic and personal detail; and, in one extraordinary sequence, solid black pages that represent the nadir of Carl's exile, reduced to a gibbering voice; a 'consciousness within a void' ([121]). As Philip Tew observes, it is at this point where 'traumatic experience expands to become the truly traumatological, a lacunary fissure widening to an ontological void' (2007: 193).

2.5 Depicting the traumatic exile of coma: towards empathic unsettlement

The range of linguistic, symbolic and structural techniques these authors employ in their portrayal of the exile of coma seem to resonate with what LaCapra calls for in the literary representation of trauma and what he terms 'empathic unsettlement'. This, he argues, is a mode of writing that will avoid fetishization of the trauma and the 'totalizing narratives' that he warns against. As LaCapra notes, 'Trauma is a disruptive experience that disarticulates the self and creates holes in existence', echoing Caruth's idea of the temporal disruption in the mind of the trauma survivor: the break in the mind's experience of time that can manifest as the inwards-turning repetition compulsion. Empathic unsettlement, LaCapra proposes, should manifest as a form of writing that avoids an appropriation of 'the traumatic experience of others' but instead uses a series of 'stylistic effects' that should render the feeling and unsettling nature of trauma without revelling in the act of writing, or fetishizing the writing itself. Such an approach should also, LaCapra asserts, avoid 'formulas or rules of methods' which have the effect of normalizing or homogenizing trauma and traumatic writing (2001: 41). In this way, LaCapra offers an ethical approach to the writing of trauma which would avoid the attempt to paint realistic and 'total' landscapes of trauma, but would instead empathically unsettle the reader through stylistic devices, such as temporal and narrative ruptures, or experimentations with form and *mise-en-page*. In her analysis of such stylistic devices, devices that are prevalent, as we have seen, throughout Garland and Welsh's novel, Anne Whitehead suggests that, 'The impact of trauma can only adequately be represented by mimicking its forms and symptoms, so that temporality and chronology collapse, and narratives are characterized by repetition and indirection' (2004: 3), embodying the haunting and possessive nature of trauma. Laurie Vickroy, in her discussion of trauma and survival in fiction, similarly highlights the, 'Textual gaps (both in the page layout and content), repetition, breaks in linear time, shifting viewpoints, and a focus on visual images and affective states' (2002: 21) which are vital in the portrayal of trauma, and upon which LaCapra's concept of empathic unsettlement depend.

This approach to writing trauma also resonates with Michael Rothberg's concept of 'traumatic realism', whereby writers 'challenge the narrative form of realism as well as its conventional indexical function' (2000: 104) in order to, as Whitehead proposes, 'make us believe the unbelievable' (2004: 84). Traumatic realism 'does not produce an imaginary resolution' (2000: 104) but 'seeks to bring forth "traces of trauma," to preserve and even expose the abyss between everyday reality and real extremity' (2000: 139). Such approaches to trauma writing might therefore constitute a 'general trauma aesthetic', a term used by Luckhurst in his discussion of Robert Eaglestone's formulation of the features of the genre of Holocaust testimony. One of Eaglestone's key components of such an aesthetic, Luckhurst goes on to highlight, is a 'resistance to closure that is demonstrated in compulsive telling and retelling' (2008: 88–9), a narrative technique that continually exposes (and repeatedly plays out) the abyss of the experience of trauma. This might be where Welsh's *Marabou Stork Nightmares* departs from the ethos of empathic unsettlement as despite its stylistic somersaults, the novel, in the end, does appear to reach narrative closure. At the moment of piecing together his coma nightmares, Roy is penectomized and killed by Kirsty, the victim of his brutal rape years earlier. At the point of his emasculation and murder, Welsh writes:

> Jamieson's facing me and he's pointing the gun and I hear it going off and it's all just one big

Z.

The large 'Z', here, refers to a famous anti-rape poster campaign in Scotland and the trigger for Roy's guilt pre-coma, as he tried to forge a new relationship with girlfriend, Dorie. Yet what seems like a moment of closure, Roy facing up to his true identity and the cause of his exile, might alternatively belie a lack of resolution. Within this ending of the novel, there is a certain element of narrative suspension or stasis. We know that the irruption of the large 'Z' indicates Roy's death, but the death itself is represented as a gap, an unfinished sentence, a non-sequitur, the full-stop attached to the 'Z' embodying finality which denies him the closure of a possible penance and atonement. In this regard, there is a complex challenge to narrative resolution and an ultimate representation of exile: consciousness is exiled, forever, from the body. This is heralded by a further representation of exile: the phallus, the physical instrument of Roy's abuse, also exiled from his body.

The endings of trauma narratives, the compulsion to repeat and resistance to closure are likewise important to consider when examining Garland's novel. At the very end of the novel, as Carl begins to 'rise out of the coma', he develops his first principle of coma-exile, which he sees as equally applicable to the world outside of coma, most notably, to the habits of sleep: 'You wake, you die [. . .] When you wake, you lose a narrative, and you never get it back' ([155]). In this, Garland touches upon a conceit within trauma and narrative theory: the notion that trauma is embodied by the structures of narrative and the reader's relationship with a text. In his essay, 'Freud's Master Plot', Peter Brooks makes the insightful connection between Freud's psychoanalytical perspective on traumatic repetition and his own narratological perspective. Brooks focuses on Freud's *Beyond the Pleasure Principle* in which, as discussed earlier, Freud attempts to hone his theory of traumatic repetition compulsion and 'haunting'. Brooks sees *Beyond the Pleasure Principle* as an 'essay about the dynamic interrelationship of ends and beginnings' (1977: 285), going on to suggest that all of the literary devices present within a text and those that keep drawing the reader back into the middle section, are indicative of the traumatic compulsion to repeat. Through the repetition of the 'unpleasant experience', the individual attempts to convert a passive subject position within a traumatic experience into an active subject position, an endeavour that can, Freud argues, 'be attributed to an instinctive urge to assert control that operates quite independently of whether or not the memory as such was pleasurable' (2004: 54). This attempt to achieve mastery over the trauma through repetition, Brooks argues, manifests itself in the process of reading a text, with literary repetition acting as a form of 'binding of textual energies that allows them to be mastered by putting them into a serviceable form within the energetic economy of the narrative' (1977: 289). Brooks therefore aligns the literary agenda with that of the victim of trauma, repeating the traumatic event in order to 'bind' it and achieve a sense of psychological and emotional control. But Brooks goes further, suggesting that, 'What operates in the text through repetition is the death instinct, the drive toward the end' (291), alluding to Freud's bold conclusion to *Beyond the Pleasure Principle*: 'The goal of all life is death' (78). In making this declaration, Freud asserted that the aim of all life was to return to the state that existed prior to the evolution of the species: the lifeless, inanimate (and ideal) state. The repetitive confrontation with the traumatic event (an event that Robert Jay Lifton refers to as the 'death encounter' (1995: 128)) reveals, Freud suggests, the drive towards death, but a death that must be achieved only on the victim's own terms. Thus the compulsion to repeat reveals a paradoxical agenda: both to come to terms with and master the death encounter but also the desire to return to a state of inertia, embodied by death itself. Similarly, Brooks argues, 'The desire of the text is ultimately the desire for the end, for that recognition which is the moment of the death of the reader in the text' (296).

This intersection of trauma and narrative theory becomes particularly evident in the conclusion to Garland's novel. By discussing, albeit cursorily, the 'loss' of self-narrative as being a form of 'death' ('you wake, you die'), Garland aligns the coma experience with this notion of the traumatic loss of story during which the element of selfhood which has been invested in that story is likewise lost. Both story and a part of selfhood dies during the reading process, creating a narrative schism, and yet the subject survives and retains this knowledge of loss. Throughout the novel, the reader and the protagonist alike are trapped within the repetitive, traumatic core of the novel and both strive towards the end through a compulsion to repeat which echoes Freud's death-drive, alongside Brooks's drive towards the end of the text. For Carl, the moment of clarity that he reaches is, paradoxically, a perplexing one as he realizes that he both desires and fears the death of his coma narrative and his role in it. In the final moments of coma, he observes, 'Now, moments from waking, the death is suddenly frightening. I want to hold it off as long as possible' ([155]). Once more, this desire to 'hold off' his emergence from coma reveals the compulsion of traumatic repetition, in the hope to master truly the death encounter. But it also reveals the conflicting desires of the reader: to hold off the ending of the novel for as long as possible, while desiring the end to come in order to gain pleasure in narrative closure.

However, as Carl begins to rise from coma, despite the fact that he will lose his coma narrative, he appears to be 'awaking' with his cognition intact, as if stirring from a bad dream. In short, he only seems to be losing a dream-narrative, not his entire pre-coma self, as is often the case with victims of coma and BI. Similarly to *The Coma*, the protagonist of Irvine Welsh's *Marabou Stork Nightmares* emerges from his prolonged coma (three years in length), seemingly with cognition intact. Neither novelist, then, is concerned with the post-coma condition of BI and the exilic nature of the coma survivor trying to forge a new life within the homeland to which they have returned. An interview Garland gave around the release of the novel helps to shine a light on this literary agenda. Speaking with *The Guardian* newspaper in 2004, Garland commented: 'I spent a lot of time wondering why dreams are so tricky in a narrative. There is something rather naff about talking about dreams. This in itself is something that pushed a button in me because it felt like a taboo or something'. This statement, significantly, omits all reference to the condition of coma, and yet this is the condition around which the novel purports to be centred. There is, however, an insightful allusion to the potential for BI and organic trauma, post-coma, within the novel. While within his coma, Carl briefly entertains the likelihood that he may have sustained a BI, proclaiming, prior to realizing that he is still in coma, that he 'was not suffering from psychological trauma' but instead 'had some sort of brain damage', optimistically considering the possibility that it 'might be reversible' and 'easier to address than psychological trauma' (2004: [39]). Taking this passage prima facie, we might suppose that Garland proposes a model of coma and brain trauma that denies the permanence of an organic neurological condition, using coma as a Sontagian illness metaphor as a means to exploring the habits of dream and sleep and their impact upon selfhood and narrative. Yet Dieguez and Annoni's approach to such texts that do not 'perfectly match scientific knowledge' – in their case, literary texts that portray amnesia – is instructive in evaluating Garland's novel. They write that, 'A different way to approach the relationships between literary and clinical depictions of amnesia is to ask how authors and readers intuitively conceive of memory and its impairment, and in turn what these intuitive conceptions tell us about the human mind and imagination' (2013: 164–5). Indeed, in his portrayal of a comatose and psychologically traumatized consciousness that lacks fixity, Philip Tew observes that Garland 'parodies the contemporary cultural obsession with the inner self' (193). For while both novels, on the surface, appear to be works of neurological disorder, in exploring the inner psychologies of the comatose protagonists, they are more closely aligned with what Marco Roth terms 'the novel of consciousness' or the 'psychological or confessional novel – the novel, at any rate, about the workings of the mind', rather than the neurological workings of the brain (2009: 3). Garland's novel, like Welsh's, may not inform us about the realities of coma and BI (indeed, the length of unconsciousness depicted, in reality, would mean both protagonists occupy the chronic VS, rather than coma) but in their very use of the C-Met we begin to learn how authors and readers conceive of these conditions. In employing the C-Met of psychological, traumatic exile, both authors explore complex ontological questions with regard to identity politics, unconscious states and psychological trauma. The novels I will now go on to discuss in the next chapter adopt a similar C-Met to portray the coma as an uncanny, nightmarish journey of exile. But they also adopt a different linguistic register altogether in order to depict both the interiority of coma, and post-coma selfhood: the language of mythological and biblical narratives.

3

Coma and the katabatic archetype

In their depictions of coma as a form of psycho-traumatic exile, both Alex Garland's *The Coma* and Irvine Welsh's *Marabou Stork Nightmares* portray the mind in topographical terms. The psyche is a landscape that must be traversed and where, at the deepest level of unconsciousness, answers regarding identity and the causes of trauma/exile may be discovered, leading to a catalyst for a return to the homeland. This Freudian model of mind, together with the uncanny landscapes through which the respective protagonists Carl and Roy travel, also bring to mind another prominent cultural trope: *katabasis*, or the narrative of descent into hell that may often be drawn upon to metaphorically describe moments of hardship, illness or trauma. This mythology of katabasis, as Hawkins observes, appear frequently within pathographies and is a 'variant of the journey myth' (1999: 79), with the illness itself 'like the hero's call to adventure' (78). Mirroring Hawkins's research into pathographies of lived experience of illness, we find that this katabatic trope is deployed in many works of coma fiction that often depict, not only the descent into the 'hell' of the comatose mind (the katabatic journey itself) but also the 'resurrection' and 'transfiguration' that occurs post-descent. This also connects with the myth of rebirth which, as Hawkins explicates, again similarly appears in illness pathographies, a myth, she writes, 'that seems as old as mythic thinking itself' and which 'appears in nearly every culture and every era' (33). Writers of coma fiction often intertextually reference archetypal tales and myths of katabasis and rebirth in order to create heroes who descend into the mind in a quest to defeat this 'psychological-hell' and to once more return to the 'overworld', to use Rachel Falconer's designation (2007) to describe the earthly world.

Iconic katabatic figures of both Judeo-Christian teachings and Greco-Roman mythology are frequently referred to in coma fiction; Lazarus, for example, from the Gospel of St John in the New Testament. We have already seen how Dennis Potter drew on this biblical tale of resurrection for the title of his pseudo-coma text, *Cold Lazarus* – his particular manifestation of the Christian katabatic traveller, Daniel Feeld, 'resurrected' from his cryogenic descent to the underworld. Robert Mawson's bestselling novel *The Lazarus Child* (1999) also openly alludes to this biblical figure who was brought back from the dead. The novel follows the Heywood family's struggle to cope with their seven-year-old son's coma following a road-traffic accident. As the title immediately suggests, the child does come back to life, though not without an intervention that crosses into the realms of the miraculous. And in the DC comic book *Batman* franchise, the Lazarus Pits have the ability to resurrect the dead once they have been submerged in them. In one particular storyline by Judd Winick, pertinent to our discussions, the second Robin, Jason Todd, within an alternative retconned timeline, inhabits coma for over a year, after a brutal beating by the Joker. While in coma (which is drawn in detail, his eyes taped down, breathing tube in place, heart monitor displaying minimal activity), two detectives discuss his situation, with one observing, 'So this kid was beaten with some kind of metal pipe, cracked his skull, shattered his sternum, collapsed a lung . . . about forty other fractures, blown up, then buried? [. . .] God almighty. Freakin' Rasputin', to which his partner replies, crucially, 'More like Lazarus' (Winick 2006: 20). Todd, now with 'brain activity [. . .]' of limited capacity', eventually emerges from his 'chronic vegetative state' (23) after a year with sustained amnesia owing to the fact that he is 'so severely brain damaged' (29), an 'unthinking, emotionless shell' who 'has never spoken' (31). When Talia Al Ghul, however, immerses him in the Lazarus Pit, his old self, lost in coma and sustained by BI, is 'resurrected'; transfigured, even. Peculiarly, there is even an intersection between science and religion in the medical term named after this katabatic adventurer of the Christian Bible: the 'Lazarus Sign'. This describes the sequence of physical movements in the brain-dead patient that occasionally occur after the life-support machine is turned off; movements that are often mistaken to be conscious and deliberate. This is a contradictory linguistic tag: a medical term that describes a set of reflex muscle spasms that offers false hope to patients' loved ones while at once evoking a biblical story that is suffused with hope: the miraculous resurrection of Lazarus.

What follows is an examination of the use of the katabatic narrative and manifestations of Judeo-Christian and Greco-Roman symbolism in key works of coma fiction.

3.1 Coma and Judeo-Christian katabasis

A *katabasis*, a word derived from the Greek, originally referring to 'any physical descent, through a cave mouth or other such entrance, into the earth' (Falconer 2007: 19), traditionally involves a journey during which the hero travels to the underworld,[1] before returning to the overworld, days or even hours later. Once back in this land of the living, the katabatic hero will have changed inexorably, their experience of the underworld impacting upon them forever. In this sense, even Christ's death and subsequent resurrection is seen as a katabatic journey, possibly the ultimate archetype of descent. The post-Jungian theorist James Hillman explores in detail the impact such religious and mythological archetypes have upon society. In discussing how the story of Christ has contributed to the development of a collective psyche, Hillman explains that, 'Christ's dying and resurrection was absorbed by the classical mythologem of the *nekyia*, now not a journey, but a *descensuskampf*' (1979: 87). Hillman describes the Christian break from classical depictions of the *nekyia* (a communion with the dead within the underworld after a katabasis has been performed) as Christ does not simply descend and return but, as Hillman goes on to explain, he 'harrows hell, and in one version, forces Thanatos to hide behind his own throne'. Rather than the classical descent heroes who, most often, experience a passive relationship with hell,

Christ *conquers* Hell: his *descensuskampf* or *descensus ad inferos* in which Christ defeats death (Thanatos) in order to save mankind and open the gates of Heaven. In this way, Hillman continues, Christ is seen to be greater than 'the greatest of man-gods, Hercules'. Despite being able to force Hades from his throne during his katabatic quest, Heracles/Hercules falls short of Christ's greatest triumph: conquering the entire kingdom of Hell, even defeating death itself for the benefit of future generations. From this point forth, Hell becomes synonymous with sin and not just a place, described in earlier mythology, where all the dead go. This, Hillman argues, has had a huge impact upon the development of archetypes within the post-Christian psyche. The notion of Christ's katabasis (and *nekyia* that takes place within the underworld) is further discussed by Northrop Frye in artistic terms, noting that the Hell into which Christ descends is 'often portrayed, especially in fresco, as the body of a huge dragon or shark, which he enters by the mouth, like his prototype Jonah' (1963: 62-63), thus linking the story of glorious katabasis from the New Testament to another tale of Judeo-Christian descent from the Old Testament.

In many works of fiction, coma is equated with a death-state, often appropriating imagery and narrative threads from a range of katabatic tales. Coma and death become synonymous because of the mysteries that surround them and the lack of empirical evidence of what occurs 'beyond' these liminal states. After all, it is only within the last fifty years, with advancements in technology such as life-support machines, CT and MRI scans, that survival from coma (the return journey of this medical katabasis) has increased. Robert P. Granacher points, in particular, to the identification of primary and secondary BI 'in the three decades from the 1970s to the 1990s' (2008: 1) as being a key contributing factor towards the increase in survival rates of the victims of coma and BI. As Couser further explicates, in writing about the rise of illness narratives, 'Modern medicine has enabled many people to survive illnesses and conditions that once would have killed them' (1997: 10).The motifs of katabatic narratives have proved a useful tool for describing this relatively recent phenomenon of coma survival, portraying the coma itself as a psychological 'underworld' into which the victim descends, occupying a 'death-state' from which an escape and subsequent survival is possible.

One of the most fascinating tales of katabasis in Christian writings, and one alluded to by Hillman, is the 'rewriting' of Christ's descent, the *Descensus Christi ad Inferos* that appears in the apocryphal *Gospel of Nicodemus* written around the fifth or sixth century. This account presents us with an early development of the figure of Lazarus, imagining and narrating his katabatic trauma, satisfying, as J. K. Elliott notes, in the introduction to his translation of the *Gospel of Nicodemus*, 'the curiosity of those who found the canonical biblical writings inadequate' (1993: 165). In this version of the *Descensus*, a conversation between Hades and Satan is imagined, with Hades, the Lord of the Dead in Greek mythology, expressing his fear at the prospect of Christ descending into his kingdom. He professes that, 'When I heard then the command of his word I trembled with fear and dread' (1993: 192), referring to the point at which he heard Jesus's order to release Lazarus from the underworld. Lazarus plays a prominent role within this text, representing the first member (as described in the Gospel of St. Matthew) of the 'walking dead' who are to arise later from the grave at the point of Christ's death on the cross. This version of the harrowing of Hell and the defeat of

Hades and Satan purportedly comes from the witness testimony of two such figures raised from the dead on the day of the crucifixion: Karinus and Leucius.

On hearing that Karinus and Leucius have arisen from the dead, several of the villagers, including Joseph of Arimathaea and Nicodemus himself, interrogate them about their katabatic journey. However, the two heroes, just returned from Hell, find it difficult to speak of the ordeal of their descent: 'Karinus and Leucius trembled in body, and being troubled in heart, groaned'. Instead of verbalizing their trauma, they make 'the sign of the cross with their fingers upon their tongues' and ask for paper upon which they can 'write what we have seen and heard' (1993: 191). Neither can express the experience of their katabasis and subsequent knowledge of Hell in spoken language. Similarly, in the biblical source material, the story of Lazarus's resurrection is conspicuous by the fact that he doesn't speak: he is denied a voice and merely passively obeys Christ's command: 'Lazarus, come forth' (John 11: 43-44). Leucius and Karinus's state of 'being troubled at heart' conveys their traumatized state and when prompted on oath to speak of their ordeal, their 'groan' reveals an anguished subversion of language itself which fully emphasizes the struggle to communicate the incommunicable: their experience of dwelling within the underworld and being wrenched abruptly out of it. They can only finally express their journey into Hell when given paper to write upon, allowing a certain distance between experience and expression. Yet Leucius and Karinus still feel impelled to narrate their experience, just as those around them feel impelled to hear their hellish trauma translated into language. For Roberta Culbertson, this 'function of narrative' allows the trauma survivor, to 'return fully to the self as socially defined, to establish a relationship again with the world' (1995: 179). This is a position supported by Susan Brison in her discussion of narrative in the role of trauma survival. 'By constructing and telling a narrative of the trauma endured, and with the help of understanding listeners', Brison posits, 'The survivor begins ... to integrate the traumatic episode into a life with a before and after' (2002: 23). This episode in the apocrypha is emblematic of this need to narrate the trauma in order to face the 'task of creating a future' outside of traumatized experience and to 'develop a new self' (Judith Herman 1997: 196). Kalí Tal observes that, for the traumatized subject, the trauma 'is enacted in a liminal state, outside of the bounds of "normal" human experience', and therefore, 'The horrific events that have reshaped the author's construction of reality can only be described in literature, not recreated' (1996: 121). For the katabatic hero, trauma occurs in an ultimate liminal space: the underworld. Leucius and Karinus 'describe' the events of their trauma, on paper, but still cannot fully 'recreate' the emotional and psychological disturbance of their katabasis, represented verbally by their collective 'groan'.

This need (and difficulty) to communicate the incommunicable in order to overcome trauma is apparent in the attempts to narrate the descent into coma in literature. This is none more apparent than in two poems that have in common their appropriation of the Lazarus motif to describe the return from a form of death-state. In Sylvia Plath's semi-autobiographical poem, 'Lady Lazarus', the narrator shares her frustrations over being successively rescued from her death-state after each of her suicide attempts. Plath's references to, 'The flesh | The grave cave ate', the 'eye pits', the 'sour breath' (1972: 16), and the 'Worms [. . .] like sticky pearls' (17) describe the corruption and decay of the body, negative effects of her descent into the underworld. The intrusive presence of the grave-worms continue to attach themselves to the narrator, a signifier of the death-state from which the narrator has been wrenched by 'Herr God' (19). Here, the spiritual command of Christ/God that allowed Lazarus to rise from his tomb is transferred to the God-*complex* of the narrator's interfering physician (in a similar vein, we see the God-complex of the corrupt media conglomerate that 'resurrects' Feeld's memories from his cryogenically-frozen brain in *Cold Lazarus*). Plath's worms are metaphorical imaginings of the narrator who sees herself as the risen 'living dead', a contemporary interpretation of the resurrected Lazarus. By the end of the poem, however, the narrator begins to imagine her katabic transfiguration, evoking a mythological archetype; that of the phoenix that will have her vengeance upon the oppressive paternalistic society: 'Out of the ash | I rise with my red hair | And I eat men like air' (19).

This adaptation of biblical resurrection, with Lazarus returning from the underworld as a reanimated corpse, is mirrored in Nikos Kazantzakis's controversial reimagining of the story of Christ, *The Last Temptation*. Kazantzakis takes Lazarus's resurrection and radically and viscerally reinterprets it, building on the notion that this is a resurrection in its truest sense: a reanimation of the dead. Lazarus, in this sense, becomes a biblical embodiment of that most staple figure of contemporary horror: the zombie. Martin Scorsese's film adaptation of the novel, *The Last Temptation of Christ* (1998), plays on this conceit by using generic conventions of horror, visually representing the stench of the corpse with even Willem Dafoe's Christ appearing disgusted at his own actions as Lazarus's rotting hand thrusts violently out of the darkened cave in a biblical 'jumping cat' moment

Kazantzakis's heightened depiction of this resurrection becomes even more apparent in the description of the aftermath of the resurrection, an event that is only touched upon in the Bible (all we are told is that Christ asks the crowd to 'loose him, and let him go': we know nothing else of this katabatic adventurer's fate). In Kazantzakis's novel, Lazarus sits 'in the darkest corner of the house', his body 'swollen and green', his face 'bloated' and exuding 'a yellowish-white liquid' like a 'four-day corpse'. Initially, he had 'stunk terribly' and any visitors he had 'held their noses'. Attached to him are 'small earthworms' (1975: 382). Kazantzakis's imagery, like Plath's, is grounded in the language of decay, detailing the degradation of the body and a physical transfiguration that is in stark opposition to Christ's only days later. Lazarus's 'stench' can only be superficially concealed with incense, the predominant scent being 'of earth'. Lazarus's process of returning to the earth (the transition from flesh to dust) has been interrupted, etched into his physical self. The stench of rot may, in time, dissipate; his wounds that have degraded his body may heal; and the worms that cling to him may eventually leave, but the memory and the feeling of his interrupted death will never leave him. Back from the grave, Lazarus is neither dead nor quite fully alive, a macabre curio at which his fellow villagers gawp and marvel in equal measures.

Like Leucius and Karinas in the Gospel of Nicodemus, the biblical Lazarus does not speak about his ordeal, but in Kazantzakis's version, Lazarus (as alluded to by Joe Bonham in Dalton Trumbo's proto-coma novel, *Johnny Got His Gun*) *refuses* to speak or narrate his trauma, as evidenced when he is visited by the blind village-chief who asks, laughing: 'Did you have a pleasant time in Hades?' before going on to warn

Lazarus not to reveal 'all the secrets of the underworld'. However, despite this caution, the old man leans over to Lazarus and says: 'Worms, eh? Nothing but worms. . .?', a rhetorical and elliptical attempt to coax some of these 'secrets' from Lazarus. When Lazarus does not answer, and after waiting 'a considerable time', the old man becomes 'enraged'. The dichotomy that all the villagers are experiencing is embodied by the blind chief: they don't want to learn of Lazarus's travails in the underworld, but at the same time are desperate for that knowledge. But Lazarus's silence, itself, provides another key motif. Unlike in the Bible, Lazarus is given the opportunity to speak but seemingly refuses: he does not have the language to express what he has witnessed and experienced. Falconer, in discussing the witness testimony of the katabatic hero, notes that, 'The wisdom acquired on the underworld journey cries out to be shared, yet at the same time it is unspeakable; it cannot be communicated' (2007: 51). The katabatic journey, therefore, is a traumatizing experience: the descent into the underworld is resistant to language and narrative structures. For both the katabatic hero and the trauma survivor, the traumatic event is insufficiently understood as it occurs and so becomes unspeakable, while simultaneously possessing and haunting consciousness. Lazarus's descent to and ascent from the underworld embodies a Freudian traumatic departure, a journey which cannot be comprehended as it occurs and which cannot be communicated immediately in language. As Caruth summarizes in her reappraisal of Freudian theory, trauma becomes 'a theory of the peculiar incomprehensibility of human survival' (1996: 58). In this particular Christian tale of hellish descent, we see both survival and incomprehensibility in extremis: the miraculous return from death itself.

Peter Redgrove's poem 'Lazarus and the Sea', similar to Plath's 'Lady Lazarus', uses the Lazarus story to specifically describe the near-death state of coma itself. Redgrove, while subjected to 'an organised programme of bullying and humiliation' during his National Service basic training, suffered a breakdown after which he was hospitalized and diagnosed with incipient schizophrenia (Neil Roberts 2012: 36). After being transferred to a civilian hospital, he underwent Deep Insulin Coma Therapy (DICT), a brutal cycle of treatment during which comas were induced in patients over the duration of five or six days a week, each coma lasting up to fifteen minutes. Within deep coma, patients would enter a state in which they lost their muscle tension and corneal and pupillary reflexes before having their system flooded with glucose to bring them out of 'the life-threatening hypoglycaemic state'. As Roberts points out, about 1 per cent of patients died from the treatment and more suffered permanent brain damage. However, it was normal practice to continue the treatment until fifty to sixty comas had been induced (45).

'Lazarus and the Sea' paints a traumatic picture of DICT in which Redgrove sees the coma as a death-state where his body is welcomed and exalted by nature. This vision is complicated, though, by the opening of the fourth stanza where Redgrove writes, 'I could say nothing of where I had been', yet goes on to assert that, 'I knew the soil in my limbs and the rain-water | In my mouth' (1999: 7). The poet acknowledges that his descent into coma triggers a void in consciousness yet at the same time he tries to navigate through this void by using the language and imagery available to him which is initially grounded in tangible concepts of burial and decay. As the poem develops,

Redgrove's imagery becomes more complex, creating a network of mythological and archetypal references which the poet knits together in an attempt to narrate and rationalize this rupture in consciousness brought on by induced coma. Redgrove continues: 'The knotted roots | would have entered my nostrils', and, 'Many gods like me would be laid in the ground | Dissolve and be formed again in this pure night' (7). The coma becomes a gateway through which one can reach a pagan ritual of death and rebirth, the narrator's body sublimated by nature in preparation for a re-forming of self or transfiguration, even a 'deification'. In this death-state, Redgrove becomes a god consumed by the earth ready to be born again. However, the use of the past conditional 'would have' reinforces this notion that he has no recollection of where he has travelled to despite the fact he asserts that he has a certain 'knowledge' of his journey into the earth. In the same way that he uses archetypal imagery of bodily decay in the earth, Redgrove now uses archetypal imagery of pagan rebirth and reincarnation, and it is the speculative past conditional that suggests that he is merely filling in the gaps of his coma experience with potential mythological concepts and stories. Redgrove creates an imagined narrative of katabasis and transfiguration in order to navigate through the trauma, not only of the cruel medical treatment, but of the void in consciousness with which he has been left. This is a particularly shattering form of katabatic 'knowledge' as it forces Redgrove to confront the fact that there may be no life after death; that the void in consciousness triggered by the death-state of coma is simply a forerunner to the eternal void of consciousness that might follow death. Redgrove explores this further when he writes: 'But where was the boatman and his gliding punt? | The judgement and the flames?' and describes being 'uprooted'. He goes on to question what brought him back from coma: 'And what judgement tore me to life?' (7). The violence of the language, the imagery of being 'torn' from the coma and 'uprooted' (literally wrenched from his re-assimilation into nature) reflects the pernicious process of the treatment (the 'judgement', as in Plath's poem) at the hands of medical staff. However, it soon becomes clear that even this sense of an interrupted metamorphosis is a construction born out of Redgrove's narrative powers in order not to face the true horror of his katabasis: that at the heart of his coma-underworld lies nothing. Both Redgrove and Plath convey Kazantzakis's notion of the interruption that occurs post-resurrection: the schism that is opened by aborting the death process, resulting in the victim coming back into consciousness but as a being that is now neither dead, nor fully living. This is alluded to in Redgrove's earlier imagery of still feeling the 'soil' in his 'limbs'. Like Kazantzakis's creation, Redgrove's Lazarus is still alive, and yet has brought back with him elements of the underworld (the soil into which he imagines he has been interred) in a similar way to how the Lazarus of *The Last Temptation* still smells of soil and still has his burial shroud 'stuck to his body', a signifier of his status of liminal being and one which cannot 'be removed' (382). Similar to Plath and her reference to the 'worms like sticky pearls', Redgrove's Lazarus merely imagines these sensations, though, using archetypal imagery.

This second half of Redgrove's poem is informative in its use of classical references, the 'boatman and his gliding punt' referring to the ferryman of Hades, Charon, in classical Greek mythology, and 'the judgement and the flames' conjuring a scene from the Judeo-Christian Old Testament. Yet these archetypes of traditional tales of death and descent are most conspicuous by their absence as the narrator descends deeper into coma (and comes closer to death). Redgrove, as narrator, steadily becomes aware that there is nothing to greet him at the end of his journey of descent into his coma, as he discussed in a 1984 interview with Cliff Ashcroft: 'I remember my last thought before nothing was, where's my soul? The universe has gone, there is nothing. Did I expect to see Charon with his punt ferrying me across the river? The thing that knew there was nothing was taken away' (2006: 154). Reading this account of Redgrove's coma descent, one is reminded of Garland's fictional account of Carl's journey into the deepest level of his coma, where he is little more than 'a voice in a void', or Hollyman's reference to the 'blackness' giving way to 'nothing' (2021: 11). In Redgrove's case, the trauma of the descent and return is not constituted as such by the visions of a hellish underworld, unlike in classical mythology where it is the experience of living within an underworld that embodies, as Falconer explains, 'The absolutely horrific experience from which no one emerges unchanged' (2007: 1). Rather, Redgrove's trauma is formed by the fact that there is no encounter with such archetypal images of Hell/Hades. At the end of Redgrove's poem, a question is posed that explores this notion further: how can a void ever be expressed within language? An absolute nothing will obviously be unspeakable, and yet Redgrove persists in trying to speak of it by using the imagery of mythology and of descent narratives which, as in the case of Leucius and Karinus, reveals an impulse to narrate. The void, the 'absolute nothing', is transformed into a tangible 'something' and so through this, Redgrove attempts to 'work through', rationalize and come to terms with the real hell at the heart of his coma therapy.

In the same interview with Cliff Ashcroft, Redgrove also referred to his comas as 'practice deaths' (2006: 154). 'Deaths', a countable noun, can only be used in relation to populations, never to individuals. While a population may encounter many 'deaths' at many different times, it does not necessarily follow that the population itself will die. 'Deaths' in a population does not mean the end. They occur as part of a continuing cycle of death and birth that allows the population to sustain itself in its environment. This idea of the cyclical nature of life is underscored by the appearance in the phrase of the word 'practice', suggesting repetition. By linking this plural in relation to the death of the individual with 'practice', Redgrove undermines the finality of death itself, so much so that 'death' is no longer an appropriate definition of his state of being: only resurrection will suffice. Plath, too, achieves a similar effect with her opening phrase, 'I have done it again', alongside her reference to the feline myth of having 'nine times to die'.

Similar language, imagery and themes of coma-katabasis and trauma are developed and explored within one particular work of mainstream fiction, Stephen King's psycho-horror novel, *The Dead Zone*. King weaves together scientific concepts and medical research with archetypal tales of descent from the Judeo-Christian canon to create the story of a victim, John (or Johnny) Smith who is transfigured, through his coma descent, into a messianic hero with the potential to save mankind. With his humdrum name (his girlfriend muses, 'With an absurd name like John Smith, could he be completely for real?' (27)), King positions his protagonist as an archetypal 'Everyman', both relating to biblical morality tales but also revealing the author's ongoing fascination with 'common Americans with whom his readers can identify' (Davis 1994: 23). As a child, Johnny sustains a BI while ice-skating, granting him psychic powers in which he has fleeting visions of the future. These powers are heightened when Johnny is involved in a road-traffic accident and he emerges from a five-year 'coma' (essentially, then, a chronic VS) to a world that has changed dramatically. Now, Johnny, through a biblical 'laying on of hands', is able to read a person's past experiences and, most significantly, predict future experiences that are yet to occur. In David Cronenberg's 1983 film adaptation, this childhood event (a call-to-adventure initiated by BI) is omitted, so that it is the coma itself which *creates* his power, rather than merely reawakening it.

Johnny's mother, a born-again, fundamentalist Christian, sees her son's power as a gift from God, insisting that he does his 'duty' when the time comes, thereby highlighting Johnny's role as a contemporary messiah. King employs a range of Christian symbolism, describing the coma itself as 'limbo, a weird conduit between the land of the living and the land of the dead' (2007: 137). Later, the Christian references become more explicit: 'He could almost see them. All the whispering voices of purgatory' (138). Johnny's former lover at one point internalizes her musings upon the derivation and implication of the word 'coma', concluding that, 'She didn't like that word *coma*. It had a sinister, stealthy sound. Wasn't it Latin for 'sleep of death'?' (86). Once more, the mythological and cultural interchangeability of sleep and death (the twins Hypnos and Thanatos) is conjured and when Johnny is referred to as the 'living corpse in the [room]' (86), the image of Kazantzakis's Lazarus is once more evoked.

King is not primarily concerned, however, with the nature of Johnny's descent itself and the topography of the underworld, unlike Redgrove's adaptation of the Lazarus story. Instead, like Plath and Kazantzakis, King is more focused upon the consequences of Johnny's traumatic return to the overworld which is described in terms of rebirth that corresponds somewhat with Redgrove's imagined experiences. As Johnny leaves the dark 'metal corridor' (178) that represents his coma-limbo in preparation for his 'resurrection', King describes Johnny being separated from the overworld 'by the thinnest of membranes, a sort of placental sac, like a baby waiting to be born'. Through the walls of this sac, Johnny sees the shadows of doctors which he concludes might be 'the shapes of angels'; this world into which he now moves as 'some sort of afterlife' (138-39). By representing the interior struggle Johnny has to emerge from coma, King attempts to metaphorically represent the physical and psychological trauma of a long-term PDoC. Johnny's emergence from his five-year 'coma' (again, in reality, a chronic VS) in Cronenberg's adaptation, however, is shot purely from an external subject position, excising any sense of struggle, with Johnny, pyjama-clad, rousing as if from slumber – a male embodiment of the sleeping beauty trope. Later, there is an overt nod to this fable, as Johnny tutors a young girl who reads from the story of *Sleeping Beauty*. In the novel, King uses the common metaphor of rebirth as Johnny leaves the clinical 'womb' of the steel hallway of his coma to come blinking, once more, into the light, fighting to break through the amniotic sac of his coma. In Christian thought, both Christ and Lazarus's emergence from their respective caves also constitutes a rebirth from the earth-mother. In his discussions of the influence of mythology, theorist of literary archetypes, Northrop Frye, analyses this image of the 'cave' as the portal to the underworld, noting that, 'The wonderful cave drawings of the paleolithic period may have been connected with an earth-mother cult in which the cave was identified with her womb' (1981: 191). Death and rebirth, then, are two sides of the same coin of the katabatic journey. Almost the first thing Johnny realizes after his resurrection is that, 'He had changed ... He had gone into the darkness with everything, and now it felt to him that he was coming out of it with nothing at all – except for some strangeness. The dream was ending' (139). This not only evokes Garland's allusion to a descent into the darkness of coma, and the eventual ascent (*anabasis*) to the overworld, as if waking from sleep, but also emphasizes the significance of the transfiguratory 'change' that occurs. Frye, when discussing tropes of the journey of descent and return, touches upon this idea of the katabatic quest-objective, observing: 'One normally attains direct knowledge or vision, but the reward of descent is usually oracular or esoteric knowledge, concealed or forbidden to most people, often the knowledge of the future' (1963: 62). It is Johnny's ability to predict the future that constitutes the quest-objective of the katabatic journey despite the fact that, in Johnny's case, he is a reluctant recipient of such a power. As Patrick McAleer observes, this initial reluctance mirrors the plight of the Baby Boomers of King's generation who were 'positioned to radically alter their social landscape and who reportedly had the necessary means to do so, yet failed to use the available resources, which were required to accomplish their ends' (2011: 1210). The description of Johnny's transfiguration, his 'strangeness', also helps to draw more links between the journey of katabasis and the post-traumatic condition. As Kalí Tal posits, 'Trauma is a transformative experience, and those who are transformed can never entirely return to a state of previous innocence' (1996: 62). This reflects earlier manifestations of the katabatic hero and the process of transfiguration that these experience, not least Lazarus's new status as the 'living dead'.

Johnny's powers of reading the future transfigure him utterly and as the narrative develops, the miracle visions he conjures become increasingly significant. Eventually, Johnny, like many of King's protagonists, 'chooses to act with good will and kindness based on morality' (Davis 1994: 43): aiding local police to identify and capture a vicious murderer; rescuing his employer's son from a freak accident at a local restaurant; and, ultimately, saving the world from a corrupt politician who will lead the country into all-out nuclear war. This hierarchy of miracles reflects the hierarchy of those performed by Christ across the Gospels, for example turning water into wine, walking on water, healing the blind, raising Lazarus from the dead, and finally saving the whole of mankind through his own death, katabasis and resurrection. In *The Dead Zone*, however, there is no final resurrection for Johnny. This being said, after Johnny has the vision of the nuclear winter that future presidential candidate Greg Stillson will help to cause, he decides to abide by his mother's final words: 'Do your duty'. Unlike the actions of Christ, accepting violence to be enacted upon him in a modern version of the Passion, Johnny decides to assassinate Stillson at a political rally.

The vision he has of Stillson is important to consider when looking at Johnny as a post-coma manifestation of Christ. It is unlike his others in that it is not an exact simulacrum of a future event. Instead, it is obscured by blue and yellow stripes, the significance of which Johnny fails to understand at the time. Johnny's assassination attempt is unsuccessful, his bullets straying far and wide as he is shot to death by Stillson's bodyguards. However, in the fracas, Stillson seizes a small child and holds him in front of him as a human shield, the photos of which are seized upon by the mass media, thus shattering his political career. The small boy wears a blue and yellow striped jumpsuit. All of Johnny's visions up until now predict the consequences of a future event or act. By paying heed to these warnings, those involved prevent these consequences from happening, shaping an alternative future and a different reality. The Stillson vision is different in that it already suggests and assimilates the alternative future, emphasizing Johnny's fate: that he was always going to die in a moment of messianic self-sacrifice in order to save mankind. For Johnny, as for Christ, the future has already been written. In Cronenberg's film, the image of Christ is visually rendered, Johnny, as he is shot, crashing through a balcony, landing on the floor below with arms outstretched and a wooden banister running the length of his body, like the upright of a cross. Realizing that, despite dying, he has still managed to stop Stillson, Johnny utters, 'It is done', a variant of Christ's final utterance on the cross: 'It is finished'. McAleer argues that, like the Baby Boomers, 'King's characters are often provided the necessary means to conquer the fears and complications that they must face, but then either whither and fade in the face of adversity, or push forward only to be met with failure in some scope, or even the ultimate failure: death' (1213). Yet in *The Dead Zone*, Johnny, in dying, achieves the ultimate success: like Christ, his self-sacrifice (which he accepts to be his fate) saves mankind.

Alongside these allusions to a contemporary Christ-figure, Johnny is frequently described as the kind of embodiment of Lazarus present in *The Last Temptation*. There is the reference to the 'living corpse' (133), and prior to his accident, because of his physical height and tendency towards slouching, he is given the moniker 'Frankenstein' by the children at the school in which he used to teach (21): another reanimated corpse. Throughout *The Dead Zone*, Johnny descends into little more than a walking corpse, his physical self gradually disintegrating and breaking apart through the physical strain of the coma and the psychological stress of the visions. His physical transfiguration post-coma can be seen as a reference to Frankenstein's monster, his body laced with scars left over from the gruelling operations he underwent in order to try and remedy the physical effects of muscle atrophy and ligament degeneration caused by the inert coma he was trapped within for nearly five years. Metaphorically, Johnny is a walking corpse, much like Lazarus, alongside Leucius and Karinus from the apocrypha.

Johnny's feeling that he has 'changed' on re-emerging from coma has a further dimension: he experiences both a psychological and physical transfiguration that exacerbates his katabatic trauma. The title of the novel, itself, is a metaphorical nod to the underworld, the ultimate 'dead zone'. At one point, Johnny's physician, Weizak, attempts to describe his patient's unusual condition at a press conference, declaring that 'a part of John Smith's brain has been damaged beyond repair [. . .] He calls this his "dead zone"'. Going on to refer to this as 'a small but total aphasia', it appears that 'all of these wiped-out memories seem to be part of a "set" – that of street, road, and highway designations' (231). Weizak then discusses how another part of Johnny's brain has been 'awakened', in an attempt to explain his patient's sudden acquisition of 'second-sight'. Weizak strives to justify a supernatural phenomenon by using language familiar to him – the language of science in an attempt to explain the unexplainable. In a pursuit that mirrors Redgrove's own biographical mission, Weizak still tries to communicate both the void of coma and the second-sight phenomenon through the language that he knows best, attempting to attribute a tangible concept to Johnny's katabatic trauma of coma. It is significant that Johnny's prophetic powers have been exchanged for topographical knowledge, a consequence of his newly acquired status as the 'living dead': like Lazarus, he stands astride the underworld and overworld, belonging to neither. But this also reveals what Jeanne Campbell Reesman refers to as King's trademark 'supernatural realism' (Strengel 2005: 12). It is this preoccupation of King that sees him rationalize Johnny's coma and the fact that he has emerged after nearly five years with language and cognition intact, despite his body atrophying and his brain injured to such an extent it reawakens his clairvoyant powers. King, in explaining Johnny's condition, writes,

> There were cases without number of comatose patients who had awakened with a dreamlike knowledge of many of the things that had gone on around them while they were in coma. Like anything else, coma was a matter of degree. Johnny Smith had never been a vegetable; his EEG had never gone flatline, and if it had, Brown would not be talking with him now. (148)

In King's 'presentation of fantastic elements as scientific reality' (Strengell 2005: 104), we again see a blurring of coma with PDoC, for instance, chronic VS, but we also see the avowal of BI in PDoC, but an attempt to explain how Johnny has avoided this. In short, King paints a largely accurate picture of the realities of deep coma and vegetative states but in the end, depicts Johnny's coma as truly 'other': a unique, supernatural coma or katabatic liminal state.

King also makes reference to Johnny's descent by comparing him to that most renowned katabatic traveller of Judeo-Christian teachings, Jonah, when Johnny (a lexical variation of *Jonah*) muses that he, 'Had been swallowed by a big fish. Its name was not leviathan but coma. He had spent four-and-a-half years in that particular fish's black belly and that was enough' (440). In this Old Testament story, Jonah's spiritual transfiguration through a katabatic journey into the belly of the whale and his restoration after three days inside the great fish prefigures the resurrection of Christ who spent three days in the 'belly' of an earthly, chthonic underworld. According to Frye, in St Matthew's Gospel, Christ 'accepted the Jonah story as a prototype of his own Passion' (1981: 191), saying to the Pharisees that: 'For as Jonas was three days and three nights in the whale's belly; so shall the Son of man be three days and three nights in the heart of the earth' (Matt. 12.40). Like Jonah, Johnny both descends into the underworld and returns, initially refusing to listen to and act upon the visions he receives until he can ignore them no longer.

3.2 Coma and Greco-Roman katabasis

These archetypal katabatic images in Judeo-Christian tradition are symptomatic of a universal and historical fascination with descent narratives in antiquity, narratives that influenced the development of the story of Christ's own 'harrowing' of Hell. In

Greco-Roman mythology, katabatic narratives are rife, depicting flawed heroes such as Theseus, Heracles and Orpheus who descend into Hades, driven by their own personal quest, only to emerge inexorably changed or transfigured.

One pertinent example of Greco-Roman katabasis, and one that has caused some controversy among scholars, is that depicted in Book Eleven (the *Nekyia*) in Homer's *Odyssey*. In this episode, the witch Circe allows Odysseus to leave her island so that he may commune with the dead in order to fathom what his next course of action should be. As instructed, in the land of the Kimmerians, Odysseus performs a ritual which summons the underworld, allowing him to seek advice from its inhabitants, not least from the blind seer Teiresias. The advice and visions of the future that Odysseus receives (prophetic knowledge akin to Johnny Smith's powers) allow him to shape his future decisions, despite the fact that he still makes errors of judgement, often ignoring these visions altogether. While some scholars, notably D. L. Page, see this not as a full *nekyia* (katabatic journey) but a *nekyomanteia* (a 'calling up' of the dead (1955: 48)), Raymond J. Clark asserts that it 'is distinguishable from regular necromantic evocations of the dead in the land of the living' (1979: 75), suggesting that what starts out as a necromantic consultation gradually becomes a full katabasis. When Odysseus first sees Hades, it does initially seem, through the use of passive verbs, as though it is a conjuration that simply appears *before* him: 'Now came the soul of Teiresias the Theban, holding | A staff of gold, and he knew who I was and spoke to me' (1991: 11.90-91). However, as Clark points out, over time it appears as though Odysseus has actually descended; that a physical journey into the underworld and a dislocation from the overworld has taken place, as seen when Odysseus is addressed by Anticleia, his dead mother: 'My child, how did you *come here* beneath the fog and the darkness | and still alive?' (11.155-56). To this, Odysseus replies, 'Mother, a duty *brought me here* to the house of Hades' (11.164 emphasis added). Such language implies that Odysseus has physically travelled to the underworld and this is emphasized later as Odysseus says that he 'descended into the House of Hades'. Circe, too, says of Odysseus, 'Unhappy men, who went alive to the house of Hades, | so dying twice, when all the rest of mankind die only | once' (11.21-23). As Clark posits, Circe's remark suggests that Odysseus, as a result of his experience, 'Will be unlike other men' which 'further distinguishes the catabatic journey from a necromantic consultation' (1979: 77). This is emblematic of the rebirth myth in pathography, a myth which, as Hawkins discusses, 'turns on the belief that one can undergo a process of transformation so profound as to constitute a kind of death to the "old self" and rebirth to a new and very different self' (1999: 33).

Odysseus's 'full' *nekyia* is a particularly instructive example of katabasis when discussing the representation of descent narratives in coma fiction. By performing the ritual taught to him by Circe, Odysseus summons the spirits of Hades to appear before him, but then there is a significant linguistic turn: he and the spirits begin to speak as though Odysseus has physically descended into Hades. Odysseus's *nekyia* embodies a genuine quest for knowledge which he hopes to gain from the underworld. Rather than Heracles or Theseus, for example, he is not looking to sack Hades, or defy the God of the underworld himself and this form of a katabatic quest for enlightenment is again a running motif throughout coma fiction. Like Odysseus, the fictional coma victim is depicted paradoxically as being stationary in space, yet simultaneously experiencing a physical journey through a psychological katabasis.

It is important to note that whereas exterior coma texts, like *The Dead Zone*, concern themselves primarily with the consequences of the return from the underworld, and the impact of this in the overworld, interior coma narratives are more concerned with the descent itself, and the journey through the underworld on the quest to acquire knowledge. Welsh's *Marabou Stork Nightmares* is a paradigm of this katabatic model. Roy's descent and journey through his various layers of consciousness eventually leads him to the monster (there are always monsters in Hades) at the heart of his psychological underworld, the Marabou Stork. After encountering the monster, a return is initiated. In Garland's *The Coma*, within Carl's psyche emerge 'Virgilian' guides that help him navigate through his own coma-hell.

Odysseus's katabasis is initiated by a ritual which requires him to dig a trench in the ground and make sacrifices and offerings within this rivulet, thus paying tribute to the infernal regions below. This concept of the gateway to Hades opening up within the earth also reflects Lazarus and Christ's re-emergence from their respective caves, their rebirth from the womb of the earth-mother and also the place into which they are laid. The cave within the earth is the departure point from which they commence their journeys into Hell. It follows that this katabasis that takes the hero beneath 'the darkness' on a journey of enlightenment also connects with another classical Greek text: Plato's 'allegory of the cave' in Book VII of the *Republic*. This extended metaphor outlines the consequences of a 'soul's earthly imprisonment' (1995: 822), discussing how we are all 'men living in a sort of cavernous chamber underground, with an entrance open to the light and a long passage all down the cave' (826). This restrictive 'cave' represents the human mind and the potential it has to stagnate, oppressing the individual within its chambers of unenlightened darkness. However, the cave image also represents the possibility the mind offers the individual to escape into the light and shed his 'unquestioning acceptance of material values' (822). If the mind is a cave, then maybe the narratives of interior coma descent symbolize a katabasis of the psyche; the 'cave' being the starting point for a descent to the underworld of the unconscious.

This Platonic concept of the mind-as-cave is exploited in another example of coma fiction, Liz Jensen's *The Ninth Life of Louis Drax*, the title immediately suggesting themes of death and rebirth and reminiscent of Plath's reference to having 'nine times to die' in 'Lady Lazarus'. The novel (adapted for film in 2016) is centred around the eponymous young hero, Louis, who lies in a coma following a mysterious 'accident'. The guardian of Louis's psychological Hades is the sinister shadow-figure, Gustave, whose face is concealed by bloodied bandages (akin to the image of Lazarus). Over time, this shadowy Other is revealed to represent Louis's murdered father, Pierre, and it is through this revelation, alongside Gustave's 'Virgilian' guidance through Louis's katabasis of coma, that the image of the mind-as-cave is developed. Gustave, when explaining to Louis how he came to reside in this hellish place, says that: 'I can't remember [how I got here]. Not completely [...] I just remember being in a dark place. A cave' (2005: 100). The fact that Gustave, to all intents and purposes, is residing within Louis's mind (the underworld of his coma) exacerbates the image of the mind-as-cave, its darkness representing the void in consciousness (akin to Johnny Smith's 'dead zone') into which biographical and experiential memory-details sink and disappear.

This cave image is emphasized further when, later in the novel, Gustave decides to guide Louis deeper into the cave, a journey that significantly involves Louis 'climbing down into the danger' (175) in a trajectory that once more evokes a katabatic, topographical descent. At the end of this journey lies the object of Gustave's mission and ultimately (because of the fact that Gustave is a projection of his psyche) the object of Louis's mission: to seek the truth of the murder of his father, hidden within the deepest layers of his unconscious. This physical landscape of the deepest level of the coma-underworld is described by Louis as, 'White stone like bone, like inside a creepy skull' (176). Louis, subconsciously, uses a pertinent simile (a Freudian 'blurt'), bestowing upon his unconscious the physical designation of the skull/cave in which his mind literally resides. Despite being cloaked as a descent into the mind of his father, into his father's 'cave', this katabatic descent is revealed to be a journey into Louis's own mind where he faces up to all of the family secrets that he has repressed in the exterior world of coma.

The image of the cave is made more complex, later, when Louis's doctor, Dannachet, learns that Pierre Drax's body has been discovered in a sea-cave cut into the cliff-side over which he was pushed. Like Christ and Lazarus, Pierre was, 'Stuck in that cave for three days' (227). Louis's katabasis of coma, with his father as Virgilian guide, thereby acts as a prophetic dream that reveals the location of his father's corpse, a katabatic enlightenment similar to Johnny's gift of second-sight in *The Dead Zone*. Through the knowledge both characters acquire at the heart of their coma-underworld, they are granted a certain vision of the future. Louis is also granted knowledge of the present: an insight into his father's final resting place; his katabasis evoking Odysseus's journey into Hades. Both are quests for knowledge that can help to alter their present predicament but which can also potentially alter and influence future actions. And though both katabatic journeys are successful in that prophetic knowledge is acquired, neither hero acts upon this knowledge. Odysseus seemingly 're-enacts' the obstacles of the future that have been predicted for him, and Louis likewise fails to act upon his newly acquired knowledge, choosing to remain within his coma and hide from his future life that awaits him in the overworld. The image of mind-as-cave is also explored in the exterior world of coma. Louis appears to 'awake' miraculously from his coma during a romantic clinch between Dannachet and his manipulative mother, the doctor rushing to the boy's bedside only to comment, 'As I looked into the dark pools of his enlarged pupils, it felt as if I were looking at holes to darkness, no more' (92). This description evokes the abyss of the mind of the coma victim, the eyes being the cave mouths through which the exterior witness can see the void of consciousness. Louis, from an external perspective, also becomes an embodiment of the sleeping beauty phenomenon with his 'soft cheeks, the waxy skin, the parted mouth, the long dark lashes'; his hair 'sleek and thick' (103). Louis is described in almost sublime terms, his corporeal self, while in coma, elevated to aesthetic, fetishized perfection. Elsewhere Jensen describes his 'luminous skin', comparing him to church carvings 'with their tiny, perfect hands and feet, their dreamily closed eyes' (27). Once more, the death-state elides with the sleep-state, but also the physical changes triggered by Louis's psychological katabasis are already becoming apparent in his physical, corporeal self: a Christ-like transfiguration that served to fill the apostle Thomas with his infamous doubt.

This proliferation of the katabatic cave motif can be more closely examined by drawing on the theories developed by the psychoanalyst Carl Jung, in particular his work on mythical archetypes and his concept of the collective unconscious. Jung's theoretical concepts of the role archetypes and mythology have in the construction of identity are particularly instructive when analysing patterns of archetypal tropes throughout biblical and mythological narratives. The conceptual cave of the mind and its potential to act as a departure point for a psychological katabasis would represent one of the 'eternally inherited' archetypes that humans, according to Jung, have stored within their psyche (1973: 38). As the father and originator of what would become archetypal psychology, Jung posits that all humans share certain images within a 'collective unconscious', archetypal concepts such as 'mother', 'God', 'hero' and 'the wise old man', but rather being fully formed, they are instead empty vessels, 'primordial images' into which the subject pours his own individual associations of 'conscious understanding' (1959: 79). As Hall and Nordby explain, the archetype is 'a [photographic] negative that has to be developed by experience' (1973: 42). For example, the Jungian archetype of 'the shadow', akin to Freud's 'Id', represents the unconscious, often constituting the subject's repressed darker side which occasionally irrupts in primal thoughts and behaviours.

Jung's concept of a shared, inherited collective unconscious is one of his more radical and controversial theories, most notably because his justifications as to how one acquires this are at best vague, attempting to attribute the cause to biological factors. He calls this unconscious a 'psychological instance of the biological "pattern of behaviour," which gives all living organisms their specific qualities' (1973: 40), yet fails to provide any real evidence of the kind which a solid biological theory would require. However, the archetypes which Jung highlight constantly occur within culture and society and are drawn upon in order to narrate and navigate through difficult, often traumatic, experiences. As in Redgrove's case, they provide a reservoir of language and imagery which allows the communication of the incommunicable through a process of codification of the trauma. Frye, in analysing the role of archetypes in narrative development, proposes that, 'Stories are told about gods, and form a mythology. The gods take on certain characteristics [. . .] The same types of characters get into legends and folk tales, and, as literature develops, into fiction' (1964: 40). Frye's narrative 'food chain' can be used to explicate the Jungian collective unconscious further, thus creating a parallel between theories of psychoanalysis and of narrative. It is through this gradual evolution of narrative and constant exposure to archetypal stories and imagery that has allowed these to become assimilated into the unconscious of the Subject. This process therefore provides us with a bank of imagery and narrative tools that can be accessed when all other attempts at communication struggle or fail entirely, constructing, as Hawkins posits in her discussion of the function of illness pathography, 'necessary fictions out of the building blocks of metaphor, image, archetype, and myth' (18).

The American psychologist James Hillman was instrumental in developing Jungian thought into what is now known as archetypal psychology, an approach that proposes the practice of discussing and analysing the influence of the varied polytheistic mythologies upon the consciousness of the individual and his psychological life. In his seminal work, *The Dream and the Underworld*, Hillman advances Jungian theory by proposing that dream represents a kind of death, a descent into the underworld or a katabasis of the mind that one experiences every time one sleeps. He writes that, 'Where do contents of consciousness go when they fade from attention? Into the unconscious, says psychology. The underworld has gone into the unconscious: even become the unconscious' (1979: 65). This underworld of the unconscious is descended into when one dreams and the dreams themselves conjure hellish images of people and places: shades or *eidola*. These immaterial spirits represent real people from the overworld but, like Jung's 'primordial image' of the archetype, they are somehow empty, devoid of the *thymos* (the body) yet craving attention of the flesh (hence the blood sacrifice that Odysseus performs). These *eidola* are described by the ghost of Achilles, in the *Odyssey*, as 'the senseless | dead men', the 'mere imitations of perished mortals' (11.475-476). Desperate to hold onto what once made them human, they nevertheless fail to understand why they possess this need, underscoring Achilles's use of the adjective 'senseless'. They have become detached from the corporeality of their human form and motivations that existed within the overworld. In short, these *eidola*, according to Hillman, refer to 'an archetypal person in human shape' (1979: 61). The image of Gustave in *Louis Drax* is one such 'senseless' *eidolon*, a shade in Louis' coma-underworld that is unable to remember the exact details of his life in the overworld, even possessing a different name, yet inextricably drawn to the fragmented memories of that world, desperate to re-unify them. Thus, for Louis, Gustave/Pierre only *represents* his father and is merely an archetype with the purpose of guiding Louis out of coma, in a similar way to how Catherine in Garland's *The Coma* is not really Carl's lover, but an archetypal Virgilian guide in the guise of Carl's lover from the overworld. Topographical *eidola* also appear frequently within interior coma narratives, the false realities of the narrator's shadow-world in Garland's novel, for example. In another work of coma fiction, Nicholas Royle's *Regicide* (2011), the interiority of the protagonist's coma (a katabatic hero, also named 'Carl', who is unaware he is in coma until the end of the novel) is depicted as an oppressive cityscape. The author implies that a map that Carl finds is actually a drawing of his coma-damaged brain, the *gyri* and *sulci* represented by the dystopian 'semi-circular streets' of the city (52). Later, Royle stresses this image as Carl muses, 'Possibly the map was as much inside my head as printed on a scrap of paper' (139). In these novels, the coma-protagonist, like Drax, must travel downwards and deeper into the nadir of their coma-underworld in order to gain katabatic knowledge and return to the overworld. In *The Coma*, this lowest point is referred to as a 'void'; in *Regicide* as 'the Dark' which 'goes on and on in all directions' and apparently lies outside the city limits (120); 'the darkness' in *The Dead Zone* (130); and in *Louis Drax*, the 'danger', all reminiscent of the tenebrosity of the archetypal Hadean underworld and Plato's metaphor of the cave. We might also think back to James B. Harris's *Some Call It Loving* and Jennifer's words in describing her experience of abuse while in her pseudo-coma, in particular the terrifying 'nothing' she experiences between the periods of violation (1973). In *Regicide*, when Carl finally locates the character of Gledhill, someone who has apparently survived a sojourn into the Dark and from whom Carl requires information as to how he can escape it himself, Gledhill says of the Dark, 'It's everywhere and nowhere' before touching his forehead and uttering, 'It's in here' (144). This once more evokes the image of the mind-as-cave and as a departure point for the hell of the mind, the dystopian city, in Royle's novel, with the nadir (the Dark) being the void of consciousness of deep coma.

3.3 Coma, the underworld and the language of excavation

Jung, among other theorists and scholars (including Frye), points towards the development of depth psychology as having a key influence in how humankind has navigated towards an understanding of the inner workings of the mind and the unconscious. Freud, in particular, mapped out a topographical model of the mind that, like Dante's vision of the cosmos, consisted of various levels to which one could travel. The very nature of depth psychology is to attempt to delve into the darkest depths of the psyche in order to confront the particular *eidolon* at the heart of the disturbance: to bring that shadow into the light and to normalize it in rational, concrete terms, thus stripping it of its mystery – its hellish qualities. Lacan went onto develop this, proposing the unconscious-as-language model, locating the traumatic *eidolon* of the Real that has evaded symbolization and attaching to it a linguistic signifier. Such psychological archetypes now occupy coma literature, as seen, for example, in *Louis Drax*. Like the depth psychologist and the katabatic hero of antiquity, the eponymous hero journeys into the deepest realms of his coma-underworld in order to excavate and retrieve what Rosalind Williams refers to as, in her analysis of underworld topographies, the 'absolute truth' (1992: 49). It is only this psychological manifestation of a geological practice that will allow him to return to the overworld. This notion of psychological 'excavation' often emerges in common parlance, as we are asked to *dig deep* or to *dredge our minds*, or even to 'get "down to bedrock"' (Frye 1963: 65), itself an archetype that metaphorically concretizes the vertical topography of the psyche. Moreover, Hillman suggests that Freud 'has returned to psycho-therapy the realm of inner space ... Through the dream, he rediscovers the underworld' (1979: 16). Freud, himself, referred to dream in geographical terms: the *via regia*, or royal road to the unconscious.

Iain Banks's novel *The Bridge* creates a multi-layered dream topography of the interiority of coma, though unlike Roy in *Marabou Stork Nightmares*, the protagonist of *The Bridge* has no real control over the transitions between layers of consciousness. Each layer also possesses its own distinct narrator, so while the layers may certainly evoke those created in Welsh's novel (the autobiographical narrative; the slips into a primal brogue of the Scottish persona; the fantasy/quest mythologem; the descent into the underworld) there is always a disjunction between narrators, causing a disruption in narrative form and flow. This implies that the Master-narrator (the victim, Alexander Lennox, trapped in coma) is for the majority of the novel unaware of the presence of his fractured alter-egos who constantly irrupt within his unconscious, jostling for narratorial supremacy and constituting the 'delayed, uncontrolled repetitive appearance of hallucinations and other intrusive phenomena' that are typical of the response to a traumatic event (Caruth 1996: 11). The complex narrative structure of the novel is scaffolded by clearly delineated, individually titled sections, themselves containing undertones of the geographical katabatic quest-narrative. The novel is split into three main sections (plus a fourth, shorter postscript, the 'Coda' section). These sections, 'Coma', 'Triassic' and 'Eocene', are then each split by another subsection, 'Metaphormosis', 'Metamorpheus' and 'Metamorphosis', respectively, which are then split into further sections or chapters, one to four or, in the case of the final 'Metamorphosis' section, split into four named parts: 'Oligocene', 'Miocene', 'Pliocene' and 'Quaternary'. There are several conceits at play within this intricate linguistic matrix. The three-part structure embodies the structure of the archetypal katabatic quest, the three stages that Joseph Campbell, writing extensively on the narrative form of mythological tales, would call the 'departure', the 'initiation' and the 'return' (1968). In this dream-like katabasis of coma, it is the coma itself, as is the case with *Louis Drax*, which proves to be the departure point, the descent from the cave-mouth of the mind into the underworld of the unconscious. As the novel progresses, each section is chronologically moving forward in terms of epoch, ending with the most recent period at the time of writing the novel: the 'Quaternary'. Each period represents significant geological and evolutionary change, suggesting that throughout his katabasis, Banks's narrator is in a constant state of developmental flux. This leads to a form of transfiguration as he gradually re-unifies his fractured pre-coma identity, an identity that will nevertheless remain forever changed. As Falconer notes, the descent into hell initiates the process of 'destruction and rebirth of the self through an encounter with the absolute Other' (2007: 1).

Each of the epochs is also marked by significant extinction events that led to radical shifts in evolution. The transition between the Eocene and Oligocene periods, for example, known as the *Grande Coupure* or 'the Great Break', was a large-scale extinction event which saw a disruption in evolutionary continuity, marked by climatic change and a dramatic turnover of mammalian fauna. This epoch is used to commence the third section of the novel, and the narrator's third stage of his journey (his 'return'), further emphasizing his metamorphosis as he battles to find his way back to the overworld. This return 'leg' of his infernal journey is integral in any katabatic quest, as Falconer explains when she writes that, 'There *has to be* a return in katabatic narrative, but it need not be the hero who returns' (2007: 45). In this statement, Falconer argues against Clark who posits that there can be no katabasis without a return to the overworld of the hero himself. However, in the case of *Louis Drax*, there is no return by the end of the novel. Moreover, Louis 'chooses' to stay within his coma rather than return to the overworld, a narrative twist that is evocative of Campbell's discussion of 'the refusal of return' depicted in several quest-narratives, whereby the hero fails to complete the 'full round' of his quest (1968: 193). However, in support of Falconer, this 'refusal' does not mean that Louis fails to perform a true katabasis. Because of the knowledge that Louis acquires at the heart of his descent, Louis realizes that the overworld has become more of a hell-state than that of his coma. As the forest fires that grip France rage on, threatening the hospital in which Louis is housed, the entire topography of the overworld is transformed into an infernal vision. At the point at which Natalie Drax throws herself into the conflagration, a final act of defiance and self-victimization, Dannachet describes her as 'hurtling into hell' (2005: 216): the irruption of Hell on earth. In this sense, and through this inversion of the physical overworld and the psychological underworld, Louis does 'return' from his hell-state, complete with katabatic knowledge, without ever actually returning from coma. He simply opts not to make the final physical (and medical) leg of the journey out of his DoC (although in the film adaptation, in true Hollywood tradition, the story ends with a close-up of Louis's fluttering eyelids before a smash-cut to black). In the case of *The Bridge*, technically it is not the hero, or in this case, multiple heroes who return but an altogether re-assimilated, re-born hero.

The use of 'Eocene' with its connotations of disruption and change is also reflected within the build-up of disruption between the various narrative threads, as the individual narrators (the 'heroes') battle for narrative supremacy. The geological references also connect with the concept of the descent to Hades through the earth as the narrator's psychological descent is described in terms of the physical world. At the point at which we meet him, Lennox is moving through the layers of the earth to get to the deepest reaches of the underworld. The novel begins in coma, the departure point for the underworld, and so as Lennox descends, he reaches the deepest part of the earth – the 'Triassic' section of the novel, from which he must attempt to return. The closer he gets to the overworld, the more recent the epoch. This structure creates another topographically vertical model of the mind and of consciousness, the layers of which the narrator must 'excavate' in order to escape the underworld and return to the overworld.

The theme of evolution and transfiguration is further emphasized through the structural designations, 'Metaphormosis/Metamorpheus/Metamorphosis'. 'Metaphormosis' implies that the entire novel is an allegory with the idea of coma utilized as an extended metaphor for hellish descent during which the mind is constantly appropriating and assimilating mythological motifs in order to cope with the trauma of the underworld of the unconscious. This is a process that exemplifies the workings of Jung's 'collective unconscious', alongside Frye's notion of the absorption of religion and myth into fiction. In an attempt to explain the phenomenological world and the trauma that caused the coma, metaphorical and archetypal 'coma dreams' are generated within the unconscious of the protagonist, forming an entire narrative of katabasis which provides the victim with a tangible coping strategy and with the *via regia* out of the hell of the unconscious. With the designation 'Metamorpheus', Banks draws a parallel between the coma-state and the sleep/dream-state, referencing the Greek god of dreams who dwells within the underworld. In the third instance, 'Metamorphosis', Banks returns to the root word upon which his other titles riff. Emphasizing the notion of change and transfiguration, the coma itself is compared to a pupal stage within which, through dream-like katabasis, the victim constantly evolves and gains the knowledge at the heart of his psychological hell before returning to the overworld, forever changed. It is significant that the very field of psychology is named after Psyche, the ancient Greek goddess of the soul and is also a word that, in one of its archaic forms, refers to a 'butterfly', a creature that experiences a profound metamorphosis, emerging from a 'katabatic' pupal stage. In *The Bridge*, the coma-psyche of Lennox, like its etymological and entomological counterpart, is forever evolving and metamorphosing with geographical and physical forms playing a key role throughout the novel in contributing to this change. It is within one such form, the sinister, oppressive structure of 'the Bridge' that the central narrator, John Orr (a pun on a geological 'ore', again representing the physical world) resides. But the structure and conceit of the novel also pays homage to a previous Scottish novel that had a huge influence upon the direction of Scottish fiction from the 1980s onwards: Alisdair Gray's *Lanark*. The split-narrative of the novel follows protagonist Lanark and his travails within the hellish, dystopian city of Unthank, together with its surrounding areas. It soon becomes apparent that Lanark is a psychological alter-ego of Duncan Thaw, a failed artist who has attempted suicide in the 'overworld' of Glasgow and since commenced his own katabatic descent into unconsciousness. In *Lanark*, we might trace the development of the oneiric motif in Scottish literature post-1980 and present in *The Bridge* and, later, *Marabou Stork Nightmares*, alongside Gray's second novel, *1982, Janine*. Cairns Craig notes in his discussion of *Lanark*, 'Such suspended animation will become a regular image of the changeless and paralysed condition of modern Scotland' (132), a Scotland that, only two years prior to the publication of *Lanark*, had lost an independence referendum. As Duncan Petrie posits, Thaw's 'cynicism, self-pity and negativity [...] poignantly embody that sense of betrayal and defeat that crystallised in the aftermath of the 1979 referendum defeat' (47).

Banks openly acknowledged the influence of Gray's novel, saying, '*Lanark* had a huge effect on *The Bridge*. I'm quite happy to acknowledge that debt' (Pattie 2013: 12) and we see this immediately in the narrative structure. Each novel moves between autobiographical narration of the *Bildungsroman* and oneiric, hellish and dystopian surrealism, worlds inhabited by a divided self on the cusp of death. There is also, as Martin Colebrook points out, 'strong thematic convergence through the representation of the cities and post-industrial spaces' that the novels present (2013: 34). Even the name of Banks's protagonist, Alexander Lennox (a name only subtly hinted at through Banks's trademark wordplay and puns) pays homage to the protagonist(s) of Gray's novel. While Orr, Lennox's comatose alter-ego, is indeed a geological pun on 'ore' (while also evoking the either/or of the divided self of Lennox/Orr), it also, Colebrook asserts, notably rhymes with 'Thaw' while the 'pronunciation of Lanark corresponds with Banks's choice of Lennox' (29).[2] In 'Alexander', we also see a reference to Lanark's son, the only person in his life with whom he feels any sense of connection and selfless love.

In the use of the split-subject, the divided self, both novels, together with *Marabou Stork Nightmares*, are yet again paradigmatic of Caledonian anti-syzygy, 'novels of damaged identity' that employ 'bifurcated narration' in order to 'focus upon the relationship between self and society' (Middleton 1999: 7). Petrie examines how, 'Lanark's narrative functions as both a reincarnation of Thaw and therefore a continuation of his life, but also as a series of repetitions or echoes that facilitate a richer understanding of the predicament of both' (47). Petrie's use of 'reincarnation' is significant, here, resonating with this chapter's interest in katabasis and the myth of resurrection/rebirth which also constitutes a central conceit in *The Bridge* but also in the other works of interior coma fiction discussed. *Marabou Stork Nightmares*, *The Coma*, *Regicide*, *Louis Drax* all represent various hellish reincarnations of the self and the 'overworld' (*eidola*) which must be interpreted and understood in order to gain deeper psychological insight which may trigger a way out of hell. In Banks's dream-world of coma, the Bridge is one such *eidolon*, an imposing, constantly-evolving structure that stretches over a seemingly endless expanse of water. The landmasses between which it stretches cannot be seen in either direction, evoking a sense of Christian limbo. Orr, the main hero trapped within the coma-underworld, has no recollection of how he has ended up in this place; he only knows that he was 'fished . . . out of the sea' (1986: 83). This reimagines classical katabatic mythologies where the descent-hero has to cross vast expanses of water to reach the edge of the world where the land of the dead meets the land of the living. The Mesopotamian *Gilgamesh* mythology and Odysseus's own *nekyia* are two examples of this archetypal narrative. Throughout mythology, the sea itself is often represented as a departure point for a katabatic journey as Frye explains: 'The lower world [is] reached by descent through a cave or under water' (1963: 59), reflecting Louis Drax's katabasis, similarly initiated by his plunge into the sea, or Jonah's katabasis in the belly of the watery Leviathan, but also Duncan Thaw whose departure into the psychological hell of Unthank is initiated by his attempt to drown himself in the 'slapping waves' of the sea into which he descends via steep 'beach shelves' (2007: 354).

Like Unthank and the city of Royle's *Regicide*, the socio-political environment of the Bridge itself is highly oppressive, with bureaucratic divisions of social class laid in vertical relation to one another, a 'totalitarian society that will take care of its occupants' needs but does so by removing their capacity for question or dissent' (Colebrook 2013: 38). The further down the Bridge you are forced to live, the lower your social class (and the more insignificant you will be), reflecting David Pike's observation that one of the chief tendencies of certain narratives of descent, such as Aristophanes' *Frogs* and Lucian's *Voyage to the Underworld*, is to create a 'transparently social or political allegory of contemporary life on earth' (1997: 7). Bethan Jones observes that in the higher reaches of the Bridge, Orr possesses a 'formality of speech and dress code (Orr "performs his toilet")' which, together with 'the use of rickshaws and wagons', produce a 'surreal image of British (rather than Oriental), antiquated elitism and urban bustle' (2013: 78). In this sense, again we see an exponent of Scottish coma fiction which, like *Marabou Stork Nightmares*, criticizes British imperialism and rule. Lennox, himself, is a working-class Glaswegian 'made good', now a rich engineer in Edinburgh who fails to be enamoured by material success. Petrie elucidates how in this, 'Lennox finds himself trapped between two world-views: the Scottish socialist tradition of his father, on one hand, and a mix of Edinburgh bourgeois gentility and Thatcherite materialism, on the other' (119). The psychological underworld of the Bridge plays out this crisis of Scottish identity; this divided self. Each of Banks's spatial divisions also reflects the delineations within Dante's topographical imagining of Hell, which itself adopts ancient archetypes of hellish society and includes satirical undertones akin to those to which Pike alludes. At one point, when Orr has been unfairly and abruptly stripped of his relatively high status as a psychiatric patient, due to the fact that he has questioned the authority of the state, he is condemned to dwell in the nether regions of the Bridge, living alongside the faceless masses. At this lowest point the environment is described as 'cold and dark' with 'grey waters' that 'crash white outside' (1986: 224). Mapping Orr's descent through the layers of the Bridge against archetypal concepts of the underworld, this lowest level becomes comparable with the nadir of Hades, Tartarus, which, as Hillman explicates, was 'in the imagination of late antiquity [. . .] a region of dense cold air without light'. Traditionally it is in this 'pneumatic region' (1979: 38) where the shades who have made some form of terrible transgression (usually against the Gods) are subjected to horrendous, repetitious punishments. Sisyphus is one such example, forced to roll a huge rock up a hill, only to have it roll all the way to the bottom before he managed to get it to the summit. Tartarus is frequently described as 'an almost bottomless pit of anguish and despair' (Harris and Platzner 1995: 200) and this is emulated by Orr's own descent into the lower depths of the Bridge where he suffers torturous punishment, stripped of all the trappings of status and position and erasing what little identity he has left.

Aside from the references to Tartarus, there are numerous allusions to Christian imagery of Hell that appear within the Bridge, infernal visions that arise out of its geological and mechanized fabric. It is revealed that Lennox once studied geology, before training and working as an engineer. Several times, this narrator's archetypal *eidolon*, Orr, encounters violent accidents within the Bridge, happenings that conjure images of mechanical suffering and hellfire. At one point, Orr inspects a sketch of the Bridge that his Virgilian guide, Abberlaine Arrol, has drawn for him. It depicts trains that are 'grotesque, gnarled things, like giant maggots' and 'girders and tubes' that 'become branches and boughs, disappearing into smoke rising from the jungle floor; a giant, infernal forest' (157). This visual interpretation of the Bridge makes open reference to it being an 'infernal' place, a sinister, smoking forest that invokes Dante's departure point for the *Inferno*. The manifestation of the Bridge, like the characters Orr encounters there, is itself an *eidolon* taken from Lennox's past life and assimilated into coma. As the novel progresses, it is revealed that the Bridge represents the Forth Rail Bridge that stretches into Edinburgh, a feat of engineering that was a source of macabre fascination for Lennox. The crash, it is revealed, was caused by him driving while drunk, absent-mindedly marvelling at that masterpiece of engineering downriver as he crosses the Forth Road bridge, leading him to take his eyes off the road and consequently follow the path of descent into his coma-underworld. As Gavin Miller observes, 'Lennox is a combination of man and machine, an amalgamation prefigured as his Jaguar crashes on the Forth Road bridge' (2007: 204) – a man who nearly died in a machine, now kept alive by machines. In a similar way to Roy in *Marabou Stork Nightmares*, these *eidola* (or 'imperfect doubles' to refer to Bethan Jones's discussion of mirror images that appear in *The Bridge* (2013: 85), employing a designation used by Banks himself in his novel) are conjurations from the narrator's unconscious. These shades that dwell within the dream-hell of the psyche represent memories from the overworld that Orr must interpret in order to return to that world. Frequently, for example, Orr is confronted with images of mechanical destruction or some 'scene of terrible disaster' (64), *eidola* that represent his crash and which need to be interpreted should a return from coma be achieved – a comatose, hellish repetition compulsion.

Like other katabatic heroes, Lennox has to keep digging deeper into his unconscious, descending further on his quest to retrieve the knowledge that will allow him to understand fully the *eidola* that appear all around him, just as Louis, led by Gustave, has to descend deeper into the skull-cave. One such *eidolon* created by Banks is the haunting vision of a man wired up to a life-support machine that keeps appearing on Orr's television set, alongside the intermittent 'bleeps' on his phone-line that he deems to be an intermittent fault but which actually represent the noise of the life-support machinery in the overworld. This image becomes an ultimate *eidolon*, representing his corporeal presence in the overworld but 'recast' as a bodiless shade in the underworld. It is an image that appears intertextually in the BBC drama *Life On Mars* (2006) and also in Royle's *Regicide* with Carl, towards the end of the novel, coming face-to-face with a 'figure in [a] bed ... tubes threaded into the patient's arm'. Carl sees 'the bruised, bloodshot eyes' staring at him, concluding, 'They were not my father's eyes, but mine' (132).

Another example of a hellish *eidolon* that is particularly significant in causing Lennox's final departure from the underworld is Abberlaine Arrol. As the various narrative threads switch between one another, she comes to represent Lennox's lover of the overworld, Andrea, the aloof object of his desire who cannot commit to a monogamous relationship and to whom the narrator is driving, drunkenly, at the time of his accident. Throughout Orr's quest, there are subtle suggestions of this connection between the underworld and the overworld, most notably in the handkerchief that Abberlaine gives to Orr. The circumstances surrounding this simple transaction are important to consider. The couple are involved in a rickshaw accident on the Bridge (another *eidolon* that references Lennox's road-traffic accident). Orr hands Abberlaine his handkerchief so that she can stem the blood running from her nose. Later, Abberlaine hands back the handkerchief to Orr – it has been washed and now bears the monogram of his initial – 'O'. Following this episode, when he is stripped of everything and condemned to the cold, isolated 'Tartarus' of his coma consciousness, the handkerchief is one of two items that he is allowed to keep. It is the monogram on the handkerchief that saves it from being impounded, due to the fact that the monogram does not fit the description of the inventory that the foreman of the search-and-seizure officiously wields. As Orr descends further into the world of the Bridge, Lennox's autobiographical narrative begins to develop and gradually reveal more information about his life leading up to the accident. In one recollection, he describes a cherished scene of lovemaking between him and Andrea. Andrea is menstruating and uses a white scarf to stem the blood-flow. Later, the narrator finds the scarf in his car, the 'blood stain, dried in a rough circle' (319). He says that this stain 'wouldn't shift', no matter how many times he washes it. However, when he hands it over to Andrea, she washes it clean with ease and hands it back to him 'monogrammed with his initials' (320).

These episodes serve to underscore the notion of hellish *eidola* of the coma unconscious that represent memories of the overworld while simultaneously depicting the interiority of coma as psychoanalytical dream-work, similar to *Louis Drax*, *Marabou Stork Nightmares*, *Regicide* and *The Coma*. The O-shaped stain in the overworld 'wouldn't shift' – in the underworld of the coma, no matter how many times Orr washes the handkerchief, it is always bloodied by various twists of fate. This *eidolon* insistently transmits and communicates memories of the overworld (the handkerchief has to be bloodied and can be nothing else), thereby presenting Orr (and therefore Lennox) with a metaphor that has to be unlocked and interpreted in order to escape from the underworld of coma. As Bethan Jones lucidly explains, 'The figure "O", resonant with possibility, repetition and the opportunity to transform, would seem to triumph over the linear, angular and totalizing perspective offered by the Bridge. But it is also this "O" (a nothing, a zero) which Lennox recognizes as a metaphor for his trapped existence; for being present in both realities' (86).

Banks' *eidolon* of Abberlaine is also reminiscent of the *eidolon* of Eurydice in the Orpheus mythology – after all, it is her lack of *thymos* (he cannot hear her footsteps) that causes Orpheus to turn around to make sure she is still following him out of Hades. For Banks's katabatic adventurer, Orr, once he finally realizes that Abberlaine is not Andrea but merely an 'ancient' and 'rotten' (232) *eidolon*, an escape from the Bridge is catalysed. He suddenly finds himself in a war between two bureaucratic armies, attacking each other from speeding trains that hurtle away from the Bridge and burrow downwards into the very centre of the earth. Through this narrative development, the geological divisions of the novel are stressed once more, reflecting the idea of physical, chthonic descent and Lennox's increasing desire to dig deeper towards the heart of his coma-hell and seize hold of the katabatic knowledge which will trigger his *anabasis* and transfiguration. The train motif is similarly used in both *Lanark* and *Regicide*, a means of transporting the divided selves of all three protagonists to, from and between liminal states. In *Lanark*, the eponymous hero's journey to Unthank (and Thaw's metamorphosis into Lanark) is symbolized by the train journey into 'the blackness' (16), a familiar designation (as we have seen) for the katabatic descent into the unconscious. In *Regicide*, the train, for Carl, is his way out of the hellish dystopia of his coma, the station itself located at the edge of a series of, 'Brownfield sites, interzones, edgelands' (167), 'Grey areas between districts' (9) that are emblematic of the blurring and competing selves, memories and places within his grey matter.

For Banks's Orr, the deeper he travels into the earth, the more extreme his visions of Hell become, but also the more traditional they become in a Catholic sense of *contrapasso*, where the 'form of retribution [is] exactly suited to the nature of each sin' (Falconer 2007: 25). Earlier, in one particular moment of clarity, Orr considers why he is trapped within this hell-state, saying, 'I do not know why I am here. Because I did something wrong' (186). The seamlessness between this call-and-response utterance, between the doubt and the certainty, echoes the notions of Hell being a place of punishment where the individual is so accustomed to their torture that they almost become senseless. They passively accept their fate, in the full knowledge that they have committed a wrongdoing and deserve their punishment in some way but forgetting the specifics of their transgression. Later in Banks's novel, captured soldiers are thrown into 'pools of boiling mud' (311) before being dragged out again, with more mud shovelled onto them so that they become 'gnarled statues', symbols of the punishment that awaits other rebels or transgressors in this psychological underworld. Betrayal constitutes the ultimate sin in this world where faceless factions go to war over an unknown cause (an *eidolon* that represents Lennox's own disgust at the senselessness of the Falklands War and oppressive British imperialism occurring in the overworld which serves to exacerbate further his crisis of Scottish/British identity). Similarly, within the ninth circle of Dante's Hell (a place that, like

The Bridge, also punishes traitors), the transgressors are punished by being turned into gnarled and distorted statues, trapped in time. However, unlike the traditional Christian image of hellfire, Dante envisions his innermost circle of Hell as being a place of utmost cold, Satan himself held in a frozen lake of blood. Once more, the symbiosis of Hell and Hades and the mythological traditions of both can be seen, Dante's ninth circle echoing the cold, pneumatic region of Tartarus, rather than the traditional Christian image of Hell. Banks, too, adopts this *bricolage* approach, developing his own vision of the underworld based upon archetypal imagery of both the Christian Hell and Greco-Roman Hades. Banks also fully simulates Dante's journey into Hell as the further both protagonists journey, the more they begin to psychologically and morally understand and judge themselves. As Hawkins posits, 'Thus for the poet Dante, the tropological meaning of his journey through Hell is a journey into the self, where what he sees in others is a dimension of what he himself is or could be' (1992: 203).

At the furthest extremity of his descent, Orr finds himself at the edge of another body of water, again the archetypal symbol, in the mythology of antiquity, of the division between the land of the living and of the dead. Here, he once more encounters an old man who whips corpses that wash up on shore and Orr asks: 'What happened here? What happened to all these people?' to which the old man responds: 'They didn't listen to their dreams'. Orr does not say anything. Instead, he sets off again 'for the distant line of light which fills the horizon like a streak of white gold' (362-33). This interchange is apposite to the entire representation of the coma descent. The words of the old man imply to Orr that the reason why he is still being punished, being psychologically *scourged* within this hell of the unconscious, is because he, too, is not listening to his dreams. It is an unconscious signpost towards the fact that he is flagrantly refusing to decode the hellish visions, the *eidola*, that are appearing all around him within his coma. It is a moment equivalent of the 'Wake Up' signs in Ubisoft's *Driver: San Francisco*, one that proves to be the final catalyst for Lennox's return and 'awakening' from the coma-underworld. Orr suddenly heads towards the light, finally beginning to understand what the *eidola* in his coma-dreams represent. The 'white gold' light takes on both physical and metaphorical connotations, constituting the bright, clinical luminescence of the hospital room penetrating his eyelids and forming a horizontal slant of light, but also representing the spiritual illumination of transfiguration that enlightens the soul and allows for resurrection and passage back into the land of the living.

As I have discussed at length, throughout *The Bridge*, Banks is preoccupied with developing katabatic dream *eidola* archetypes, 'enigma codes' that Lennox must 'crack' in order to unravel the mystery at the heart of the novel. Banks therefore bestows upon Lennox the role of Jungian psychoanalyst who has to draw out the dream-images of the underworld and make the connections between these and their equivalent manifestations in the overworld. It is a similar conceit to that which appears in Jeremy Dyson and Andy Nyman's 2017 film adaptation of their hit stage play, *Ghost Stories*. Their protagonist, Professor Goodman (Good/Man being a variation of the 'Every/Man' archetype), in attempting to debunk a series of paranormal experiences, must act as both analyst and analysand in decoding the dream-images of his own underworld of the unconscious that lead him to confront the fact that he occupies his own liminal state: locked-in syndrome. The 'ghost stories', therefore, are figments of his fevered dreams, *eidola* from his past and from the overworld that are assimilated and work against Goodman's screen memories in order to force him to psychoanalytically confront both the trauma of his childhood and the current trauma of his locked-in syndrome which his physicians, significantly, confuse for coma. Goodman's moment of realization comes when he is led to his hospital bed by one of his *eidolons*, the decaying corpse of a boy from his childhood past for whose death he feels responsible. As the ghoul inserts his fingers into his mouth, Goodman exclaims, 'No, not again!', implying a looping, circular trauma that is replayed within his hell-state of locked-in syndrome. The fingers are also an *eidolon* of the breathing and feeding tubes that are inserted into his mouth and throat to keep him alive. This end sequence sees one of his Virgilian guides lead him to a confrontation with the corporeal self, a trope in so many works of coma fiction discussed herein.

For Banks, his position as novelist writing within the 1980s, an era of psychoanalytical revisionism, is further exemplified by one of the other narrative threads that he creates: the folkloric narration of an illiterate, Scottish barbarian. Written in a thick brogue, rendering him, as Petrie notes, a 'Gothic manifestation of the Scottish hard man' (119), this fantasy-narration persistently intrudes upon both Orr's journey of katabasis and Lennox's biographical revelations, drawing on archetypes of descent mythology and overtly so. In one sequence, in a hybridization of fairy tale and myth, he is set the task of travelling into the 'Underwurld' [*sic*] in order to rescue the 'Sleepin Byooty', following the model of the archetypal katabatic quest in the vein of Orpheus or, more pertinently, Heracles. Like that man-god, instead of passively interacting with the shades of Hades, the Barbarian battles against them. Within this subplot, Banks explicitly draws a parallel between the coma descent and the katabasis of antiquity, the Barbarian encountering such mythological figures as the ferryman of the river Styx, Charon (here pronounced 'Karen') and Sisyphus, the doomed transgressor who keeps rolling 'this huge fuckin chuckie right tae the tap aw the hill' (212). Truly Herculean in his aggression, the Barbarian disrupts this repetitious punishment, helping Sisyphus with the boulder by leaving it at the top of the hill, a dream action which implies that Lennox, too, has the power to put a stop to the repetitious nightmares that grip him and sustain his coma-hell. These archetypal dream-images of the underworld allude to the possibility that, like the greatest of man-gods Heracles and even Christ, Lennox has the power to conquer the underworld (to *harrow* the Hell of his unconscious) and rise again.

At the end of this quest into the underworld, the Barbarian finally locates the goal of his katabasis, the 'Sleepin Byooty', a designation that immediately resonates with the Wijdicks' identification of the sleeping beauty trope in coma fiction and examined throughout this volume. However, this particular fairy tale 'princess' turns out to be no such thing, as we see when the Barbarian finally meets the object of his quest: 'A man lyin in bed, all white-faced an asleep . . . metal chests on theyre sides all clustered around him' with 'wee bit things like strings attached tae him' (217). The *eidolon* of Orr's narrative (the bed-ridden coma patient) also makes an appearance at the heart of the Barbarian's own story and in both cases, he represents the knowledge at the heart of all katabatic quests. The Barbarian represents both the Freudian 'id' and the Jungian 'shadow', encapsulating deeply primal, violent and sexual urges that have the potential to result in self-destruction. In contrast to this, the old man on the beach conjures Jung's archetype of the 'wise old man'. After all, it is this archetype that initiates Orr's final journey out of coma, an escape which is a paradoxical and oxymoronic journey: an inversion in which Lennox can only move up and out of coma by going deeper into its hellish landscape. This psychological manifestation of a topographical inversion that occurs at the deepest point of the descent journey is reminiscent of the Dantean model of escape from Hell during which there is, in Falconer's words, a 'turning upside down at a zero point and a return to the surface of some kind' (2007: 45). In the *Inferno*, Dante travels down through Hell until he re-emerges on the other side of the earth. He and Virgil climb down Satan's body, reaching the deepest point of Hell at which point the inversion occurs: 'I raised my eyes, believing I should see | the half of Lucifer that I had left; | instead I saw him with his legs turned up' (1995: 211, lines 88-90). He has descended into the earth via one hemisphere and ended his katabic journey emerging into the other hemisphere. In *The Bridge*, a similar inversion occurs. As Orr further traverses the world of the Bridge, the deeper he journeys into its geological landscape, burrowing into the volcanic layers of the earth and so therefore delving deeper into his unconscious. In moving towards the 'core' of this world, he comes closer to the surface of the waking overworld, a paradox represented by the increasingly modern geological epochs used as section-titles for the novel. Falconer suggests, 'Katabatic inversion thus inverts the hero's sense of entrapment into one of liberation or insight' (53). Such depictions of hellish inversions are rife within the literature of the mythological underworld. Hillman, for example, discusses how in the Egyptian underworld imagination, 'The dead walked upside down so that stuff of their bowels came out through their mouths' (1979: 183). In another one of Orr's many visions of hell, he imagines that, 'The bridge is part of a circle', Banks again drawing on Dante's topographical model of the nine circles of Christian Hell. However, Banks also employs archetypes from ancient mythology, not least this hellish inversion of faecal matter. At one point, Orr dreams of being trapped in a different manifestation of the Bridge, staring at macabre sexual orgies on the shore opposite where the women, in an image reminiscent of the sirens in the *Odyssey*, call to him to join them. He cannot cross the water, though, because of the 'carnivorous fish' which inhabit the water, embodying the monstrous guardians of the underworld inherent in mythology (the Greco-Roman hellhound of the underworld, Cerberos, being one such example, and one that appears in the Barbarian's own descent). Orr details his frustrated revenge upon these 'Hell-bags': 'I waited until I needed a crap, then threw the turd at them. Those obscene brats *used* it in one of their filthy sex games' (187). In a scene that harks back to Hillman's discussion of Egyptian inversion within the underworld, faecal matter, a symbol of unwanted waste, becomes a symbol of sexual desire and virility reassimilated into a fertility ritual. The excrement, to refer to Julia Kristeva's work on abjection, 'Signifies the other side of the border' (1980: 3), reminding the Subject that it is not a stable, fixed system – that its borders are constantly being breached. The fact that an Other assimilates the abjected waste into their own borders exacerbates this feeling of disgust within Orr, even subconsciously reminding him that the border of his psyche has also been breached within coma, a crisis of post-traumatic identity.

Within this 'inverted' world of both hell and coma, time, too, becomes inverted. In archetypal manifestations of the underworld, there occurs at once the impossible re-running and collapsing of time (the repetitious punishments of Sisyphus and Ixion, for example, that never reach a conclusion) and yet the descent-hero must move through time and space in order to fulfil their katabasis and return to the overworld. The *Inferno* is a paradigm of the dichotomy of Hell-time whereby Dante perceives *eidola* trapped in time and yet his own journey is framed by a time-scale, descending at 6.00 am and re-emerging at 6.00 pm. Juxtaposed against this contradictory inversion of time is again the other inversion of place: the return to the overworld by climbing further into the underworld. It is this sudden inversion in katabatic narratives that can also be seen in coma literature, *Louis Drax* being another such example, as discussed earlier.

In another example of Greco-Roman descent literature, the *Aeneid*, Virgil writes, 'The way that leads down to Avernus is easy to tread [. . .] But to retrace thy steps, to merge once more | In the upper air – that is a wearisome task' (2004: 6.127-130). However, this depiction of the difficulty of the katabatic return is contentious, as explicated by Falconer in her discussion of Eduard Norden's work on the hellish inversion of return, when she writes that the difficulty of return 'is only true in a limited sense . . . The return journey in most cases occurs swiftly and with little hindrance' (43). Virgil's use of 'retrace' implies that a return involves travelling back over the hellish lands already covered, yet this does not occur in the *Inferno*. Dante travels *through* Hell to come out on the other side, a return he describes in less than seven lines. Odysseus, too, at the end of his own katabasis, seems to find the return easy, simply turning away from the teeming, tortured souls of Hades and returning to his ship. A process of wearisome 'retracing' is avoided. Even Theseus's return from the labyrinth at Minos is easy (in a version of the descent myth occurring within the overworld). He does retrace his steps, yet his passage is made effortless through the gift of Ariadne's thread. Contrary to Virgil's statement, katabatic return seems to be not so difficult and this model is likewise exploited in coma fiction. In *Marabou Stork Nightmares*, no sooner has Roy faced up to his inner demons than a return is triggered; in *The Coma*, a similar transition occurs, the return triggered by confronting the simple contents of a briefcase, and in *The Bridge*, the return is entirely in Lennox's hands. Like Carl, at the deepest point of the hell of coma, all the hero of Banks's novel has to do is to make the cognitive decision to return, and a return will be granted. As Lennox says, evoking the language of Garland's novel, 'The choice is not between dream and reality; it is between two different dreams' (380). In the end, return from the underworld is all about choice, an active decision that is in itself an inversion of Orr's passive helplessness within the hell-dreams of coma. In *Louis Drax*, return from Hades is similarly a matter of choice, as perceived by Louis in the novel's final lines: 'I know that one day, if I want to, I can do it. I can take one step forward. And then another' (2005: 227). Crucially, Louis describes moving forward; not backward.

3.4 Coma and the restitution narrative

Rosalind Williams, in her work on the archetype of actual and imaginary subterranean worlds, observes that, 'Since the nineteenth century [. . .] excavation has served as a dominant metaphor for truth-seeking [...] In this respect scientific inquiry retains an aura of the mythological, since the heroic quest for scientific truth has the pattern of a descent into the underworld' (1992: 49). This elision between the language of mythology and the language of science reveals how embedded cultural archetypes are within human consciousness: we use such archetypes in order to help us to explain the inexplainable, such as the medical term 'Lazarus Sign', discussed earlier. Judith Greenberg, in discussing the role of narrative in trauma survival, draws an explicit parallel between the victim of trauma and katabatic mythologies, writing, 'The post-traumatic victim and "storyteller" occupies a kind of Orphic role, having descended into the depths of horror and a form of "death" and returned to the world of the living' (1998: 325), here alluding specifically to the descent of Orpheus. Similarly, Hawkins observes that for the writer of illness narratives, 'The "pathographical act" is one that constructs meaning by subjecting raw experience to the powerful impulse to make sense of it all, to bind together the events, feelings, thoughts and sensations that occur during an illness into an integrated whole' (1999: 18). Paul Ricoeur highlights, in his appraisal of Frye's ideas about the longevity of mythological narratives, that, 'If an archetype designates a stable conventional order, this order can be established in terms of its correspondence to the order of nature and its recurrences – day and night, the seasons, the years, life and death'. Ricoeur attempts to explain why these archetypes are still in existence: that no matter how distant they now are from their original mythological source material, they have over the centuries helped to form 'an already existing order of words [that] is not pure chaos', therefore allowing humankind to attempt to make sense of the world (1985: 9). Ricoeur's redevelopment of narrative theory highlights a link between the Jungian concept of the archetype and narratological discussions of the role of mythological archetypes in the creation of selfhood. Ricoeur, in development of Aristotelian theories of emplotment and narrative, asserts that, 'Fiction contributes to making life, in the biological sense of the word, a human life' (1991a: 20), mirroring Frye's observation that, 'Literature [...] has a lot to do with identifying the human world with the natural world around it, or finding analogies between them' (1964: 49). Literature, therefore, is not just a record of human experience with which the reader has a passive relationship. Instead, it actively informs one's knowledge of the world and helps to develop one's understanding of the self. Thus, as Ricoeur proposes, 'Narrative fiction, is an irreducible dimension of *self-understanding* ... An *examined* life ... is a life *recounted*' (1991a: 31). Ricoeur points towards the interplay between the analyst and the analysand in psychotherapeutic sessions, with the latter encouraged to draw out 'story-fragments' into 'a narrative which would be at once more bearable and more intelligible' (30). In Jungian practice, this unification of story-fragments would be encouraged by tracing them through archetypal imagery and narratives, mythologies, fables – that which forms the collective unconscious. Ricoeur's concept of 'fragments' is mirrored by Jung's concept of the 'fragmented' self which needs to be fully 'individuated'. It is also a term that Jung would perhaps have found more acceptable than Freud's designation 'archaic remnants' which he used to describe the 'dream-images' that Jung consistently argued were 'analogous to primitive ideas, myths, and rites'. Jung heavily criticized Freud's use of 'remnants', arguing that this contributed to a 'prevailing depreciation of the unconscious as a mere appendix of consciousness [. . .], a dustbin which collects all the refuse of the conscious mind' (1977: 206). Ricoeur's 'fragments', rather than Freud's 'remnants' (things left behind) is suggestive of something that can be potentially re-formed into a cohesive form once more, a concept central to the Jungian approach to 'dream-work' in which the symbolic and archetypal language of dreams is translated from its cultural form into one that speaks of the truth at the heart of the unconscious. Similarly, central to Ricoeur's work on the importance of narration in the formation of selfhood is the idea of 'sedimentation' and 'innovation', concepts that correlate with Jungian concepts of the 'archetype' and 'translation'. The 'sediment' (universal historical archetypes) are the 'models that constitute, after the fact, the typology of emplotment which allows us to order the history of literary genres' (1991a: 24). 'Innovation' is the assimilation and redevelopment of such archetypal tropes (the sediment), allowing the possibility for 'a later experimentation in the narrative domain' (25). In other words, individual creativity and reinterpretation of the 'sediment' allow the development of individual, personal narratives. Frye, too, observes, 'Everything is new, and yet recognizably the same kind of thing as the old', alluding to how a new baby is 'a genuinely new individual' while simultaneously 'an example of something very common, . . . linearly descended from the first human beings there ever were' (1964: 45). Frye's use of the image of biological 'inheritance' to describe how literature constantly assimilates and reinvents what has gone before once more evokes Ricoeur's concepts of 'sedimentation' and 'innovation'. However, while Frye uses biology and genetics as a metaphor for how literature has developed, in Jungian terms, such a 'literature' has been biologically 'inherited' through the collective unconscious. The 'sediment' can therefore be seen to be the conceptual, literary equivalent of the Jungian collective unconscious. As both Ricoeur and Frye suggest, the sediment is a constant reinvention and innovation of literature and this has its equivalent in the Jungian collective unconscious that also perpetually evolves. Literature holds the 'sediment' of all historical human experience, emotions and attempts to understand the world. This allows the individual both to assimilate and innovate the sediment in literature, allowing him to continue to try to make sense of the world and thereby continue to develop 'new-but-different' literature. This process helps to further elucidate Ricoeur's assertion that, 'Fiction contributes to making life'. In this way, Jung's collective unconscious is not necessarily unlocked by literature, or by tracing the links between literary or mythological archetypes and the mind. Instead, the collective unconscious *is* literature. In his discussion of the katabatic journey (one particular aspect of the 'sediment'), David Pike observes that, 'It requires the descent through hell to teach the protagonist allegorical interpretation' (1997: 113). Perhaps writers of coma fiction are consistently using and innovating sedimentary archetypes from the mythologies of descent to try and come to terms with the fear and chaos that the coma itself represents: that they are creating allegories to help rationalize coma. In doing so, coma fiction, in particular, fills in the gaps of experience with archetypal narratives and imagery in an attempt to navigate through an incomprehensible concept (a total void in consciousness) by equating it with a vastly more comprehensible concept (a semi-conscious state – sleep and dream and the hellish descents this state can initiate). As with Redgrove's poem, an *absolute nothing* cannot be communicated, so it has to be narrated through the medium of a near-tangible *something*. In this sense, authors, like the creators of mythologies and religious stories before them, attempt to express the unspeakable by grounding it in archetypal images – the 'order of words' to which Ricoeur refers.

During a seminar talk given in London to the Guild of Pastoral Psychology, Jung observed that, 'Now, we have no symbolic life, and we are all badly in need of the symbolic life. Only the symbolic life can express the need of the soul' (1977: 274). The need of the Jungian soul (*psyche*), contemporaneously associated with the mind, evokes Ricoeur's insistence upon the self's 'genuine demand for narrative' (1991a: 29). These human needs and demands become a fundamental desire for the human mind to comprehend the incomprehensible and to strive continually to find ways to communicate the incommunicable. By concentrating on the dwindling of Christianity and religious faith in the West, Jung neglected to acknowledge that the symbolic life also resides within literature. It is literature that both reveals authors' concerns and obsessions with unanswered questions, but which also exposes their need to try and answer those questions in an attempt to alleviate the inner fears of the unknown – to translate the unknown into language and to maintain, as Ricoeur states, the 'stable conventional order'. Frye further suggests, 'When a system of myths loses all connexion with belief, it becomes purely literary' (1963: 32). This does not necessarily mean that it loses all of its power and influence upon the individual and upon society. Instead, it provides one with the tools with which one can narrate, 'work through' and comprehend the world in which one lives. Couser, in discussing illness narratives and life writing, also alludes to this need to comprehend and communicate illness, often made more complex by the fact that often, the patient and his illness is communicated through his physician who may 'reinterpret patients' pasts and literally pre-script their futures' (1997: 10). Couser further explains, 'Just as patients wish to vanquish the illness that alters their lives, they may also wish to regain control of their life narratives' (10) and such use of myths and archetypes (or 'master plots' (216)) help to achieve this. As Hawkins explores, such 'mythic thinking of all kinds becomes apparent in that delicate autobiographical transition from "actual" experience to written narrative' (1999: 18).

Coma fiction is one manifestation of the 'symbolic life' and 'myth-making', though with a key departure from that which occurs in illness narratives and pathographies of lived experience. Baldly, coma fiction does not necessarily concern itself with the realities (the 'actual experience', to use Hawkin's designation) of the illness or condition itself – in this case, the void of coma; the various PDoC to which the chronic vegetative state can progress; prognosis of PDoC; and the potential for BI and long-term neurological conditions. Instead, the coma, the condition, is narrated and mythologized to examine and rationalize a wider existential threat: the potential void of death. This use of mythological narratives of katabasis is sharply satirized by Richard Dooling in *Critical Care*, his darkly comic novel of bioethics and the law in the caring of patients in PDoC. In considering the vegetative patient known impersonally as 'Bed Five', cynical ICU physician Dr Peter Werner Ernst ('Werner') ponders, 'He looked like any other septuagenarian who had endured seven surgical procedures in as many months, was crucified, died, was buried, descended into hell, and on the third day was coded again, strapped down in bed, and seated at the right hand of a Bennett MA-2 ventilator' (1992: 107). For Werner, there is no redemptive mythological narrative that helps stave off the fear of death; there is only science and science is God. This cynical intersection of science and religion is visually rendered in Sidney Lumet's 1997 film adaptation. The ICU in which Bed Five is treated is cavern-like, akin to an ossuary, with each patient housed in low-arched ante-rooms that are lit so brightly with stark white lighting that it almost bleaches out the screen: a representation that calls to mind the 'white tunnel' of the near-death experience, or of purgatory.

Sontag's hypothesis that 'part of the denial of death in this culture is a vast expansion of the category of illness' (1991: 57) is pertinent to this discussion. Through the C-Met, and literary licence that is taken by authors, the 'category' of coma is 'expanded' into other categories of consciousness and states of being (sleep and dream, for example) from which the patient 'awakes', seemingly with no long-term effects. Sontag's concept of a 'denial of death' resonates with Arthur Frank's work on patient and illness narratives, most notably his assertion that the metaphorical restitution narrative of recovery from sickness allows one to 'deny' and therefore 'conquer' death. In this way, the use of the C-Met contributes to what Zygmunt Bauman refers to as 'deconstructed mortality' (1991: 131), a concept that Frank explores in analysing the various narrative archetypes employed in stories of illness. Examining, from a sociological and philosophical perspective, death and dying and how modern societies deal with these 'taboo' subjects, Bauman argues that such a process of deconstruction 'does not abolish death' per se, but instead allows death to be 'stripped of significance' in the light of medico-social rhetoric and promises of hope of survival. As Frank explicates in his discussion of Bauman, modernity 'exorcises the fear of mortality by breaking down threats, among which illness is paradigmatic, into smaller and smaller units' (1997: 84). Superficially, this appears to contradict Sontag's notion of the 'expansion' of illness, but in fact these two theoretical positions dovetail neatly into each other, as we see in the case of the C-Met. As coma is 'expanded' into other 'categories' through the use of metaphor, myth and archetypes, coma itself starts to become demystified and broken down into smaller, more manageable associations and meanings. Coma is 'expanded' into the category of what Frank terms the 'restitution narrative', that is, a narrative told by the sick that 'displays a heroism in the face of bodily breakdown' (1995: 93). It is a narrative which 'attempt[s] to outdistance mortality by rendering illness transitory' (115). It is, as Frank posits in further developing Bauman's concept of deconstructing mortality, the 'culturally preferred narrative' whether it is told by 'television commercials, sociology, or medicine' (191). This narrative type is preferred precisely because it offers hope of conquering death and in the case of coma fiction, it allows the incomprehensible notion of a void in consciousness to be broken down into the 'smaller units' or stages of a journey into the unconscious which the protagonist must complete in order to reach an almost inevitable point of return, allowing authors and audiences to defeat the fears they may possess surrounding their mortality.

In his work on the dead, and his explorations of the places where the dead co-habit the world of the living, Robert Pogue Harrison explores the human need to delineate and 'contain' space. Asserting that, 'Places are located in nature, yet they always have human foundations', Harrison observes that places 'do not occur naturally but are created by human beings through some mark or sign of human presence'. Harrison therefore suggests that out of the abstract notion of 'space' humans craft more tangible embodiments of 'place' by creating concrete, delineated 'landmarks'. It is this process that allows nature to 'become bounded', thus granting man the power of 'human containment' (2003: 18–19). This creation of place as a form of human containment of an abstract concept is at the heart of traditional tales of katabasis. The construction of subterranean topographies is an attempt to concretize and rationalize the abstract concept of death and the afterlife. By attributing physical, traversable landscapes to the underworld and, moreover, by allowing their heroes to return from these places, authors of katabatic narratives are able to 'contain' death by describing it in terms of tangible, imaginable and topographical imagery. Similarly, the pursuit of depth psychology was to 'contain' the somewhat abstract concept of the mind within a more 'bounded', perceptible model: a physical and geographical landscape. And many writers of coma fiction, too, in their creation of such interior, psychological landscapes of the underworld are attempting metaphorically to harrow the hell of a liminal space. By 'binding' the unconscious state of coma within topographically concretized and archetypal depictions of a physical underworld, writers attempt to contain and comprehend coma.

In Liz Jensen's novel, the interior space of Louis's unconscious becomes concretized and 'bounded' in the form of his own cave which, in turn, increasingly maps onto the subterranean topography of Hades. At the deepest point of descent, and shortly before reaching the point of katabatic enlightenment, the cave is described as 'a freezing mouth breathing out' (2005: 174). Here again, a comparison with the deepest part of Hades – Tartarus – can be made through the reference to cold air, expelled from the cave mouth. Banks's novel borrows topographical motifs from traditional representations of both Hades and Hell to represent a vertically-structured hellish society, the layers of which the coma victim must travel through in order to return to the 'waking' overworld. At one point, when Orr is cast down to the lowest reaches of the Bridge, he wakes from a nightmare and believes he is 'encased in ice' (194). This not only stresses the allusion to Tartarus, through the depiction of a sub-zero landscape, but also chimes with Dante's own nadir of Hell in the *Inferno*, itself influenced by various strands of Greco-Roman thought as dramatized in the katabatic works of Homer and Virgil. Banks even openly alludes to katabatic descent in the narration of the Barbarian alter-ego, who has to travel through the Hadean topography of the 'Underwurld' [*sic*], and is at one point told to, 'Beware Lethe, the waters of oblivion' (21). The 'containment' of the space of the mind in a physical place is once more emphasized, this particular reference to Lethe, the river of forgetfulness within Hades, acting as a warning to Lennox to battle against the potential oblivion of coma. Ultimately, the language and imagery of underworld topography attributed to the interior state of coma allows authors and readers alike to rationalize the terrifying prospect of a violently-induced DoC. Through literature, through the exploration of the 'sediment' and the process of 'innovation', authors strive to narrate through the void of unconsciousness. In this way, and to return once more to Ricoeur, we are constantly 'applying to ourselves the plots that we have received from our culture . . . [in an] . . . attempt to obtain a narrative understanding of ourselves' (1991a: 33).

Arthur Frank writes that, 'Any sickness is an intimation of mortality, and telling sickness as a restitution story forestalls that intimation' (1997: 85). Much of coma fiction embodies this principle and in particular, by adopting the ultimate archetype of the restitution story, the katabatic journey and return from the underworld, such literary works articulate a disavowal of mortality. Significantly, in all of the works of fiction discussed, the protagonist returns from his coma-underworld (or at least, gains the knowledge of *how* to return). In this way, by allowing their protagonists to travel through and return from a physical underworld, both writers of coma fiction and of katabatic tales of antiquity are, in turn, allowing humankind to 'translate' and 'work through' incidents of trauma and the Liftonian 'death encounter'. These attempts to overcome this confrontation with mortality (which, Frank argues, 'cannot be part of the story' of restitution (1997: 95)) ultimately leads to a sense of hope and the promise of survival. As Frank further argues, 'Turning illness into story is a kind of meta-control' (32), an attempt to overcome the confrontation with the fragility of life that is acquired, often, through experiencing serious illness. In essence, all of these novels translate the neurological condition of coma into a psychological condition in order to contain the fear of death and explore deep questions of trauma and identity, even despite the huge swing from psychology to neurology during the 1990s: the 'decade of the brain'. The next chapter, however, examines texts that are very much products of this swing; examples of what Marco Roth terms the 'neuronovel'. And the representations of coma and brain injury couldn't be more different.

4

Selfhood and the post-coma condition

As we have seen with Stephen King's *The Dead Zone*, not all works of coma fiction are interested exclusively in depicting the imagined interiority of the DoC itself. This novel, too, is peculiar in that, despite its fantasy credentials, King portrays factual symptoms of the post-coma condition and ensuing long-term neurological disability: muscle atrophy, for example, and Johnny's aphasia. Despite the fact that Johnny emerges from a five-year coma with cognition and identity immediately intact, his prophetic powers, and the affect they have upon him, seem to be, to return to Joseph J. Fins's description of the portrayal of coma and brain trauma in Almodóvar's *Hable con Ella*, 'metaphorically powerful' (2007: 80). Johnny's visions themselves become a metaphor for long-term BI: every time he has a vision, they are described as having a physical and emotional impact upon him, leading to a growing deterioration of his neural functioning – symptoms that are emblematic of secondary BI. Developing this line of investigation, this chapter will continue to explore exterior narratives of coma survival and the representation of permanent BI, examining patterns of language and imagery used to depict post-coma identity and long-term neurological conditions.

4.1 Authenticity, plasticity

Tom McCarthy's novel *Remainder* portrays an unnamed narrator's recovery from coma and his difficulties of coping with a TBI that was caused by 'something falling from the sky'. The accident has left, 'A blank: a white slate, a black hole' (2010: 5), a physical and psychological consequence of the accident that is exacerbated by the fact that the Enactor, to use Zadie Smith's designation to refer to *Remainder*'s protagonist (2008), is not allowed to talk about the accident. This is a constrictive condition of the £8.5 million pay-out he receives from the shadowy organization that is indirectly responsible for his plight, and a caveat that seems strictly academic as, by the Enactor's own admission, he 'never had any memory of it in the first place' (8).

Since the accident, the Enactor no longer feels 'authentic' (a crisis of identity reflected in McCarthy's refusal to name him): his 'movements are all fake. Second-hand' (23). He comes to the gradual realization that he had 'always been inauthentic' (24) and, moreover, that everyone that inhabits the world around him are plagued with the same affliction, seeing them as 'self-conscious' and 'false' characters that put in 'amateur performances' (27). This concept of authenticity of selfhood is highly complex and exemplified by Freud's identification of the 'split-subject'. Freud's denomination of the id, ego and super-ego called into question exactly which one of these multiple, competing 'selves' residing within the subject was the truly 'authentic' self. As Charles Guignon posits in his extensive work on selfhood and authenticity, the discovery of the 'heart of darkness' that the id represents called into question the 'placid assurance that human beings are fundamentally good at heart, their natures having been distorted only by socialization' (2008: 280). Freud saw the id as the truly authentic self, its dark desires only tempered by the ego and super-ego, concluding in *Civilization and Its Discontents* that, 'Human beings are not gentle creatures in need of love'. This primordial aggression is summed up, by Freud, in the Latin phrase: '*Homo homini lupus*' (2002: 48) – man is a wolf to man – and because of this propensity to enact violence, humans have developed the super-ego, an 'internalized sense of a moral authority that promises punishment for infractions of a moral code' (Guignon 2004: 102). This identification of a tripartite model of selfhood meant that if the id (the 'real' self) was controlled by the super-ego (a product of socialization and moral control) as well as the ego (an 'appendage that is added on to the id in the course of its development' (2004: 98)) then in psychoanalytical terms, authenticity of selfhood was constantly being compromised. As Guignon concludes, 'Seen from this angle, to be authentic is to openly express all the rage, raw sexuality and cruelty within you' (2004: 105).

We have seen how this concept of the 'split-subject' has been exploited in many works of interior coma fiction, with the protagonist often having to relocate his so-called 'authentic' self in order to emerge from coma: Roy in *Marabou Stork Nightmares*, for example, forced to accept his 'true' barbaric and id-like nature that he consistently tries to repress. But even before Freud came to prominence, the American psychologist William James proposed that a 'normal' individual may contain many selves, all operating on multiple levels and achieving different purposes according to the needs of the individual at any given moment. The subject, according to James, is constantly 'adopting different masks appropriate to different contexts' (1890: 294): father, husband, work colleague, friend, lover. If the individual is no longer an autonomous, cohesive and unitary 'soul', but an 'unfolding, centerless play of persons', as Guignon notes (2004: 113), it follows that there is also a 'decentring' of what it means to be authentic. Despite the fact that the individual constantly adopts different masks of subjectivity for different purposes, it does not necessarily mean that each one is inauthentic or that any particular one of them is the true 'authentic' self that is concealed by the other masks.

This postmodern 'play' of selves and of authenticity refutes the Platonic notion that the actor, in engaging with the identification and appropriation of different characters (or masks) jeopardizes the authenticity of his soul. This is a concept that Jean-Jacques Rousseau further developed through his own theories of authenticity and of his conception of the one 'true' self of a 'naturally occurring' individual 'that is preyed upon and entrapped by society' (Mansfield 2000: 18). In his seminal work, *Sincerity and Authenticity*, Lionel Trilling explicates Rousseau's position with regard to the performance of the actor: '[B]y engaging in impersonation at all the actor diminishes his own existence as a person' (1972: 64). While this is a rather arcane concept, it resonates with the Enactor's distaste for the inauthentic 'actors' he sees all around him in *Remainder*. Yet, it is precisely this fluidity of subjectivity and authenticity, the movement between different masks of identity, which resonates most with modern, neurobiological models of selfhood and which is represented in several works of coma literature, not least McCarthy's novel. Moreover, real-life cases of post-coma brain trauma, whereby the identity of the victim is changed inexorably, expose the huge problems inherent in Rousseau's entire concept of authenticity and his promotion of individualism. Michael Paul Mason, in his pathographies of BI and the impact upon identity and personhood, writes, 'A tap on the head, and anything can go wrong. Anything usually does go wrong [. . .] You may not know your name, or you may think you're someone different every hour. Everyone you know and will ever know could become a stranger, including the face in the mirror' (2008: 6–7). Brain injury, then, is an ontological crisis that causes a rupture in one's sense of self and authenticity, leading to 'a mass of mutually constraining dualities, a complex of contrary truths [. . .] forever in tension' (Ben Platts-Mills 2019: 91).

Thomas Docherty, in his discussion of Gilles Deleuze's theory of selfhood and authenticity, points towards the importance of the concept of 'becoming' which connects with current neurobiological concepts of a self that is constantly evolving according to changes in its environment. Docherty writes that, 'For Deleuze, [. . .] one is never in a state of being (a being that would allow me to give an account of 'my identity') but only becoming (in which 'I' never quite coincide with myself)'. This means that selfhood (and therefore the possibility of achieving authenticity) is always elusive; for Deleuze, Docherty observes, to be human is to be 'necessarily always in flux' (2012: 30), thereby reflecting the 'decentred subject' of postmodernity. But it also reflects the neurobiological model of the pre-conscious 'proto-self' (Damasio 2000: 153) proposed by the influential neuroscientist Antonio Damasio. This proto-self, Damasio writes, is 'a coherent *collection of neural patterns which map, moment by moment, the state of the physical structure of the organism in its many dimensions*' [original emphasis]. This unconscious process of mapping such neural patterns, or 'signals', occurs, according to Damasio's tests, across multiple regions in the brain and points towards a constant state of development 'in the process of regulating the state of the organism'. This biological pre-conscious functioning is a 'ceaselessly maintained first-order collection of neural patterns' (154) that sets in motion an entire chain of 'becoming' and flux within the ongoing construction of selfhood and identity. The proto-self is born out of the non-conscious neural signalling of the organism, which then allows the development of the 'core self' and 'core consciousness', which, in turn, gives rise to the possibility of an '*autobiographical self* which permits '*extended consciousness*'. At the end of this chain of 'becoming', '*conscience*' is finally reached (230). The subtlest unconscious shift or change in the proto-self has huge ramifications for the chain of becoming, affecting the organism's development of selfhood and, consequently, its sense of authenticity. As Catherine Malabou summarizes, 'From one end of the chain to another, Damasio explains, one must assume that the brain somehow recounts its own becoming, that it elaborates it in the form of an "account"' (2008: 58). Again, Malabou refers to this process of 'becoming'; selfhood forever based upon what it will be rather than what it is.

This sense of becoming and authenticity is thrown into extreme crisis, as in the Enactor's case, when the brain suffers a severe injury: when a huge rupture in the conception of one's identity occurs. As Mason explicates,

> The survivor's life emerges as an ongoing pull between the changes that occur within an altered brain and the outward repercussions that follow. It is this tension between being and becoming that begs the intimate, soulful questions posed by every BI. What are we other than our brains? Is there a part of me that can't be changed by brain injury? (11)

Tom McCarthy explores such a crisis of identity and authenticity par excellence: the decentring of an already decentred subject – the postmodern man. Ultimately, for McCarthy, 'becoming' seems to depend upon one's understanding of who one once was and so he examines the struggle to regain authenticity when the anchor-points of a previous identity are detached by coma and TBI.

This central conceit of a 'shattered' post-BI identity (to use Luria's descriptor of his patient, Zasetsky's, condition) is explored across numerous works of fiction, to greater or lesser degrees of accuracy. We have already seen King's metaphorically rendered depiction of BI in *The Dead Zone*, whereas novels like *Marabou Stork Nightmares*, *The Bridge* and *The Coma* do not seem to entertain the possibility of permanent injury at all. And while Carl, in Nicholas Royle's *Regicide*, seems to come back from coma lasting 'more than two months' (184) with no obvious signs of permanent injury, he mentions that his girlfriend Annie 'was happy to look after me until I felt myself again' (185), suggesting that Carl has come back from coma 'changed'. The vagueness of this timeline of recovery also suggests that a full recovery may not take place. Umberto Eco's *The Mysterious Flame of Queen Loana* similarly depicts the ontological crisis of BI. It follows antiquarian book-dealer Yambo who attempts to piece his life together following a massive stroke. The 'incident' (2006: 11), an equivalence of the 'accident' of McCarthy's Enactor, leads to him losing his 'episodic memory' (or, as his physician explains, the 'episodes of [his] life' (13)). Similar to novels discussed earlier, his initial coma is described in terms of obscure blanks, replacing the paradigmatic 'dark' or 'nothing' with a 'fog' (3) that erases memory and selfhood. But his emergence from coma is also described in terms of other common tropes of wider coma fiction: it is as if he 'had awoken from a long sleep' (3) and akin to a 'reawakening' (7). Like the plight of BI survivors outlined by Mason, Yambo sees his wife as a 'stranger' and at one point, he recollects, 'I saw myself in the mirror. At least I was fairly sure it was me' (9). His dislocation from his self and environment is profound, only retaining memories of his books and work through which he narrates his trauma, at times intertextually referencing pioneers of BI research such as Oliver Sacks and Anton Luria to allocate language to his own predicament. As Yambo reflects, 'I don't have feelings, I only have memorable sayings' (18). Again echoing Mason's observation of the crisis of being and becoming for the BI survivor, Yambo's wife says, 'You can't stretch towards the future because you've lost your past' (29), with Yambo describing himself as 'like a stuck record' (37).

Desperate to regain control of his life, Yambo returns to his childhood home, spending days searching through books, comics, magazines, vinyl records and old newspapers, an archive of memorabilia and personhood which, he hopes, will help him recover his past and episodic memory. This frenzied search seems to hinge on his pursuit of the face of his old flame, the name of which, Loana, is all the information Yambo retains. Stylistically, every time Yambo uncovers an artefact from the archive, Eco includes a visual facsimile: frames from *Phantom* and *Flash Gordon* comics; plates from history books; illustrations from adverts or magazines; screenshots from films, thereby simulating Yambo's act of recovery of memory. Early on in his search for his lost self, Yambo makes an ominous declaration: 'Not only am I amnesiac, but I may be living out fictitious memories' (63) and this deep concern is played out in the latter half of the novel when he realizes that the object of his romantic pursuit, the memory he feels sure will unlock his entire past self lost to BI, is actually the name of a Tim Tyler comic: 'The Mysterious Flame of Queen Loana'. The story itself turns out to be 'the most insipid tale ever conceived by the human brain [. . .] a ramshackle story' (251). In the end, he concludes, 'What seemed to have fertilized my slumbering memory was not the story itself, but the title' which had 'bewitched' him (253), instigating the detachment of a signifier and its reattachment to a different signified of the lost love of his past. In this, Yambo finds himself trapped by his own confabulations, common to BI survivors, often owing to the amnesic condition.

Such an ontological crisis of BI, a rupture between past and present selves, is similarly depicted in Roy Hutchinson's *Head/Case*, a stage play based upon the lived experience of BI survivors. At the play's heart are two survivors, Tracy and Julia, who both experience a crisis of identity. Hutchinson portrays the range of traumatic behaviours each character exhibits, from the compulsive, repetitive actions of Tracy who sits on a chair before immediately springing to her feet over and over again (21), a repetition compulsion born out of injury; to Julia's emotional 'flattening', speaking with an uninflected voice. Julia speaks of a certain separation of selves after her car accident, narrating her trauma in third person and seeing the accident as happening to someone else 'other' than her, a rupture in pre- and post-BI identity, creating two senses of self (31). Tracy, too, speaks of this fracturing of self, reflecting, 'I've had a bit taken away from me, you see, I'm never going to get back' (34). In this, she acknowledges the permanence of BI and traumatic dislocation of personhood, echoing again Platts-Mills's concept of the 'mass of mutually constraining dualities'.

Craig Clevenger, in his hallucinogenic novel *Dermaphoria*, approaches this ontological crisis of BI from a unique perspective, depicting a protagonist, Eric Ashworth, emerging from coma with amnesia after he is caught in an explosion which he may or may not have caused at a drugs laboratory. A chemist for a Los Angeles drugs cartel and awaiting trial, Eric ingests his own hallucinogen in order to try and retrieve memories that were lost within the 'eight-second black hole' in which he technically died (2007: 207). Significantly, Eric muses, 'Everything prior to this second is a blank' (207), once more conjuring the coma-as-void image. The dizzying and surreal language and imagery of Eric's condition blurs the boundary between reality and hallucination but also between the borders of memory itself. As Eric seemingly begins to recover memory traces through more and more drug use, seemingly depicting the 'soap opera' model of BI recovery, the memories themselves become increasingly questionable and suspicious. At one point, his employer, Manhattan White, desperate for Eric to remember the formula to his most potent hallucinogen, comments, 'It sounds as though your memory's returned [...] You got hit on the head but you're all better now' to which Eric replies, 'I was not hit on the head. I overdosed. I was brain dead for eight seconds' (184). Here, Clevenger subtly yet knowingly rejects and subverts the soap opera model of BI recovery – the metaphorical second blow to the head which allows for a return to a pre-amnesic, former self. In the end, there is no such miracle recovery for Eric, discovering that all of the 'memories' the drug has unearthed are in fact fabrications – confabulations (a commonality among BI survivors, as I will explore) that serve to fill the blank void of memory that is so terrifying for him, in much the same way the void of Peter Redgrove's coma has to be filled by archetypal narratives of descent and resurrection.

But such a duality is not always depicted as inherently traumatic in coma and BI fiction. In Abby Kohn and Marc Silverstein's 2018 romcom *I Feel Pretty*, Amy Schumer's Renee, struggling with low self-esteem, hits her head while in an exercise class, after which she suddenly begins to perceive herself as magically changed, thrilled by her 'new' body shape in a depiction of reverse body dysmorphia syndrome (RBDS). This instils in her the confidence that sees her begin to carve out a highly successful career and personal life. Unlike other magical realist films of physical transformation, *Big* or *Vice Versa*, for example, the 'miracle' arises out of BI, not from a spell or wish. At one point, Renee's new-found partner, Ethan, comments, 'You are so yourself – you know who you are!', a comedic reading of what is actually a crisis of identity and dislocation of selfhood. It is inevitable that this 'spell' must be broken, and not surprising that this break in the illusion must occur through an inversion of the spell itself – a second brain 'injury' when Renee walks into a glass partition; the 'soap opera' model of BI recovery, mentioned at the start of this investigation. Renee 'returns' to herself and all of the past insecurities this includes, until she realizes that the confident behaviour she exhibited while living with her BI came from the same person she has always been. The BI which is eventually erased informs Renee of how she should now behave as her future self, a depiction that conflicts with the lived experience of BI whereby a reclamation of the lost self is often impossible.

The Enactor's emergence from coma acts as an immediate reminder of his struggle to feel 'authentic'. His 'no-space' of coma (another variant of the darkness motif) gradually becomes his 'no-past' of post-coma cognitive confusion, sitting in bed but failing to remember anything about himself. He then metaphorically describes the eventual recovery of 'memories' with the majority of his past returning 'in instalments, like back episodes of some mundane soap opera' (6). This depicts a sense of detachment from his own memories as he stands as isolated witness to the gradual piecing together of a fragmented self: identity re-edited. McCarthy later extends this metaphor. Caught in a slapstick repetition of journeys between a phone-box and his London flat (due to the fact that he keeps forgetting items that he needs to remember in order to break this cycle), the Enactor reaches a heightened state of self-awareness. Caught in a pattern of stuttering movement, turning towards his flat a couple of steps, then turning back, he realizes that two men are staring at him from across the street, seeing him 'jerking back and forth like paused video images do on low-quality machines' (15), an image that resonates with Yambo's description of himself as a stuck record. By his own admission, this eventually becomes a 'performance' that allows his movements to 'come across as more authentic' (15). He becomes an actor in his own 'video images'. The importance he places upon authenticity seems based upon his desire for others to see him as being 'authentic' and 'real', leading to a double-bind: 'performing' authenticity so that others can see him as being authentic yet this very process of performance exacerbates his feeling of being inauthentic.

Throughout the novel, McCarthy renders his protagonist's crisis of authenticity using the metaphor of technology, as seen when the Enactor, making an over-enthusiastic grab for his landline telephone while being told of his 'pay-out', yanks it out of the wall socket, referring to how the 'connection had been cut'. He stands 'holding the dead receiver', staring at the hole in the wall that 'looked kind of disgusting, like something come out of something' (9).This mishap serves immediately as a metaphor for the Enactor's plight: the connection has been cut between his pre-coma and post-coma selves. It is an image similarly and repeatedly arising in Nicholas Royle's *Regicide*: a phone line to the world outside of coma, but one with a 'connection that had been severed' (2011: 131). The Enactor's emotionally neutral behaviour reflects a common symptom of BI and long-term neurological conditions; what Moyra Williams refers to as a 'flattened' emotional condition whereby mood 'fails to move at all' (1979: 26), similar to Hutchinson's character of Julia in *Head/Case*. Trevor Powell explains how such 'emotional blunting or flattening' can be attributed to damage to the 'neural pathways' that link the Limbic System (which includes the amygdala and which is a 'primitive emotional centre' at the heart of the brain) and the Frontal Cortex, responsible for 'rational thinking' (Powell 1994: 117–18). Mark Sherry, too, draws attention to the personality changes associated with BI as identified by Ownsworth and Oei, highlighting the potential for 'apathy' and 'loss of ability to show empathy' which as Gratton and Eslinger highlight 'may also reflect compromises in cognitive flexibility' (2006: 35, 37). As the Enactor states prior to this incident with the phone socket, 'I didn't feel like doing anything. I wasn't doing anything' (7), reflecting Rose and Johnson's discussion of 'psychological problems' (1996: 119) with BI, again acknowledging the blurred line that can appear between functional and organic diagnoses. As they further point out, apathy and tiredness, again key indicators of long-term neurological conditions post-BI, can lead to the survivor 'no longer hav[ing] the imagination or initiative to explore alternatives to leisure activities that they enjoyed pre-injury' (55). The Enactor embodies the 'dead receiver', taking in external signals and impulses, but neither knowing what to do with them or, most importantly, not really caring what he does with them: a functional failure of his non-conscious neural signalling, to return to Damasio. Even the 'settlement' fails to arouse him; he is more concerned with the irksome half-a-million (the point-five decimal 'remainder', which the Enactor describes as a 'messy . . . shard of detritus' (9)) that corrupts the perfection of the circuitous whole integer of the 'eight'. In the same way that he is disgusted by the mess that his broken phone leaves, he is similarly disgusted by the person he is 'becoming'. The Enactor is the 'something' that has come out of 'something', the repetition of this abstract pronoun not only a subtle allusion to his post-TBI aphasia but also to the neutral incomprehension of both who he once was and who he is now and is to come. Malabou notes that, 'Coolness, neutrality, absence and the state of being emotionally "flat"' indicate wounds of the brain that 'have the power to cause a metamorphosis which destroys individual history' and which 'cannot be reintegrated into the normal course of life' (2012: 53). Omer Fast, in his film adaptation of the novel (2015), represents this emotional blunting and destruction of a previous self through the visual language of mise en scène, using a palette of desaturated colours of cool blues, greys and browns, the landscape populated by large, minimalist, glass-fronted buildings to represent a sense of clinical alienation. Populating these buildings are impassive, inscrutable inhabitants, the most inscrutable of all being Tom Sturridge's Enactor who speaks in a measured, dispassionate monotone, only ever moving beyond the emotional coolness of his damaged brain when, battling against his aphasia, he reaches for, and attains, an elusive word that perfectly embodies what he is struggling to describe.

In her overview of BI recovery and the brain's resistance to injury, Malabou examines further this instant metamorphosis of selfhood through the brain wound by explicating the neurological concept of brain plasticity, that is, 'A form's ability to be deformed without dissolving and thereby to persist throughout its various mutations'. It is precisely this 'strange sculptural power' of lesional plasticity, Malabou argues that 'produces form through the annihilation of form' (2012: 58). This dichotomy of creation through destruction is sharply observed by McCarthy, and consistently explicates the crisis of authenticity. The Enactor's re-formed self has been born out of his 'remoulded' brain; while it is still made out of the same *material*, it has now metaphorically taken a new 'shape'. The very notion of plasticity suggests that the brain is malleable, resistant, yet by its very definition it can never fully return to its original form because of the permanent damage that has been caused. This being said, in the Enactor's case, some of his memories alongside his 'biographical self' have returned but to a newly formed 'brain' or 'shell'. In this regard, lesional plasticity creates two senses of self shaped from the same material yet conflicting through their difference in form. From a neuropsychological perspective, Gronwall, Wrightson and Waddell observe that, 'The majority of the improvement which is seen after a head injury is due to reorganization of the brain which is undamaged [. . .]. Functional areas take over from the areas which are no longer functional' (1990: 16). As Powell further explicates, 'In effect new pathways are being created and opened up' (37), a process also alluded to by the Enactor when describing his 'memories' of the accident and subsequent time in hospital: 'Who's to say my traumatized mind didn't just make them up, or pull them out of somewhere else, some other slot, and stick them there to plug the gap?' (5), a notion that echoes Yambo's distorted and invented memories.

The neuroscientist David Eagleman further explicates this concept of neural plasticity and its implications for authenticity of selfhood, observing that, 'We're not fixed. From cradle to grave, we are works in progress'. (2016: 36). Referring to a study by University College London that scanned and examined the brains of London black cab drivers, Eagelman notes how in the drivers, the posterior area of the hippocampus (crucial for spatial awareness) had grown physically larger than those in the control group (19). The Knowledge that all black cab drivers have to acquire if they wish to attain a license to operate in London, has a physical, ongoing impact upon the brain. But Eagleman points towards a further confusion with regard to authenticity of identity, observing that physically, we constantly become a new person ('Within about seven years', Eagleman writes, 'Every atom in your body will be replaced by other atoms'), so in the end, we tend to think of memory as being the real seat of identity and authenticity. But this in itself is complicated as memory is 'a reconstruction, and sometimes it can border on mythology'. This is no surprise, as Eagleman points out, due to the fact that there are a 'finite number of neurons, and they are all required to multitask' and so neurons become 'co-opted in other memory networks'. Eagleman concludes, 'The enemy of memory isn't time; it's other memories' (22–5). As the mysterious Jack observes in Clevenger's *Dermaphoria*, '[E]veryone forgets how seldom our memory is accurate. Having more memory is just a way of distorting a greater amount of the past' (193).

This notion of post-coma/TBI plasticity and the crisis of authenticity, memory and identity is examined in close detail by McCarthy in one particular sequence of the novel that describes the Enactor's physical rehabilitation. In a passage that echoes Gronwall, Wrightson and Waddell's discussion of the reorganization of functional/non-functional areas of the brain, the Enactor speaks of his physiotherapist who had to 'route the circuit that transmits commands to limbs and muscles through another patch of brain – an unused, fallow patch' (19). McCarthy paints a picture of 'becoming' a future self that is both physically and mentally frustrating; that is forced to compartmentalize every subtle manoeuvre involved in an individual movement. He describes the 'seventy-five manoeuvres involved in taking a single step forward' (21), each of which the Enactor has to learn in order to 're-route' his damaged brain, a painstaking process that seems to be inherent in the growing fissure between mind/body unity. The Enactor observes that this process of 'learning' how to walk is itself inauthentic: 'In the normal run of things you never *learn* to walk like you learn swimming, French or tennis [. . .] you stumble into it, literally' (21), leading him to the devastating conclusion that, 'My movements are all fake. Second-hand' (23). Omer Fast's film adaptation pays meticulous attention to these physical effects of BI, Sturridge's Enactor initially walking with a crutch and thereafter stumbling or tripping, often banging his head in attempts to lift himself off the floor, representing the potential for secondary BI. There are shots of the Enactor holding a pen, awkwardly gripped between middle and ring finger, the camera particularly focusing on this as he signs the non-disclosure agreement that releases his settlement – a vivid close-up of his 'second-hand' movements, born out of his accident.

The whole question of authenticity becomes even more complex when the Enactor begins to see the authentic in the inherently fake – when he takes a trip to the cinema with his friend, Greg. Watching a screening of Scorsese's *Mean Streets*, the Enactor is struck by just 'how perfect De Niro' is, seemingly executing each action perfectly. He is, as far as the Enactor is concerned, 'perfect, seamless' [. . .] He's natural when he does things. Not artificial, like me"' (23). It is ironic that the Enactor sees authenticity and spontaneity in cinematic performance and, in particular, in an actor who is famous for his meticulous adherence to 'the method', that painstaking process of making a performance seem real and 'authentic'. But McCarthy's role as postmodern novelist is also at work, drawing on Jean Baudrillard's concepts of the 'more real than real' (1997: 30) and cinema becoming 'more cinema than cinema'. In *The Evil Demon of Images*,

Baudrillard refers to certain exponents of the American new-wave of the 1970s, and the obsessive preoccupations to capture the 'real' that are all 'a little too good, better adjusted, better than the others'. In being charmed by the 'more real than real' of *Mean Streets* and De Niro's performance (themselves arising out of the realist movement of the New-Wave), the Enactor is duped by cinema's 'ever-increasing perfection, absolute reality' (Baudrillard 1997: 33). It is this illusion of the real that heightens the Enactor's sense of inauthenticity all the more, despite the fact that De Niro's 'authenticity' is clearly rehearsed. Ultimately, for the Enactor, anything he does now in his pursuit of becoming a new self will be forever superimposed over the trace of a former self he had become prior to coma.

4.2 Self, coma, the trace

The turning point for the Enactor comes when, at Greg's behest, he attends a party. Meeting the Enactor at the door of his flat, the party's host exclaims, '"Oh! Hello! [...] I heard you were ... you know, better"'. As he utters this somewhat normalizing greeting, the Enactor observes that, 'His eyes were scanning my forehead above my eyes; Greg must have told him about the plastic surgery on the scar' (57). Earlier, when the Enactor meets his friend, Catherine, at the airport, the first thing she says is, '"You don't look like – oh yes, you've got a scar right there"' (28). The plastic surgery represents the attempt, on behalf of medical staff, to conceal the rem(a)inder of the accident, yet the 'trace' of it both remains and reminds. This trace signifies both who the Enactor once was and who he is not now. In terms of Derridean deconstructive analysis, the scar represents the 'absent-presence' of the trace of the accident and of the Enactor's pre-coma self. Collins and Mayblin, in discussing Derrida's concept of the trace, refer to the figure of the zombie in culture as being a paradigm of undecidability conveying the ultimate play between absence and presence. The zombie occupies the uncertain space between the living and the dead and may be 'either' alive 'or' dead. However, it is 'neither' alive 'nor' dead since neither of these existential states fully describes the state of the zombie. Therefore the zombie is *both* alive *and* dead. Cutting across these categories of existence, the zombie is a paradigm of undecidability: 'Cinematic inscriptions of the failure of the "life/death" opposition ... [marking] the limits of order' (Collins and Mayblin 2012: 21). Coma constitutes a real-life paradigm of this Derridean and existential undecidability, the victim neither dead nor fully alive: an absent-presence of who he once was (interestingly, Adrian Owen uses the description of 'zombies' in describing vegetative patients he has worked with (2017: 3)). Malabou's definition of post-lesional plasticity can likewise be seen in light of Derrida's philosophical notion of undecidability: a phenomenon that is *both* destructive *and* creative that leads to a person, like the Enactor, who is the same-but-different.

Damasio, writing on the survivors of BI, makes a particularly pertinent observation in regard to this 'same-but-different' concept: 'The distinction of the patients with damage to the retromedial sector of the frontal lobe is that their problems seem confined to their strange social behaviour. For all intents and purposes, they "look the same"' (2003: 143). This misconception is illustrated by McCarthy through both Catherine and the party-host's very real need to look for the difference in the Enactor, and their sense of disappointment at not finding the difference. Malabou similarly examines the persistence of the trace in BI survivors, asking: 'How can one deny, even in cases of very serious damage, that something like a psychic structure or profile remains intact? [. . .] Even if a subject no longer recognises us, don't we always recognise him within his very metamorphosis?' (2012: 68). From this standpoint, the absent-presence of the BI survivor may manifest itself in the perceptions and the remembrances of who he once was, archived within the minds of his loved ones. Because of their need for him to 'return' to himself, and their insistence on him not being 'changed' in any way, the survivor both 'lives on' as his 'old' self, while having to become his new. Looking across case studies of BI survivors who seem to demonstrate traces of their pre-injury selves, Malabou insists that, 'Something remains [. . .] that resists the ordeal of trauma', going on to ask, 'And doesn't this prove that, regardless of the apparent metamorphosis, the victim of brain damage or trauma has not entirely become someone else?' (2012: 69–70). To Malabou, this 'trace' is a presence of who this person once was. However, the presence of this trace can be questioned from a Derridean perspective that would see this trace not as a full presence, but rather as, 'The simulation of a presence that dislocates, displaces, and refers beyond itself' (1973: 156). The 'original' self has been lost through BI so all attempts to reassimilate such a trace will only lead to further dislocation and fracturing of the subject – a reminder that one can no longer be who one once was.

The shadow of the trace affects the Enactor acutely. As he proposes, on multiple occasions, 'Everything must leave some kind of mark' (11). Like Freud's reference to the 'mystic writing pad' (2008), a child's toy that was rather like the modern Etch-A-Sketch (and an analogy that Derrida, himself, refers to), despite the fact that one element is seemingly wiped off the plastic cover sheet of the pad to make way for a new inscription, there will always remain the indelible print in the wax layer of the toy below the sheet. There will always be the trace of the Enactor's pre-coma self, lying beneath his future 'inscriptions' of post-coma selfhood. In his navigation between theories of selfhood and Derridean deconstruction, Edward E. Sampson insightfully argues, 'The trace, which is absent from consciousness, forms the basis of consciousness itself' (1989: 11). This is a conception of selfhood that reflects Derrida's postulation that, 'There are only, everywhere, differences and traces of traces' (1981: 26). For the Enactor, though, while he is aware of these traces of his pre-coma self, through coma and BI, they are fragmented and inherently alienating, creating a schism in his chain of becoming and leading to his crisis of authenticity which denies the possibility of a future self.

It is at the party when he is offered the lifeline, he thinks, that will allow him to once more feel 'whole' and 'real'. Wandering restlessly through the flat, he realizes he is following a circuit that has 'the pattern of an eight' (11). Since the accident, the Enactor sees patterns and circuits in everything, akin to Carl in *Regicide* who is obsessed with his map, figure-skating and the grooves in records. Patterns provide comfort for the Enactor as they represent unbroken systems and feedback loops, authentic totalities that temporarily distract him from confronting his own fractured selfhood. The Enactor's obsession with closed circuits also reflects his traumatic compulsion to repeat and his inability to come to terms with the traumatic event that was erased even as it happened. McCarthy, in a 2008 interview, himself draws attention to his representation of the erasure of the traumatic event and the gap that 'demands to be substituted or supplemented', leading to a 'kind of stuttering, repeating, looping logic' (2008: 2). However, despite the Enactor's security in his figure-of-8 movement at the party (a 'perfect' 8 as opposed to the settlement that includes the 'messy' (9) point-five-million remainder), it is within another 'remainder' that he finds something like true security: an 'extra room' that 'seemed to have just popped up [. . .] like the half had in my settlement: off-set, an extra' – a remainder. This room is a bathroom, and inside it the Enactor has 'a sudden sense of déjà-vu' (60). He sees a crack in the wall beside the mirror and bathtub, images that he remembers seeing before, but it is the crack that seems to be most vivid, most 'crystal-clear, as clear as in a vision' (61). This begins to evoke other traces, an entire signifying chain: his room in a flat; a building opposite with red roofs, black cats lounging on them; the smell of liver cooking in the flat below, the 'spit and sizzle' loud in his ears; a pianist rehearsing; an old woman taking rubbish out of her flat, saying something to him as he passes her, him saying something back; iron banisters; a patterned, tiled hallway; marble floors. He 're-remembers' every little detail or more precisely (and by his own admission) he *mis*-remembers these details as he later admits: 'I don't think this was a straight memory. It was more complex. Maybe it was various things all rolled together: memories, imaginings, films' (76). Similarly, in Bigley's *Comaville*, the geography of Josh Husk's coma-dream (his collage of memory) is not just built from the real-life places he has seen and inhabited throughout his life but also 'from television, and from imagination' (2019: 6). This echoes Eagleman's assertion that memory is a 'fragile brain state', leading to identity and authenticity encapsulating a 'strange, ongoing, mutable narrative' (2016: 23, 29), a phenomenon depicted in Eco's novel also. Omer Fast visualizes this notion of the amalgam of recollection in the moment the Enactor has his first full flashback to the building. The inhabitants he 'remembers' appear at first to be clothed in 1950s fashion, yet a little boy sporting a 1970s tracksuit also haunts the 'memory'. The interiors, too, seem to exhibit the design tastes of the middle of the last century, yet the Enactor interprets the look of the building as being much later – the 1980s, around the time when he would have been born and been inside this building – if the building ever existed at all. Fast's visual language of the mutable memory echoes Eagleman's discussions of the human capacity for confabulation, again like Eco's Yambo – inventing or embellishing memories, alongside the brain's willingness to adopt false memories or the memories of others (2016: 25–6).

Armin Schnider and his team examined how the mechanism of both spontaneous and provoked confabulation commonly occurs within the brain-injured patient and especially those suffering from amnesia. Referring, in particular, to one research patient who suffered a TBI in a motorcycle accident, they observed how, 'He would tell true stories . . . and entirely invented stories', occasionally acting 'according to his confabulations' (1996: 1368). They concluded that for this confabulator, 'This disturbance leads to recollection of elements of memory that do not belong together, hence the production of false memories' (1373). For McCarthy's Enactor, though, regardless of this possibility of him faking this memory, he realizes that in this other place all of his 'movements had been fluent and unforced. Not awkward, acquired, second-hand but . . . seamless, perfect. They'd been *real*'. He also asserts, 'I'd been real – *been* without first understanding how to try to be' (73). The Schnider study further clarifies, 'Because spontaneous confabulations reflect a confusion of memory traces from diverse events rather than a lack of traces, they are not associated with a feeling of deficient memory' (1373). And so it is for the Enactor, taking this memory trace that feels real and which makes his whole sense of selfhood feel authentic. In the end, he decides to use his settlement money to 're-enact' this memory trace by recreating it as a fully-operational, 1:1 scale *Wunderkammer* (literally a 'wonder chamber' where curiosities and rarities are exhibited), despite the fact that this may lead to the ultimate paradigm of an absence: false memories. McCarthy's image of the crack is particularly germane to the Enactor's re-ownership of the trace: it is, itself, an absent-presence, a trace of what used to be there with the plaster falling away and the paint around the aperture chipping and flaking. The crack is only understandable through its difference from the whole and the crack becomes a counterpoint to the Enactor's scar. The plastic surgery is an attempt to conceal the rem(a)inder of the accident and who the Enactor has become. But the trace still remains, reminding him that he is no longer who he once was: the same-but-different. By re-creating a memory trace around a crack, a gap, he embraces this schism in selfhood and accepts the need to reassimilate these fragmented absent-presences, these remainders of a previous iteration of selfhood, if he is to feel 'whole' again.

4.3 Trauma, simulation, assimilation

Jean Baudrillard's seminal essay 'The Precession of Simulacra' opens with a reference to Jorge Luis Borges's short story, 'On Exactitude in Science', that 'finest allegory of simulation'. In it, Baudrillard explains, the cartographers of the Empire create a map that is so meticulously detailed that it 'ends up covering the territory'. Now, Baudrillard argues, 'The territory no longer precedes the map, nor survives it', with 'the real' disappearing in a precession of simulations, thus 'substituting signs of the real for the real itself' (1983a: 1–2). For Baudrillard, signs have become fractured, with an almost viral production of 'floating signifiers' infecting the world; signifiers that have broken away from their corresponding signifieds, thus no longer corresponding to any objective 'reality'. Within this system, reality quickly disappears and becomes a simulation or, more accurately, becomes a simulation of a simulation: a copy of a copy. This is what Baudrillard refers to as the breakdown of the reference principle of images: the basic reality that the sign represents and then distorts is already a simulation in itself, thus it has become impossible to 'recognize' reality as it now no longer exists. As Madan Sarup explicates, for Baudrillard, society now functions within a postmodern world 'in which all we have are *simulations*, there being no 'real' external to them, no 'original' that is being copied' (1993: 144). Tony Thwaites, in his discussion of Baudrillard's 'four stages' of simulation, refers to the fourth stage (in which the sign has no relation to any corresponding reality and has become 'its own pure simulacrum' (1983a: 4)) as 'an involution that swallows its own tail' (2000: 273), a comment that refers to the ancient symbol of the Ouroboros (Figure 4.1).

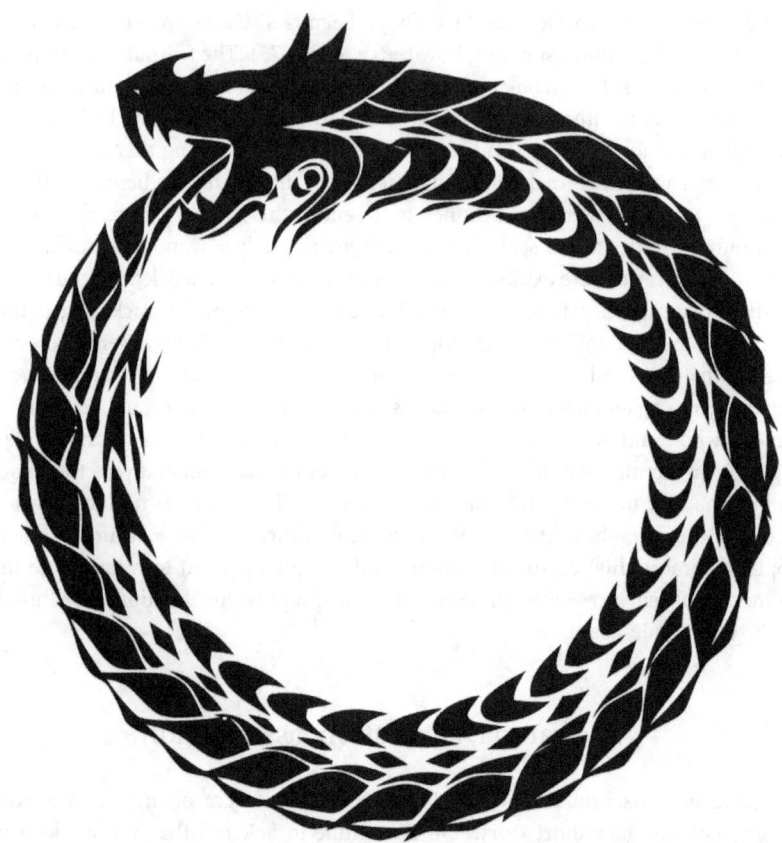

Figure 4.1 Image of the ancient symbol of the Ouroboros.

Such a system of production, re-production and simulation (and therefore a loss of the real) is clear to see in *Remainder*, with the Enactor embarking upon a mission to re-create the building (and its inhabitants) 'awoken' in his unconscious. By the Enactor's own admission, his recreation, like Yambo's Queen Loana, is not necessarily based upon an objective reality, a 'straight memory'. Instead, it is based upon a *bricolage* of fragmented images and senses that may have come from many different sources that have been re-edited. In this regard, the Enactor's simulation has no reference principle: it is the copy without an original, not a 'mirror of being and appearances, of the real and its concept' (Baudrillard 1983a: 3). However, for the Enactor, it is of no concern to him that his simulacrum (and simulacra within his building) represents reality, thereby inadvertently privileging 'a real without origin or reality: a hyperreal' (Baudrillard 1983a: 2). All that matters to him is his memory of being in this place and feeling real – itself a simulacrum of who he once was and once felt. As soon as the Enactor leaves the party, he embarks upon a frenzied attempt to capture what was 'recovered' from his 'memory', manically sketching 'diagrams, plans, layouts of rooms and floors and corridors' on every spare piece of paper he can find, sometimes running images over onto 'three or four or five' sheets to create 'a big block' (68). This description of frenetic sketching and commitment to paper of memories, while not reaching the extremity of Borges's cartographers, resonate with the image of the expanding map: the cartographic exercise out-of-control. In his critique of modern society, Baudrillard points towards the 'hysteria of production and reproduction of the real' in order for society to restore 'the real which escapes it' (1983a: 44). In trying to simulate a non-existent real, the Enactor becomes caught up within such a postmodern hysteria, a frenzy of production and re-production in order to recapture the elusive lost real.

This hysterical obsession with reproducing and simulating the lost real on behalf of the amnesic, brain-injured patient is similarly represented in Jonathan Nolan's short story 'Memento Mori', later to be adapted by his brother, Christopher Nolan, into the feature film *Memento* (2000). Both story and film have at the heart of them a protagonist profoundly affected by anterograde amnesia (the inability to form new memories) stemming from a BI incurred while trying to prevent the brutal rape and murder of his wife. It is a crime that both protagonists are trying to solve despite their severe incapacity of memory. In Jonathan Nolan's short story, reproduction and simulation are represented in the repeated passages describing the daily routine of his protagonist, Earl, waking up in the same room, opening 'one eye after another to a stretch of white ceiling tiles' (2002: 85, 87). Like Tracy in Hutchinson's play, writing notes and notes on notes to remind her to perform everyday actions, Earl uses Post-Its to prompt his own course of action to keep him on-track: aides-memoires that help him to move forward with his life (and his investigation). But as Earl reflects in his internal monologue: 'You've only got about ten minutes, in fact. Then it starts all over again' (89), acknowledging that ultimately, he is forever trapped within a looping, inwards-turning pattern of behaviours, actions and thoughts that are forever reproduced. Earl makes a pertinent observation with regard to the process of 'becoming' when he muses, 'So the question is not "to be or not to be", because you aren't' (88). Taking Hamlet's fundamental philosophical question of becoming (Hamlet, himself, being that great procrastinator, trapped within the moment of *being*), Nolan deconstructs the proposition, his protagonist unable to 'become' because he isn't even 'being' who he once was, trapped in a stuttering feedback loop. As Earl observes, in the aftermath of seemingly achieving his revenge in the action of killing his wife's murderer, and in the face of the memory of it already fading, 'The only thing that matters is this moment. This moment a million times over' (96), evoking a similar internal logic to that of McCarthy's Enactor: finding selfhood and authenticity in repetition, reproduction, simulation.

Christopher Nolan's film adaptation exploits further the concepts of simulation within a feedback loop, not least in his inventive use of narrative structure. One plot strand moves backwards, with each scene not fully making sense until contextualized by the following scene (representing the dizzying confusion of his protagonist, Leonard's, anterograde amnesia); and one strand, the monochrome scenes, move forwards chronologically – with both strands meeting towards the end of the film, creating a perfect loop. Leonard prides himself on his 'system' that allows him to carry on with his life and his investigations. It is a system that is even more intricately conceived than his literary ancestor, Earl: post-its, again, but used in conjunction with polaroid photographs with notes written on them; clues placed strategically in pockets; tattoos; police files – a system designed to help him move beyond his BI by 'conditioning' other parts of his brain through rote behaviours. Early on in the film, Teddy, a policeman who apparently facilitates Leonard's investigation, aiding him in finding and killing his wife's murderer, says ominously, 'You don't even know who you are – what you've become'. This again is a key reference to brain plasticity and 'becoming' and one germane to our discussions. At once, Teddy reflects upon the fact that Leonard cannot *become* because he has no idea who he *is*; yet simultaneously, he implies that he *has* become someone else – but that he just can't remember this, trapped within the feedback loop of his inability to produce short-term memories. Becoming is therefore profoundly negated by his particular BI. The real ramifications of this are seen in Nolan's narrative twist when it is revealed, at the moment Leonard finally kills his wife's murderer, enigmatically known as 'John G', that he has already killed John G months before. This particular act of revenge was just the murder of a random criminal who happened to also be a 'John G' provided by Teddy. Teddy accuses Leonard of jeopardizing his own 'system': removing pages from the police file, redacting information, failing to tattoo himself when the initial act of revenge was achieved – even falsifying pre-BI memories of his wife, creating a constant enigma, a looping investigation, in order to give him a never-ending narrative of revenge. As Roger Luckhurst discusses, Leonard's 'subjectivity thus renders him frozen in the timeless time of the post-traumatic condition, where time seems arbitrary but is in fact undergirded by a repetition compulsion that he cannot know or master' (2008: 206), highlighting here another work of fiction which links brain injury to traumatic neurosis. In the end, angered by this confrontation and revelation, Leonard biases his system further by burning the polaroids of both of his revenge murders he has committed and jotting down Teddy's car registration number, making a note on the Polaroid that Teddy cannot be trusted. Teddy, himself, is another 'John G' (Teddy being a moniker his mother uses for him). In this, the Ouroboros of simulation is complete, the film effectively ending where it began: with the murder of Teddy – a simulation of a simulation of a simulation of revenge.

Sallie Baxendale, in analysing the representation of amnesia in feature films, notes that Nolan's representation of anterograde amnesia in *Memento* is a rare 'exception' to most films in 'accurately describ[ing] the problems faced' by such patients (2004: 1482). She particularly points towards Nolan's narrative structure in achieving this, the 'fragmented, almost mosaic quality to the sequence of scenes in the film [that] cleverly reflects the "perpetual present" nature of the syndrome' (1483). This 'perpetual present' constitutes this stuttering, looping condition of 'being' and the need to reproduce and simulate the lost real of the brain-injured patient, clearly also present in McCarthy's novel as well as Clevenger's *Dermaphoria*. To aid his own reproduction of the lost real, McCarthy's Enactor, like Christopher Nolan's Leonard, has his own 'facilitator' – Nazrul Vyas, or Naz, employing him to act on his behalf to help him realize his simulations. In the end, though, it is the Enactor himself who locates 'his building', the 'reality' of which is confirmed by the fact that it is close to a sports track, one very *similar* to hallucinations created within his lightening coma, the *realness* of this building, then, seeming to be a direct correlative to the unreality of his coma.

This paradox of the real in simulation appears throughout the novel, represented by the Enactor's continuing faith in the principle that reality and 'realness' lies within rehearsal. However, during discussions with Naz over the people the Enactor needs to populate his building (the old 'liver' lady; the pianist; a motorbike mechanic), he balks at the use of 'performer' to describe these people: "'Performers isn't the right word . . . Staff. Participants. Re-enactors'" (95). This notion of 're-enactment' again invokes the notion of simulation, and the simulation of simulations which, according to Baudrillard 'transforms the real into the hyperreal' (1983a: 50). This concept of hyperreality (in which all that is left of the world is a 'reality' that is made up of endless simulations) is sharply realized by the Enactor's simulations of the gaps and voids in his consciousness and in the pre-coma memory. Like Redgrove describing an intangible 'nothing' in terms of a tangible 'something' in his poem 'Lazarus and the Sea', the Enactor tries to embody the 'non-spaces' of his consciousness. When trying to 're-remember' the building, he had left blank spaces in his diagrams. In translating these absences into physical, architectural spaces, the Enactor creates what he calls 'neutral space' with 'doorways papered and cemented over, strips of wall left bare' (113), although these forgotten parts 'should be blank in reality', according to the Enactor (realized filmically by Omer Fast by objects and spaces wrapped in brown paper). The principle of this architectural approximation of the void is fully represented by the crack in the bathroom wall (the kernel of the whole building simulation based upon an absence) and also extends to some of the re-enactors within the building whose faces the Enactor cannot remember. These people (including the concierge of the building) wear blank hockey masks (body suits in Fast's film) and the Enactor makes a point of justifying this decision: 'Her face had never come back to me – or to be precise, it had come to me, but only as a blank – so I'd decided she should wear a mask to blank it out' (128). Here, again, is a total loss of the real, with a simulation of voids in consciousness that become more real than the objects and places and people to which they refer.

The Enactor's hunger to recapture the lost real does not just stop at simulating absences; he also assimilates and simulates memories that were never of his 'reality', as seen in his simulation of the building's courtyard: 'Swings were being installed that day. I hadn't seen swings in my original vision of the courtyard – but they'd grown there later, as I thought about it further' (115), once more resonating with the peculiar tendency towards embellishing even confabulated memories. In the installation of swings, the Enactor appropriates a childhood memory of his friend, Catherine, yet he does not acknowledge the source of his new 'memory', demonstrating that the image has become detached from its referent, and so by becoming part of the Enactor's so-called real memory, it no longer refers to his real. This process of assimilation and simulation is an attempt to create 'an uninterrupted circuit without reference or circumference' (Baudrillard 1983a: 11). In this, the image of the Ouroboros is once more evoked and it becomes increasingly significant that the Enactor is fascinated with the '8' of his £8 million settlement and with performing 'figure of 8' circuits. It is also the reason he is disgusted with the .5 'remainder' of the settlement. The figure of 8 is not only seen to be a perfect unbroken loop (a seamless form that the Enactor wishes to adopt with regard to his identity) but also, laid horizontally, it represents infinity (Figure 4.2) and is also identified, in modern mysticism, with a variation of the Ouroboros:

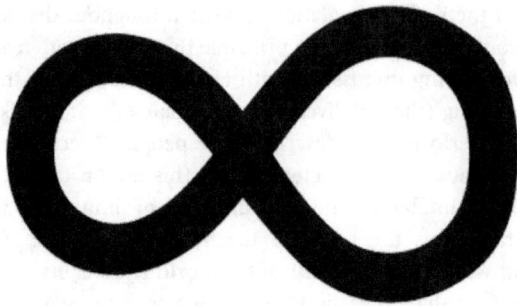

Figure 4.2 Image of the mathematical symbol for Infinity.

Yet the constant haunting of the 'remainder' of his pre-coma self (again represented metaphorically by the 'ugly' half-a-million pounds of his settlement) suggests that the Enactor's quest to feel real again is doomed from the very outset, and this fate becomes immediately apparent in the first re-enactment within his building.

The first suggestion of a problem comes when the building is initially put into 'on mode' and the cooking of liver downstairs begins. To the Enactor, the liver smells 'a bit like cordite' (131), while not really knowing what cordite is. It is the trace of a signifier that has become detached from its specific signified (the smell of a discharged gun) but re-attached, in the Enactor's mind, to the sensation of a non-specific unpleasant smell. But McCarthy also subtly references a common dysfunction arising from BI or neurological disorders: parosmia, or the inability of the brain to properly identify an odour's 'natural' smell, often replacing it for an unpleasant aroma – most commonly one of a burning, rotting or chemical nature. It is striking, too, that such an odour of 'cordite' occurred in some of the shell shock patients treated by Charles Myers during the First World War and written about in his research study for *The Lancet*, referring to the 'subjective sensation' of one patient who complained of 'the odour of cordite' (1915: 320). And in Royle's *Regicide*, Carl, too, has frequent olfactory disturbances, encountering the spectre of industrial odours: 'Railways or diesel oil. Engines' (35).

The Enactor's failure and dissatisfaction with simulation and repetition is manifested when, during the first re-enactment, he encounters one of the re-enactors: the old 'liver' lady who, as he passes, is tasked with placing a bag of rubbish outside her flat. The Enactor re-remembers the fact that she says something to him, although he cannot remember what. It is then decided that she should make something up on the spot, and this is precisely what she does do: 'Harder and harder to lift up', to which he immediately replies, 'Yes. Every time'. The words just 'come' to him in a moment of spontaneous confabulation and it is at this point when he feels a tingling and lightness in his body, granting his physical self the ability to 'glide fluently and effortlessly through the atmosphere around it' (135). It is the same feeling that he describes in the moments just before the disaster, as though all of his simulations (unbeknownst to him) are actually to try and re-create the moment before the disaster: the last time he felt real, inhabiting his lost, pre-coma self in a looping identity of being in order to screen out the trauma of becoming of the post-BI survivor. It is an attempt to recapture what Maurice Blanchot refers to as 'the disaster, unexperienced' (1995: 7). However, this sensation soon fades and he quickly has the desire to recapture this 'new' moment, once more halting the process of 'becoming' by simulating that already absent-presence of dialogue that occurred within the lost moment of the immediate past. The second re-enactment instils the same sensation; the third fails, the old lady re-enactor inadvertently introducing a different parabola through which she lifts the bag of rubbish and the bag itself leaving behind a 'sticky-looking patch on the floor' (147), yet another motif of detritus (of a remainder) that runs throughout the Enactor's life. McCarthy, in the writing of this first 're-enactment', presents a puzzling dichotomy once more: the Enactor wishes to recapture his lost 'real' through rehearsed production, re-production and simulation, yet he seems to get the greatest pleasure and sensation when the genuinely spontaneous occurs. As Daniel Lea cogently posits in his analysis of the anxieties of authenticity in *Remainder*, 'Such re-enactments are attempts to access the authentic through the profoundly inauthentic process of endless recreation, robbing the moment of its spontaneity through forensic aestheticization and examination' (2012: 467).

It is this pursuit of the impossible that leads to the growing dissatisfaction with all of his simulations, even his re-enactment of a gangland shooting in which he replaces the murdered man with himself. In this scenario, he slows down the re-enactments of the shooting to greater and greater degrees, in a desperate attempt to become at one with the event itself and which evokes the Freudian death-drive: the need and desire to return to the perfect state of inert matter once more. After all, as Malabou asserts, there is an inherent contradiction within this drive: its 'tendency towards restoration', leading the organic life back to the inanimate state, working in conjunction with the 'tendency toward destruction'. Significantly, Malabou notes, this characteristic dichotomy of the death-drive is the same that occurs within moments of destructive plasticity in brain trauma: a restoration of the brain (and selfhood) that occurs through destruction (2012: 71–2). The Enactor clearly exhibits this confusion, employing his technique of slowing action down throughout his building, resulting in his instructions to his extremely confused concierge to 'do nothing even slower' (207). In Fast's film adaptation, this is developed further, with his reenactors being set 'on pause' for hours at a time mid-action, another evocation of the death-drive and the pleasure gained from life, in effect, returning to inert matter. But despite the 'performance' of meticulous slow-motion (or, in the film, no-motion) re-enactments, he can never fully incorporate or assimilate the trace and can never be at one with the lost real. Thus, the Enactor's mania of simulation threatens to become over-saturated and implode, a consequence of which Baudrillard is all too aware. Douglas Kellner, in his critical appraisal of Baudrillard's theoretical positions, explains how this proliferation of simulation presents a '"cool" catastrophe for the exhausted subject, whose fascination with the play of objects turns to apathy, stupefaction, and an entropic inertia' (2009: 22). As his simulations increasingly begin to spiral out of control, the Enactor sinks into entropic fugue states, 'waking comas' (203) that, like his actual coma, begin to blur the boundaries between the 'real' and authentic and the 'fake' and inauthentic. The Enactor becomes addicted to the 'panic-stricken production of the real and the referential' (Baudrillard 1983a: 13) leading to periods of catatonic inertia: an implosion of simulacra. This frenzy comes to a head in the Enactor's final act of simulation, and one that constitutes McCarthy's most obvious reference to Baudrillardian theory: a re-enactment of a bank robbery.

One of Baudrillard's most notable claims in 'The Precession of Simulacra' is that if you were to stage a 'fake' hold-up within a bank, there would be nothing to separate this from the real as the signs of this simulated robbery would inevitably be the exact same signs of a real theft: 'The web of artificial signs will be inextricably mixed up with real elements'. Thus, by staging a fake bank robbery, 'You will unwittingly find yourself immediately in the real' (1983a: 39). Taking the image of the Ouroboros once more, the production, reproduction and simulation of reality has a profound affect and influence upon reality itself. As Mark Poster advances, for Baudrillard, 'The simulacrum is also real but of a different order from everyday life [. . .] the hyperreal' (2009: 81). For the Enactor, the re-enactment of a bank robbery seems the perfect way to feel real once more, the rules and patterns and signs inherent in a hijack promising the perfect opportunity for his skewed vision of 'rehearsed authenticity' and for him to re-invoke 'realness'. Hiring an ex-bank-robber-turned-author, Edward Samuels, the Enactor is charmed by his observation that all bank robberies have a 'preset pattern' (231). When asked by his consultant-thief if he wishes to re-enact a particular bank robbery, the Enactor says: 'No, not a particular one. A mix of several ones, real and imaginary. Ones that could happen, ones that have, and ones that might at some time in the future' (233). At once, this evokes Baudrillard's concept of the hyperreal while also communicating the Enactor's post-coma plight. Baudrillard's 'indefinite reproduction' (1983b: 112) of the bank robbery certainly seems to demonstrate what he famously describes in 'The Orders of Simulacra': 'The real is not only what can be reproduced, but *that which is always already reproduced*. The hyperreal' (146) [original emphasis].

The Enactor's crisis of identity and authenticity becomes clear when the Enactor, under the guidance of Naz and Samuels, hires re-enactors to simulate the robbery with the Enactor 'directing' each move, once more borrowing from the conventions of the film industry to rehearse realness and authenticity. At one point, Robber Five trips on a kink in the carpet, much to everyone's amusement. But the Enactor responds with, 'Do that each time' (238), a moment that is reminiscent of his improvised dialogue with the old 'liver' lady in his building. He even gets one of his facilitators to slip a piece of wood under the carpet, so that the kink does not smooth over. The Enactor, in his perception of an absence of 'fluency' in his own movement post-coma, finds great pleasure in the genuinely spontaneous and authentic 'real' events that occur; the original spontaneity of action that is then consumed by his obsession with simulacra. This 'hypersimulation' (38) leads to his most dangerous simulacrum yet, as he restages the simulation within an actual bank, but without informing the staff (or even his re-enactors). Accordingly, the Enactor, to return to Baudrillard's analogy of the simulated bank robbery, finds himself 'unwittingly' and 'immediately in the real, one of whose functions is precisely to devour every attempt at simulation, to reduce everything to some reality' (1983a: 39). This seems to be the perfect solution for the Enactor, to feel real again, allowing him to 'insert' himself 'back into the world' and return his 'motions' and 'gestures' to 'ground zero and hour zero, to the point at which the re-enactment' would finally merge 'with the event'. The simulation of the bank robbery, therefore, will allow him to inhabit, finally, the real and 'penetrate and live inside the core, be seamless, perfect, real' (244–5).

Initially, this 'echo of an echo of an echo' (259) seems to be going well, the Enactor gaining pleasure from the fact that the re-enactors are looking for 'some kind of boundary' between the simulation and the real, but as Baudrillard postulates, no such boundary exists in a simulated hold-up. The Enactor's pleasure comes from the fact that, 'There was no edge, that the re-enactment zone was non-existent, or that it was infinite, which amounted in this case to the same thing' (260), once more evoking the image of the Ouroboros, an infinite loop of 'being'. McCarthy calls upon Baudrillard's theory of the simulacra when the Enactor refers to the markings on the surface of the road outside of the bank, as the getaway car pulls up: '[They were] perfect reproductions of the ones outside my warehouse'. The Enactor views his simulacrum of the bank as being 'more real than real' (the hyperreal) with the 'real' road markings constituting 'copies' of his simulacrum, again placing under threat the very principle of reality. As the Enactor observes, when discussing the impact of the 'scripted' lines of dialogue that are now spoken by the re-enactors: 'Now, though, they were more than accurate: they were *true*' (261). The 'real' begins to 'devour' the simulations.

As the robbery commences, the Enactor begins to feel his (re)immersion into the real: 'I was right inside the pattern, merging, part of it as it changed and, duplicating itself yet again, here, now, transformed itself and started to become real' (264). In this frenzied moment of realization, he is finally becoming at one with the world, wiping out the trace of his former self alongside the memories of the 'false' and 'second-hand' processes of post-coma rehabilitation that caused him to feel inauthentic. However, it is another 'trace' that comes back to haunt the robbery, making it at once a 'fuck-up' and 'a very happy day' (260): the kink in the carpet. As Robber Re-enactor Five feels for the kink (the 'ghost-kink', an 'absent-presence' that haunts the 'real' of the bank), he applies the same force, the trip transformed into a full-blooded pratfall that causes him to collide into Re-enactor Two who, in turn, discharges his shotgun into Re-Enactor Four's chest, accidentally killing him. The Enactor, however, rather than being dismayed at such a 'disaster', revels in the confusion and gradual realization of the other re-enactors. He is finally able to experience and sustain the sensation of feeling 'real' and 'weightless' at the moment when one of the Re-Enactors exclaims: '"*It's real!*"' (270). The Enactor becomes caught within a trance-like, transfiguratory and hallucinogenic reverie, glorying in the spontaneous act of violence, in this confrontation with the real: with *death* and the death-drive. As he and his fellow Re-Enactors flee from the scene of the crime, he is serene in the face of their panic and horror at the fact that this 'had been real and not a re-enactment'. To this, he responds: 'But it was a re-enactment. That's the beauty of it. It became real while it was going on. Thanks to the ghost kink, mainly – the kink the other kink left when we took it away' (273). This, again, seems to be another direct nod to Baudrillard, this time to his own reflections upon 'The Remainder' when he writes: 'When everything is taken away, nothing is left. This is false. The equation of everything and nothing, the subtraction of the remainder, is totally false' (Baudrillard 1994: 143).

The concept of death and the real is also at play in McCarthy's denouement of the novel. In his discussion of Baudrillard's position on death and simulation, Ryan Bishop posits that, 'Death resists modelling, the simulation [. . .] Death is the event without compare and which must be elided at all costs' (2009: 65). For the Enactor, all sense of feeling authentic and real had been damaged by his accident and subsequent coma: his unwitting 'death encounter'. This encounter constitutes a 'failed' simulation of death.

Thus, McCarthy implies that his protagonist has been trapped by an 'incomplete' simulacrum – the simulacrum that, Baudrillard argues, resists modelling. Thus, from this point onwards, the Enactor cannot feel real because of the rift that this failed simulation has driven between his pre-coma and post-coma selves. It is significant, therefore, that the Enactor appears to feel real once more when he is witness to a 'complete', non-simulated death that occurs within a simulacrum of his own creation and that becomes real within the context of the real setting of the bank.

McCarthy makes subtle allusions to this realignment and re-assimilation of his pre- and post-coma selves (to the Enactor's 'merging' with the real) by implying that his pre-coma memory is coming back to him. Most significantly, as he takes his seat on his getaway jet, the Enactor reflects upon the other jet on which his re-enactors and staff of 'simulators' have been booked and which he and Naz have arranged to be blown up to eliminate more remainders of his simulacra. The Enactor wonders if 'their plane [has] already exploded', and muses: 'I wondered if it would be over sea or land. If it was land, perhaps a bit of debris might even fall on someone and leave me an heir' (281). At this point, the trace of the Enactor's accident (which he has always explained has been lost) is finally reawakened and brought back into consciousness. By the subtlest of suggestions, the death encounter in the bank has brought him back to the moment when he last felt real, just before a rogue fragment (maybe a 'remainder' that had broken away from a damaged aeroplane) fell from the sky.

4.4 The self, the trauma, the model

While McCarthy clearly adopts various strands of deconstructive and postmodern theory, he takes a rather playful approach in order to explore their manifestation in a real-world setting: the trauma that arises from coma and BI. This literary agenda seems clear, immediately, in his acknowledgements at the end of the novel, thanking two individuals in particular for 'generously sharing their experiences of (post-) trauma' with him (285). This interest is also supported in several interviews McCarthy has given, the author citing various cases of brain trauma and their aftermath as profound influences upon the novel. In an interview given for *The White Review*, McCarthy discusses the case of the cricket commentator Henry Blofeld, a promising young practitioner of the sport whose prospects were cut short when, as a teenager, he was knocked off his bike by a double-decker bus, causing him to slip into coma. After emerging from coma, he discovered that his hand-eye co-ordination had been lost. Blofeld, instead of playing the game, commented on it, 'Watching his own past-future that never happened' (2011: 11), reflecting the stuttering narrative logic of *Remainder*: the difficulty in becoming a future-self based upon a schismatic past-self. In another interview, McCarthy refers to the two individuals he thanks in the acknowledgements of the novel, while also referring to cases of 'traumatized [Vietnam] veterans' who, likewise, suffered with his protagonist's syndrome – of the constant feeling of 'nothing being real' (2008: 2). He goes on to discuss cases of such post-trauma victims who 'would also reconstruct events', for example one veteran who became a bank-robber, his crimes often recreating the layout of the battlefield on which he'd lost all of his friends. As McCarthy points out, he 'reconstructed and replayed the battle that he could not actually remember' (2008: 2). This is an obsession with recreation in an attempt to recapture and confront a lost event (or identity) of the past shared by the fictional Enactor of McCarthy's novel.

Remainder is an example of what Marco Roth terms the 'neuronovel', an exponent of a 'set of neurological novels in which the author inhabits a cognitively anomalous or abnormal person' (2009: 12). Stephen J. Burn, in developing Roth's designation of this new genre which has moved away from the 'novel of consciousness' (Roth 2009: 3) sees such works as 'a kind of neurofiction, a work that absorbs and carries on a dialogue with the contemporary sciences of mind' (2015: 211). Roth, however, is more critical of the neuronovel, concluding that 'novelists have ceded their ground to science' (19), disparagingly aligning the neuronovel with the '"research novel" – novels stuffed with facts, names, things, impressing the reader with the author's store of "nonfiction" knowledge' (14). Yet as Burn highlights, Roth's 'account of the neuronovel's timeline depends on a shallow chronology that is tied to millennial pop science rhetoric and Ian McEwan's recent fiction' (213), ignoring texts, such as *Remainder*, that detail the long-term neurological condition of BI in an enigmatic, alienating mode through an affectless narrator. It is McCarthy's fascination with how simulation manifests, not just as a theoretical paradigm, but within the psyche of the postmodern, post-coma survivor that perhaps matches Roth's call for neuronovelists who 'describe and mimic traits of cognition that neurology can't yet experimentally confirm' (19) and it is this concept of simulation as a path to 'feeling real' once more that Pieter Vermeulen calls McCarthy's 'signature logic'. Throughout the novel, Vermeulen explains, 'A residue is generated through the friction generated by an attempt to cancel one reality by the imposition of another', created through a process of hypersimulation (2012: 561). At its most extreme, this 'residue' is the Enactor's former self over which he tries to superimpose another self. As part of his physical rehabilitation, for example, he has to imagine lifting an invisible, imaginary carrot to his mouth. However, when it comes to lifting a real carrot (the imposition of one reality over another in an attempt to cancel it out), the whole process fails, the real carrot being 'more active' than the imaginary one. Not only is the real carrot a superimposition over a visualized carrot, but the entire exercise is a superimposition over how the Enactor *once* performed this movement, without even thinking about it: fluently and 'real-ly'. Thus McCarthy's 'signature logic' of post-coma, post-trauma simulation creates a perpetual chain of residue. As Lea explicates, '[The Enactor's] attempts to reconstruct unreliable memories and re-enact the coalescence of the sublime moment of individuation all fail in the face of the materiality of matter' (2012: 467).

Significantly in *Remainder*, despite the fact that the Enactor seems to finally feel real again in the aftermath of the robbery, in the final coda to the novel, the reader learns that he has not really changed after all. As his plane is recalled back to the terminal, he forces the pilot at gunpoint to continue on their flight-path, the plane banking to-and-fro in a figure-of-8 pattern thus granting the Enactor a new pleasure as part of a new systematic 'loop': an illusion of 'infinity' (the Ouroboros). We have here another interesting link to Christopher Nolan's *Memento*. As mentioned, by the end of the film (despite being confronted with the truth about his biased, corrupted 'system'),

Leonard inserts himself back into the loop of being by setting up his next mission of revenge on the hunt for John G – his next target being his facilitator, Teddy. The film ends, like McCarthy's novel, with a reinstatement of the Ouroboros. Yet also like *Remainder,* despite ending on an image of the infinite feedback loop, beyond the events of the novel, the system is destined to break – the Enactor's plane *will* run out of fuel, and without Teddy, Leonard's looping mission *will* eventually be halted: both men, by initiating and embracing their respective final feedback loops are also accepting a potential end to their predicament. Omer Fast's film adaptation of *Remainder* creates the perfect, unbreakable and most enigmatic feedback loop as the narrative truly does end where it begins. It is revealed that the event leading up to the Enactor's disaster and ensuing BI was a bank robbery in which the Enactor was involved, but a bank robbery that, post-BI, the Enactor learns about and the robbery which he goes onto re-enact – a narrative twist that truly constitutes the Ouroboros: the involution that swallows its own tail.

This need for simulation and reproduction, it appears, is not just a peculiar condition born out of destructive brain plasticity or catastrophic brain trauma but is entrenched within the human psyche. In their discussion of the reconstitution of selfhood post-BI and coma, Biderman and team cite Erik Erikson's concept of the formation of 'ego-identity', one stage of which is 'identity as imitation' (2006: 356). As they discuss, this first crucial stage of development is the child's inherent mechanism to imitate others and to 'simulate' the habits and mannerisms of parents and peers. As it reaches adolescence, the child gradually fuses these imitations together and consolidates them into a unitary sense of self or 'ego-identity'. Over time, these imitations/simulations become more subtle, from dress codes to music tastes to political affiliations. Turning once more to neurobiology and its explication of how we 'see' and process the world around us, this capacity and desire for simulation can be seen to be even more deep-rooted. The things that one sees are mapped in neural patterns that are created according to an object's design. As Antonio Damasio concisely posits, 'The images we experience are brain constructions *prompted* by an object, rather than mirror reflections of the object. There is no picture of the object being transferred optically from the retina to the visual cortex' (2003: 199). In this sense, everything is simulated. This process of simulation, however, can enter into crisis when the ego-identity's sense of continuity becomes ruptured in some way, either through physical or psychological trauma, leading to what R. D. Laing calls 'ontological insecurity' (2010: 39). Within this state, the individual 'may feel more insubstantial than substantial, and unable to assume that the stuff he is made of is genuine, good, valuable' (42). Developing this existential and psychoanalytical model further, Laing goes on to suggest that, 'If the individual cannot take the realness, aliveness, autonomy, and identity of himself and others for granted, then he has to become absorbed in contriving ways of trying to be real, of keeping himself or others alive, of preserving his identity' (42). While Laing is primarily discussing cases in which there are ruptures in psychological identity, the language that he uses can be adopted to further elucidate the Enactor's pursuit of 'realness' in *Remainder*. From Laing's psychoanalytical perspective, the Enactor's increasingly manic 'contrivances' promise the possibility of reinstating a continuity of selfhood and 'substantial' identity post-coma. These contrivances take the form of simulations, futile attempts to get back to and 'preserve' the ego-identity that existed prior to the accident and the subsequent BI. As Biderman et al. discuss in their appraisal of various theories of the rebuilding of ego-identity post-BI, one aspect of rehabilitation should be to help the survivor to 'rebuild his or her sense of identity based on exploring the individual's new possibilities and capacities, rather than focusing on attempts to restore the pre-injury ego-identity of those individuals' (358). Through the lens of Thomas Docherty's discussion of Deleuze, this is an approach that favours 'becoming' (a new individual) rather than 'being' (an older individual or lost-original). Certainly, McCarthy clearly depicts the Enactor falling into the trap of the latter approach, of 'ontological insecurity', and therefore caught in a perpetual simulation of the lost real.

The intersection between cultural, neurobiological and psychological theories of simulation can be seen most prominently in Jeff Malmberg's compelling documentary *Marwencol* (2010), an example of 'documemoir', to refer to Couser's designation for such films (2011: 235). Later adapted by Robert Zemeckis into the Hollywood biopic, *Welcome To Marwen* starring Steve Carrell (2018), the film explores the simulation compulsion of the post-coma, BI survivor. It tells the story of Mark Hogancamp who, after undergoing a brutal attack at the hands of five youths outside his local bar, went into a nine day coma, after which he had to undergo a rehabilitation programme similar to that of McCarthy's Enactor. This programme, Hogancamp's friend makes clear, involves him 'literally [having] to learn everything over'. Hogancamp, himself, states that, 'When the teenagers kicked my head to pieces [. . .] they wiped everything'. Hogancamp and Shellen expound on this in their book, *Welcome To Marwencol*, writing, 'He'd lost most of his adult memories – his alcoholic past, his former marriage, friendships. And he'd forgotten how to do simple everyday things, like tying his shoes, going to the bathroom, or eating with a fork' (2015: 42). In figurative language that chimes with McCarthy's depiction of the return of the Enactor's memory, Hogancamp explains in the documentary that, 'My memories that I do get, they come back in stills, single shots but no context'. This intersects with McCarthy's imagery of the Enactor's memory coming back as soap opera episodes, within a context that has changed inexorably. Hogancamp's image of snap-shots, likewise, can be connected to McCarthy's reference to the Enactor's memories being like 'wrong holiday photos back from the chemist's' (23).

Losing his ability to sketch and draw (his 'depth perception was off. And his right hand – his drawing hand – shook badly' (Hogancamp and Shellen 2016: 42)), Hogancamp finds respite from the frustrations of rehabilitation in another artistic hobby – the creation of 6:1 scaled models. These intricate simulacra, created out of meticulously-realized buildings, action figures and *Barbie* dolls, have given birth to an entire fantasy world, set within the fictional Belgian town of 'Marwencol' during the Second World War. Within this model-town, he has created his own alter-ego, but more than this: he has alter-egos for all of his friends and family, all interacting, all involved in the action of the complex narratives that he invents and plays out within the town (Figure 4.3).

What he creates, therefore, are not just tableaux of simulated scenes but a series of 're-enactments' in which he fully immerses himself, to the point whereby when he discusses 'his life', there is frequently a blurring between his 'real' life and the simulated

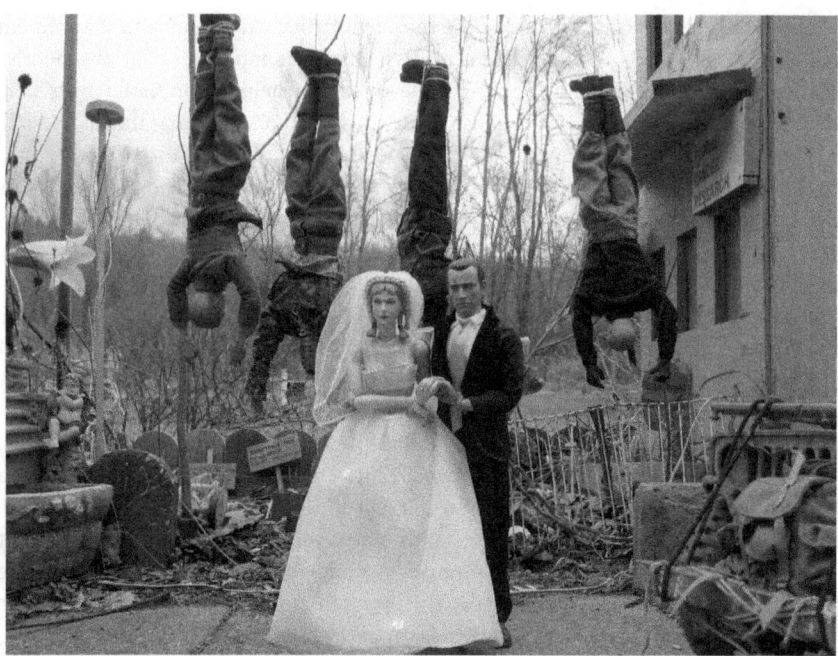

Figure 4.3 Photograph 'Anna and I Get Married' by Mark E. Hogancamp. Courtesy © Mark Hogancamp / DACS 2019.

life in his town. When we first meet Mark, he is holding 'his' doll and proclaims: 'This is me, after the attack of course. Always smoking [...] I used to carry one revolver. Then General Patton gave me his other revolver, so now I have two'. Initially, the viewer, in this introduction to Hogancamp himself, thinks he is talking about his life in the 'real' world (with his reference to the attack) but it soon transpires that he is talking about his simulacrum. This confusion is heightened when it is revealed that Hogancamp's simulacrum is not just based upon his fantasies, but that he incorporates and translates his own experiences into these simulations, the most notable of which being the trauma of his attack. In this sense, when Hogancamp refers to 'him' after the attack, he is talking about both his 'real' self and his 'simulated' self: blurring the line between the real and the simulacrum, like the Enactor's road markings outside the bank. This blurring and ultimate loss of the real is further voiced when Hogancamp, demonstrating a tiny toy gun belonging to one of his model re-enactors, says, 'Everything's real. The slide on the 45. The hammer. The clip even comes out. So that adds to my veracity of getting into it, of getting into the story'. This is realized fully in Zemeckis's adaptation, with the models coming to life in animated scenes of violent confrontations and shoot-outs that dramatize Hogancamp's fantasies, these scenes often spilling over into the real world when he is reminded of his attack thereby representing the intrusive past of Mark's ongoing trauma – like *Remainder*, the line between the model and reality, between simulacra and the real, becomes blurred. The models, when they come to life, also become simulations of Mark and his acquaintances – in his case, an action figure that looks like Steve Carrell, emphasizing Mark's position both inside and outside the model. Hogancamp's ardour for the simulation of the real has its fictional counterpart in McCarthy's Enactor, with his absolute attention to detail essential in order to recapture and recreate the lost real. Indeed, in his book, Hogancamp reflects, 'Those guys don't know what they took from me. I figured I'll never get those memories back, so I'll just make new ones' (2015: 56) – just as the Enactor 'makes' new memories from 'imaginings', and Yambo inadvertently creates memory amalgams.

The loss of the real and the creation of the hyperreal is rendered no more powerfully than in one particular anecdote, regarding Hogancamp's neighbour. Despite his neighbour already being married, Hogancamp reveals to her that she is about to get married to him within his town Marwencol. She clearly balks at this news, exclaiming, 'There comes a time when you just have to *stop!*'. This reaction causes Hogancamp to recreate her rejection of the marriage within the simulacrum. The rejection of the marriage (a 'real-world' rejection of a proposed 'simulation' of marriage that has no reference to a 'real' marriage between them) then leads to a second, simulated rejection of marriage within the simulacrum of Marwencol. But it is even more intriguing and complex than this. His neighbour in the real world reacts to the prospect of a simulated marriage *as if it were her real marriage to him in the real world*. Thus, to return to Baudrillard, the 'simulation envelops the whole edifice of representation as itself a simulacrum' (1983a: 11). The simulation of marriage in Marwencol is not simply false but is of the order of the more real than real: it influences the reality that precedes it. Here we see Baudrillard's theoretical paradigm manifesting itself in real-world terms, arising out of severe physical trauma – coma and BI. It appears that there is something within the human brain that has an inherent propensity for simulation. As humans we are constantly drawn into acts of simulation and we are likewise fascinated by that which is simulated: dolls and doll houses; model vehicles, railways and villages; building blocks; actors; impressionists; impersonators. The proliferation of social networking sites has given rise to another frenzy of simulation, the simulacra of our 'online selves' interacting within the hyperreal of hyperspace, what Ruth Page, in her discussion of Sherry Turkel's work on the blurring of boundaries between 'simulation and human relationships', refers to as 'the performance of identity through online interactions' that can 'become more "real" than offline experiences' (2012: 166). These all generate pleasure and the more exact the simulation (the more 'real') the more pleasure that is created. This 'more real than real' is seen in Hogancamp's photographic work in which he commits the actions and narratives of his re-enactments to celluloid and is highlighted further by the proclamation of the magazine editor who commissions his work: 'I was astonished by the realism'. He later comments that Hogancamp is 'in the work [. . .] A very authentic feeling', resonating with the Enactor's pursuit of feeling authentic again through re-enactments, rehearsals and simulations.

Just as the Enactor finds comfort in loops and circuits so, too, does Hogancamp find comfort in routine and, in particular, in 'patterns'. It is revealed that his reintegration into the work environment involves working at his local bar for a few hours one day a week where he makes meatballs. The camera shot focuses on the repetitious and precise movement of his fingers and hands (movements that, like the Enactor, he has had to 'relearn') as he instinctively moulds the meat into orbs, laying each one next to each other: near-perfect simulations of each other. In a similar system of repetition, Hogancamp constantly re-enacts the trauma that he experienced outside his local bar within his simulacrum: gradually, his attack is confronted again and again through the re-enactments and simulacra that take the form of violent attacks by 'SS Guards' (re)enacted upon his alter-ego. In one attack, he scars one side of his alter-ego's face, the side that corresponds to his 'real' scarring: the 'remainder' of the attack. In another, even more evocative simulation, five SS Guards kick his alter-ego to a pulp (the visceral nature of the violence made clear in the bloodied doll-simulacrum he creates), at which point Hogancamp closes his eyes and utters, 'And then it all comes back to me' in a moment of traumatic reverie akin to the Enactor's trance-state in the bank as the violence unfolds around him.

Even his photographic and artistic praxis seems to reveal the desire to produce and reproduce. When asked by another photographer how he captures perspective and light so perfectly so that the models no longer look like models (another slippage into the domain of the hyperreal), he admits that it is trial and error and that his light meter does not work. He says that if the photographs come back from the commercial developers as over- or under-exposed, he just re-enacts, re-shoots and re-sends them until they come back correct. This frenzy of simulation and reproduction is encapsulated in a moment in Zemeckis's film when Mark's carer, seeing that he is using a doll in one of his simulacra who has died in a previous narrative, asks whether she has come back, to which Mark replies, 'No, no, she's never coming back, I just resurrected her for an old picture I wanted to fix'. Like the Enactor, the past is constantly replayed and simulated but is never enough and always has to be re-edited before once more being re-played.

All of the people in the documentary view Hogancamp's use of simulacra as a clearly therapeutic praxis: his lawyer comments on how the violence his alter-ego enacts upon his simulated attackers in Marwencol is a positive way to deal with the trauma; his magazine editor sees the simulacra as a way to 'regain something that is lost'; and Mark, himself, sees the model as a 'safe' place, proposing that, 'I created my own therapy'. Yet, like McCarthy's Enactor, the rem(a)inder will always be there for Hogancamp, haunting his reformation of selfhood, resulting in a simulacrum that is self-perpetuating. This is exemplified when, in the coda of the film, Mark's alter-ego likewise begins to create simulacra, even smaller, more intricate scaled models, in order to re-enact and simulate the traumatic attacks at the hands of the SS: a copy of a copy of a copy. It is a narrative twist omitted from *Welcome To Marwen*, Zemeckis's Hogancamp, at least, able to find some respite and escape from the infinity loop of simulation although, interestingly, this mise-en-abyme pattern of simulation is portrayed by McCarthy in *Remainder*. The Enactor is not just compelled to create re-enactments in his life-size models (the building, the gangland shooting, the robbery), but also in scaled-down versions, most notably a scale-model of the building-simulacrum. Crucially, 'The figures of the characters were moveable' (152), the Enactor picking them up and making them do his bidding – playing the role of a Greek god in an old Harryhausen movie. As the Enactor moves the figures around this model, Naz radios down to the re-enactors in the building, instructing them to replicate, reproduce and simulate the miniaturized movements that the Enactor has performed in the model. In a reversal of Hogancamp's post-coma world, actions are created in the model then played out in the 'real' world.

For both the Enactor and Hogancamp, the simulacra are ultimately ways to recover control that was lost in their respective disasters of their physical traumas, and the trace-echoes of trauma in their new post-coma lives. Yet the simulacra, in the attempts to re-assimilate the remainder and to feel whole again, may always be haunted by the irruptions of violence and the trace of trauma. This being said, for Hogancamp, there is a possibility of escape from the fate that McCarthy bestows upon his protagonist. Against the cycle of simulation and stuttering condition of 'being' is the hope of moving forward and 'becoming'. This comes in the form of his new narratives of self that he is gradually developing. In this process of affirmative self-storying, Hogancamp refers to his 'second life', in contrast to his 'first life' (Hogancamp and Shellen 2016: 23), an image that has undertones of the miraculous and which resonates with imagery of resurrection discussed earlier. At one point, he holds up a photo of his pre-coma self and proclaims, 'I never want to see this guy again'. Hogancamp almost re-codes the trauma of his attack with a positive nucleus. Despite the trauma and violence of the attack, his 'second life' is one free of alcohol, thereby constituting a full, irreversible recovery from the addiction that plagued his 'first life', pre-coma. As his friend and boss at the local bar says, 'After he got out of hospital it was like somebody turned a switch. He had no interest in alcohol at all'. This is in line with many clinical studies of the reconstructing of self-narratives in BI survivors, with patients often revising, according to Masahiro Nochi, 'their self-narratives by changing the appearance of their past and future' (2000: 1797). Hogancamp's positive interpretation of his post-traumatic self can therefore be equated with what Nochi would call the 'grown self'. This manifestation of the reconstruction of post-BI identity leads to patients suggesting that TBI had at least one positive outcome for their lives. Significantly, Nochi cites an example of one participant in his research study who stated that, 'When I had my accident, it was kind of a balancing because it stopped my drug use and alcohol use for a while'. Despite the fact that Nochi goes on to point out that in actuality, his substance abuse was not halted 'immediately after the accident', he does concede that, 'He certainly considered the accident a fundamental step toward abstinence, however' (1798). For the Enactor, though, no such option of a 'grown self' is available as he possesses no satisfaction with his post-coma identity, rendering his ability to move forward, to 'become', null and void.

4.5 Reality, unreality, realism

In examining the human propensity for simulation, theories he would go on to fictionalize in his own novel, *The Mysterious Flame of Queen Loana* discussed earlier, Umberto Eco's work on the cultural phenomenon of simulacra and the hyperreal is particularly instructive. In his pseudo-travelogue, 'Travels in Hyperreality', he suggests that, 'The pleasure of imitation, as the ancients knew, is one of the most innate in the human spirit', suggesting that when one takes pleasure in a perfect imitation, one 'also enjoy[s] the conviction that imitation has reached its apex and afterwards reality will always be inferior to it' (1987: 46). Eco is therefore more critical of simulacra than Baudrillard, suggesting that the 'Absolute Fake' (31) is more preferable than the lost original. Rather than seeing the real as being merely supplanted by the simulacrum, Eco proposes that the division between the real and the simulation is no longer recognizable. Eco's allusion to the innate pleasure of imitation connects with the theories of the formation of ego-identity and the neurobiological notion of neuronally-constructed representations or simulations. When trauma strikes, the compulsion to repeat, reproduce and simulate seems to arise. In the texts I have discussed, the physical trauma of BI, leading to the sensation of not feeling real any more against the trace of a former self, awakens a further compulsion to simulate. The fact that both the Enactor and Hogancamp create dioramas in their process of simulation emphasizes their need for some kind of reality, as Eco hypothesizes when he writes that, 'The diorama aims to establish itself as a substitute for reality, as something even more real' (8). This seems crucial for the Enactor and Hogancamp, in the face of the disappearance of their 'real' and authentic pre-coma selves.

This notion of post-coma/TBI simulation is a particular preoccupation with several authors of coma fiction in their attempts to emulate the crisis of authenticity and simulation that occurs in many neurological cases of brain trauma patients. A further example is Richard Powers's 2006 post-coma novel, *The Echo Maker*, which follows the travails of Mark Schluter who, after being involved in a major road-traffic accident, emerges from coma with severe brain damage. Like McCarthy, Powers is meticulous in his depiction of the trauma of coma and rehabilitation. In writing about the degradation and dehumanization of Mark Schluter's body, describing Mark as 'a face cradled inside the tangle of tubes, swollen and rainbowed' (7), a 'felled mannequin' (15) with a 'slit throat' and 'bolt [in] his skull' (9), Powers also deconstructs the 'sleeping beauty' trope. Throughout the first section of the novel, while Mark is still in coma, Powers frequently shifts from third-person focalization to first person, depicting Mark's comatose consciousness. Powers focuses on Mark's struggle to regain his identity and, chiefly, his reacquisition of language, speech and mental lucidity: 'He has to work some, with time come back. Up and attic, there and bath again. Have him living in a boxcar now. Old train with others orphaned like him. He's lived in worse. Not easy to say just where he is. So he says nothing' (49). Powers creates approximations of the coma consciousness as Mark moves through other DoC in order to achieve 'full' consciousness in the 'overworld'. Powers describes a vague awareness of Mark's physical entrapment that collapse into distant, fractured memories of the past. Powers depicts traumatic aphasia and the breakdown of language signification, a technique similarly employed by Alex Garland at the point whereby, as discussed earlier, Carl reaches the nadir of his coma consciousness, the broken signifying chains of language eventually flooding his consciousness as his brain 'reboots'. Mark's linguistic slips and trips metaphorically represent the impact of his BI upon his personhood, memory and language skills. Luc Herman and Bart Vervaeck in their analysis of Powers's 'effort to imagine the basic level of Mark's consciousness' (2009: 442) refer to 'the narrator's fabulating presence' that constitutes 'a shining illustration of poetic illusion' (427). At the moment at which he begins to gain full consciousness, he sees himself as a beached whale rotting on the beach with his 'skin' peeling off 'in sheets of blubber' until 'his parts come back to him, so slowly' (42), metaphors of rebirth and metamorphosis that are common motifs in coma fiction with Powers also describing a 'rising' that is taking place (32) which implies a katabatic resurrection, further stressed by the description of Mark coming 'back from the dead' (61). These staccato and disjointed imaginings of the cognitive process during which Mark, 'Makes a list of himself, like old rebuilt machines' (42) embody the painstaking and traumatic return to consciousness and reacquisition of mental faculties. It is a process that is once more depicted by McCarthy in writing of the gradual return and re-ordering of memories of his Enactor, or even by Redgrove, when writing of his induced comas, describing the sensation of the 'pieces' of his selfhood being 'taken away like a stage-set being dismantled' (2006): 154). These pieces ('parts', to refer again to Powers's novel) are gradually reassembled post-coma. While Herman and Vervaeck contend that such representations of the interiority of coma 'for some readers run counter to the rather elementary brain activity of which Mark gives proof elsewhere in the early depictions of consciousness' (427), I would argue that Powers creates an approximation of the lightening of coma, akin to what Hollyman describes as a 'surfacing' in *Lairies* (2021: 11) and which will be examined in more detail in the following chapter when discussing the lived experience of coma survival. Powers therefore depicts the survivor's struggle with the impact of BI, while simultaneously conveying the chaos of cognitive impairment and confusion that will continue throughout post-coma rehabilitation.

But Mark's BI has also led to a further complication: the long-lasting neurological condition of Capgras Syndrome and this is where the peculiarity of post-BI simulation lies. This disorder is concisely described by V. S. Ramachandran in his work on rare neurological conditions. With Capgras Syndrome, he writes, 'The patient, who is often mentally quite lucid, comes to regard close acquaintances – usually his parents, children, spouse or siblings – as impostors' (1998: 161). John M. Doran, in his overview of various perspectives on Capgras, also observes, 'Through the ages, there has come a wealth of evidence that humanity has been preoccupied with the double as an ideational theme' (1990: 30), a statement that evokes Eco's concept of the 'innate' tendency within the human condition to simulate. In the case of Mark, the impostor or 'double' is his sister, Karin, much to her great frustration and despair. This crisis of simulation is two-fold. On the one hand, for some reason unknown to all around him, Mark's brain can only see Karin as a simulation: 'Kopy Karin', an 'actress who looked very much like his sister' (2006: 86). On the other hand, for Karin, Mark, too, is a kind of simulation. He is someone who looks like her brother, but is not quite him; a loved one who seems 'almost healed' (89) and is 'almost there' (44): the same-but-different. It is a description which embodies Ben Platts-Mills's designation of the BI survivor as an 'inexact replica' (2020) and which also seems indicative of Malabou's discussion of destructive plasticity during which 'the permanent dislocation of one identity forms another identity – an identity that is neither the sublation nor the compensatory replica of the old form' (2012: 18). This is a common feeling held by the loved ones of BI survivors as Pachalska et al. allude to, the family of one particular patient feeling 'his presence as a stranger among them', despite looking the same (2011: CS23). Ramachandran, too, discusses this notion of the physical invisibility of BI when referring to a particular case of Capgras that he worked with where the patient seemed 'to all outward appearances' to be back to normal (1998: 159).

Like McCarthy, Powers focuses on his protagonist's post-coma rehabilitation with Mark having to re-learn everything, eventually appearing to be 'one hundred per cent [. . .] Back together' (41). Nevertheless, from both Mark's subjective perspective (and Karin's external, objective perspective) this is not the case. Both of them know that something is not right, a feeling that is generated and exacerbated by the fact that this 'new' Mark and his 'second life' (to quote Hogancamp) is not quite the same as the 'old' Mark, leading to the trauma that stems from superimposing the new self over the trace of the old. As Mark tries to continue the life he led prior to coma, 'Kopy Karin' prevents a full return to 'normality'. Not only does her presence remind him of the fact that something is not quite right, it also reminds him that Karin is absent and has not even visited him in hospital which would be anathema to his 'real' sister, thus exacerbating his sense of post-coma trauma, alienation and unsettlement. Karin is a perfect example of the Derridean trace. She is an absent-presence for Mark and is 'both' his sister (physically) and is 'not' her (emotionally). It is this haunting paradox that Kopy Karin represents that causes Mark to enter a crisis of post-coma simulation in order to explain and narrate through this rupture in selfhood which he is experiencing and of which he is reminded every time he sees Karin. Powers's neuroscientist Gerald Weber (a character loosely based upon the neurologist Oliver Sacks) highlights the medical profession's fascination with the syndrome while invoking Derrida's philosophical position when, ruminating on whether Mark's Capgras is a product of neurological (organic) or psychological (functional) damage, concludes: 'It's the kind of neither-both case that could help arbitrate between two very different paradigms of mind' (105). In this, Mark's liminality and existential undecidability is emphasized. His Capgras confabulations create narratives that attempt to logically explain the Karin-simulation and in turn resolve this undecidability in order to preserve his ego-identity that has been shattered through coma and BI. Many case studies of Capgras detail the creation of such extremely complex narratives in order to explain the simulations that are created, occasionally leading to disturbing and tragic consequences. One of the most infamous of these is the case of one patient who believed his father to be a robot and proceeded to decapitate him so that he could locate the batteries and microfilm in his father's head. In other cases, patients have deemed their pets to be doubles (Silva et al. 1989), a simulation that also occurs in Powers's novel, Mark failing to recognize his beloved pet and explaining the exuberant affection the dog shows for him by suggesting he has 'rabies or something' (86).

Ramachandran, in line with other studies, has looked at how Capgras more than likely arises from damage to the limbic system, which is concerned with the generation and processing of emotions. Ultimately, for Ramachandran, the syndrome is caused by a disconnection between the part of the brain that is responsible for facial recognition, and that part that is responsible for emotions, a position supported by John M. Doran: 'The Capgras patient "recognizes" the significant other in every sensory way an organically intact person would, except that the Capgras patient does not recognize him emotionally!' (1990: 37). However, the novel also examines another aspect of Capgras, exemplified by the two physicians Professor Weber and Doctor Hayes. As Christian Knirsch explicates, in the representation of the doctors' 'shifting evaluation of Capgras as either a neurological or a psychological phenomenon' (2014: 48), Powers perfectly encapsulates the raging, wider controversy between competing schools of scientific thought. Hirsten and Ramachandran observe that, 'Although frequently seen in psychotic states, over a third of the documented cases of Capgras syndrome have occurred in conjunction with traumatic brain lesions, suggesting that the syndrome has an organic basis' (1997: 437). In line with this diagnostic conflict, Weber muses, 'True Capgras resulting from closed-head trauma: the odds against it were unimaginable' (102)'. *The Echo Maker* is one of the texts Roth cites in his critique of the neuronovel yet interestingly, in name only; he offers no specific analysis or criticism of the novel itself, overlooking the complexity of the debates and issues Powers explores. As Knirsch posits, in Weber's fear that Mark's organic/functional diagnosis could be a 'neither-both case', the novel 'clearly transcends the epistemologically narrow boundaries of a neuronovel as defined by Marco Roth. The neuro-empirical worldview *is* articulated, but certainly not perpetuated – on the contrary, it is called into question' (Knirsch 2014: 56). Knirsch concludes his analysis of *The Echo Maker* (together with his refutation of Roth's unevidenced criticism of the novel) by postulating that the novel 'ties the epistemological discourse of the neurosciences into a general epistemological and ontological discourse as it can be found in postmodernist theory' (61). It is a summation, I suggest, that can be similarly said of *Remainder* in its portrayal of the crisis of identity post-BI and its evocation of postmodernist theory in depicting the shattering of an already decentred Subject.

In his discussion of the representation of trauma and selfhood in *Remainder*, Pieter Vermeulen argues that, 'The novel is an attempt to debunk the customary pieties of trauma fiction' by remaining 'conspicuously indifferent to the weighty ethical issues that normally mark our engagement with the extreme violence and the psychological suffering that characterize trauma' (2012: 550). Using an affectless protagonist, with anti-realist plot, lack of psychological depth and 'readerly empathy and sentiment' (549) are a few of McCarthy's techniques Vermeulen picks out in order to demonstrate that, while employing the characteristic tropes of repetition and re-enactment, *Remainder* is not a 'typical' trauma novel. Furthermore, going on to discuss how McCarthy's anti-empathic approach leads to a refreshing lack of psychological realism, Vermeulen argues that, 'Trauma, far from registering as a psychological event, is merely mobilized as a structural plot element' (551). However, in what Vermeulen sees as constituting McCarthy's absolute lack of psychological realism lies the foundation of realism itself. It is exactly McCarthy's depiction of behaviours stemming from both organic and functional post-trauma that connects theories of simulation and the trace with medical theories of the human capacity for simulation, manifested post-coma, that constitutes a nucleus of realism within the novel and which refutes Vermeulen's notion that McCarthy 'merely' uses trauma as a narrative device. What Vermeulen (alongside other critics) might see as a lack of psychological realism (and a general criticism that is often directed at the novel) actually conveys the lack of empathy and emotional intelligence so often present in the survivors of coma and brain trauma. At one point, the Enactor is told that all of the black cats have fallen off the red roofs of the building opposite as they lack the ability to cling onto the incline. When asked what he wants to do about the rate of loss of the cats, he simply replies, 'Get more' (146), a comment that again emphasises McCarthy's sharply observed representation of a damaged brain.

It is overly simplistic, therefore, to suggest that *Remainder* is an anti-realist novel. Certainly, it may lack the psychological and emotive depth of traditional trauma novels but this is indicative of the specific type of trauma that McCarthy portrays. It is this trauma, the trauma of coma and BI, both psychological and physical, that allows the novelist to explore complex literary and cultural theories by looking at how these manifest in real-world situations and crises. The following chapter will examine such real-world crises: narratives of the lived experiences of the coma and BI survivor, and the language and imagery such survivors adopt to express their personal trauma and tales of survival.

5

Coma, brain injury and lived experience

As we saw in the previous chapter, certain works of coma and BI fiction often reflect and portray the lived experience of these conditions, albeit within heightened or extreme scenarios. What texts like *Remainder, Memento* and *The Echo Maker* manage to uniquely achieve is a portrayal of the post-coma condition, the trauma of living with BI and the permanent impact this has both upon the conception of a future self and the maintenance and context of a past self. Nevertheless, across all works of fiction discussed, there exist patterns of language and imagery that arise throughout narratives of lived experience of coma and BI. And conversely, there simultaneously exist plot devices, narrative techniques and imagery that obfuscate the lived experience of coma survival, as well as negate the potential for BI.

This chapter will seek to explore narratives of lived experience of coma and BI, drawing links between the language and imagery used in fictional works while also interrogating some of the mythologies created by such portrayals. As part of this, I will draw on my own work with coma and BI survivors, referring to writings developed within writing classes that I run in Sheffield. The membership of this writing group, The Write Way, consists of survivors of coma and/or BI, with members having sustained either a traumatic brain injury (TBI, caused by an external trauma, e.g. car accident, violence etc.) or acquired brain injury (ABI, caused by internal trauma, e.g. stroke, brain haemorrhage etc.). Over the course of running this group, I have published two chapbook collections of their work under the title *Head-lines* and it is to these published works that I will refer. But before I look at these contemporary autopathographies of lived experience, I would like to look at two famous cases of BI survival from the nineteenth century, highlighting commonalities in aetiology and sequelae of the injury.

5.1 Anatomy of a brain injury: two early case studies

The first case, and one that is widely referred to as neuroscientist's most famous patient, is that of railway worker Phineas Gage, a case of BI survival, Christian Jarret notes, which has entered 'neuroscience folklore' (2015: 37). On 13 September 1848, Gage was foreman in charge of a gang of workers blasting rock in preparing the roadbed for a new train line. While using his tamping iron to pack inert material around the gunpowder payload, he became distracted, the tamping iron sparked against the rock and set off an explosion which propelled the rod (around 1 metre long and 3 centimetres in diameter) upwards, entering the left side of Gage's face, passing straight through his left eye and left side of the brain, and completely exiting the top of the skull through the frontal lobe. The rod fell some distance behind him, 'smeared with blood and brain' (Harlow 1868: 333). Despite the severity of the injuries, and coming close to death on several occasions, Gage survived – but he was irrevocably changed. In the words of his physician, and the second doctor to attend the scene, Dr John Harlow, Gage's 'mind was changed, so decidedly that his friends and acquaintances said he was "no longer Gage"' (340). Harlow details some of the specific behaviours that indicated this rupture in identity: Gage's hitherto unheard-of propensity for 'indulging in the grossest profanity'; or how he was 'impatient of restraint' and 'pertinaciously obstinate', 'capricious and vacillating' – concluding that Gage had become 'a child in his intellectual capacity [with] the animal passions of a strong man' (339–40). These are some of the earliest observations of brain damage to the prefrontal cortex, this frontal lobe, as it was later to be discovered, being responsible for regulation of emotions, judgement, social behaviour and impulse control. Despite referring to claims made at the time that this case was 'one of complete recovery', Harlow was more cautious: 'Mentally the recovery certainly was only partial, his intellectual faculties being decidedly impaired, but not totally lost' (345). Nevertheless, there was much resistance to this diagnosis, as in the age of phrenology, Harlow's identification of post-trauma symptoms (and the localization of the injury that led to these, alongside a lack of full recovery) did not make sense in phrenological terms, nor in the prevailing belief in the duality of mind theory that judged both brain hemispheres to be identical. In other words, *theoretically*, Gage should have made a full recovery – and so it was perceived to be the case by the lauded thinkers and scientists of the time. Harlow's considered, empirical appraisal of Gage is one of the earliest examples of observations of permanent changes to personality and identity after injury to the prefrontal cortex, even though at the time, it wasn't accepted as such. Moreover, he foreshadowed David Ferrier's experimental program to determine how brain functions were hierarchically organized. Experimenting on a number of animals, commencing in 1873, Ferrier was instrumental in identifying the fact that injury to the prefrontal cortex of the frontal lobes of the brain can cause profound personality changes, without other apparent neurological deficits (O'Driscoll and Leach 1998: 1674).

The case of Phineas Gage not only gives us a useful example of the early fascination with the brain but also the resistance to neurological theories of mind that would, a century later, prove to be accepted by the medical profession. It is also a very early example of the stigmatization of the brain-injured patient. Gage became as much of a mythic figure as he was a paradigm of pioneering neurological studies. Appearing for a time at P. T. Barnum's *American Museum* in New York City, the 'new, aggressive Gage, rod in hand, became a circus freak and wanderer' (Jarrett 2015: 38). Malcolm Macmillan further notes that both popular stories and so-called scientific reports 'misrepresent the changes to [Gage's] behaviour, and fabulate a subsequent history that, rather than having him work in a reasonably normal way, turn him into something like a drunken liar who drifts around as a circus freak' (2002: 304). In reality, the truth is a lot more benign, discovered, as Jarrett points out, through a 'dramatic re-evaluation' of the story. Gage's 'stint as an exhibition piece' was short-lived, eventually emigrating to Chile where he embarked upon a successful career as a coach-driver, a very demanding career, requiring him to 'pick up new vocabulary, deal politely with passengers, control the horses, and navigate a treacherous route over hundreds of miles' (38). As Macmillan and Lena posit, in their reappraisal of Gage, his 'post-accident employment may have provided him with just the kind of structured environment needed for rehabilitation, consistent with temporary accounts of brain-damaged patients who have recovered well' (Jarrett 2015: 38). Yet the image of the brutish recidivist, drastically transformed through tragic misadventure, savagely wielding an iron bar, takes precedent. Macmillan even writes how 'at least one "scientific" source actually has Gage surviving for twelve years with the tamping iron embedded in his skull' (2002: 304), a narrative, Macmillan supposes, influenced by a sensationalist Ripley's *Believe It Or Not!* cartoon panel of 1947 which showed the iron bar still inserted into the skull alongside the details of 'the most amazing accident that ever happened'.

Another equally high-profile case of a survivor of frontal-lobe damage is that of the innovator of photography, Edweard Muybridge (1830–1904). In 1878, using a battery of twenty-four automatically operated stills cameras, Muybridge proved conclusively that horses, running at pace, would at periods have all four legs off the ground simultaneously. This cemented Muybridge's reputation as a pioneer in photographically capturing motion. However, four years before this groundbreaking moment, Muybridge was in the public spotlight for an altogether more nefarious reason. In 1874, Muybridge was arrested for the murder of his wife's lover, and potential father of his child. What is particularly informative in this case, and germane to our current discussion, is the evidence that was presented in defence of Muybridge at his trial, and the contextual background to this evidence that unfolded fourteen years prior to the murder. In 1860, Muybridge was involved in an accident while travelling from San Francisco to St Louis. En route, his stagecoach lost control and 'started down the hill, swerving, the horses running for perhaps half a mile'. Muybridge, himself, reflected that, 'The best plan would be ... to get out of the back of the stage', predicting that, 'An accident would take place'. He took out his pocket knife to cut the canvas and escape when, and again in his own words, 'The stage ran against a rock or stump and threw me out' (Ball 2013: 242). The next thing Muybridge remembered was waking up in hospital.

What is fascinating about this incident is that, despite being in a DoC for several days, most accounts avoid using the designation 'coma' to describe this disorder, including Muybridge himself who, interviewed for the *San Francisco Chronicle* after his accident on 6 February 1875, merely referred to his return to 'consciousness' (Hendricks 1975: 10). This provides a useful example of how, in that period, 'coma' as a diagnostic term was often unacknowledged or overlooked, and we even see this avoidance in some contemporary accounts. Clegg, in his biography of Muybridge, describes the incident using Muybridge's own language: 'Muybridge was thrown free of the wreckage. His head hit a rock and he lost consciousness' (2007: 26). However, most modern accounts do acknowledge, given the length of his state of unconsciousness and the level of permanent TBI sustained, that Muybridge did lapse 'into a coma that lasted more than a week' (Horspool 2010). Edward Ball takes the most diplomatic approach in his biography of Muybridge by declaring that he 'was taken from the scene unconscious, perhaps in a coma' (242). Nevertheless, all accounts are united in their observation of the significant, permanent brain damage sustained in the accident: 'There was a small wound on the top of my head', Muybridge himself recollected, continuing, 'When I recovered, each eye formed an individual impression, so that, looking at you, for instance, I could see another man sitting by your side. I had no taste nor smell, and I was very deaf' (Clegg 2007: 26). Muybridge's eyesight never recovered, leading to what David Horspool has referred to as 'a premonition of the multiple image-making that made him famous' (2010): creativity arising from a devastating injury. Yet something else was to come out of this injury, and a consequence that was to be raised at the murder trial in his defence: a different Muybridge.

Friends and colleagues were called to Muybridge's defence who all commented upon his 'changed' character: that prior to the accident 'he had been "genial" – not to mention "pleasant and agreeable", but that afterward he was "irritable", "surprising and wavering", "more careless in his dress", and "not so good a businessman"' (Clegg 2007: 94). Ball notes, too, that one of Muybridge's colleagues commented, 'He was eccentric, peculiar and had the queerest of odd notions, so much so that he seemed like a different man' (252). In this early example of language used to describe the effects of the observed phenomena of BI, we are reminded of Harlow's words, a quarter of a century earlier: that Gage 'was no longer Gage'. Arthur Shimamura, in revisiting Muybridge's injury, observes that his double vision, loss of taste (hypogeusia) and smell (anosmia) are all symptoms that 'can occur as a result of damage to the orbitofrontal cortex or to nearby nerve fibres' (2002: 348) – the same area of the brain that was damaged in Phineas Gage and which had such a profound effect upon his identity. In the end, Muybridge was acquitted of murder based upon the evidence of his changed identity, and so began his pioneering work in the photographic studies of motion.

What these two case studies demonstrate is a very early fascination with BI and their contribution to informing and understanding the brain and the effects of injury upon it, as detailed in Chapter 1. But they also provide us with an early acknowledgement of the indelible change of personhood that occurs with BI, a change encapsulated by McCarthy's metaphor in *Remainder*: 'like something come out of something'.

5.2 Coma: the void; the dream

I have discussed, at length, the schism that exists within coma literature between two models of representation of the interiority of coma: those narratives that posit the coma as a complex dreamscape and those that present this DoC as a void. In *The Echo Maker*, Powers details the void of his protagonist's coma, writing, 'First he's nowhere, then he's not'. This 'nowhere' is, 'Not even a place until feeling flows in' and at the moment when feeling returns, when Mark Schluter begins to emerge from his coma, 'He loses all the nothing he was' (2006: 41). Later, Powers explicitly describes this void in coma consciousness, writing, 'He [Mark] remembered nothing of the accident' (62), echoing McCarthy's empty, senseless vacuum of coma in *Remainder*, referring to the Enactor's 'no-space of complete oblivion' (McCarthy 2010: 6).

Similarly, returning to Steve Hollyman's *Lairies*, coma is depicted immediately as a void, as the author describes a character's emergence from coma: 'There was the blackness, and it blanketed me, and then there was nothing. Nothing for days, and then the wall clock tick-tocking. And here it comes, The Surfacing. This is how it felt to be born. Unwombed and taking the first breath' (2021: 11). As discussed at the start of this book, Hollyman employs the imagery of (re)birth also present in Ruthann Knechel Johansen's biographical account of her son's coma. Yet like Powers, Hollyman simultaneously draws a fascinating distinction between the 'blackness' and the 'nothing' of coma. The first denomination suggests the slippage into coma (the 'nowhere' to which Powers alludes); the second the coma itself (when Mark, in Powers's novel, becomes 'not', equivalent to McCarthy's 'oblivion'). Like McCarthy, Hollyman was chiefly interested in presenting the lived experience of the post-coma condition and the traumatic process of rehabilitation, conducting interviews with coma survivors and victims of TBI. Speaking in an interview with me in 2013, Hollyman discussed these literary aims, reflecting, 'I wanted the novel to be realistic, and no one I spoke to had any memory of being "inside" the coma'.

These fictional texts that present coma as a void (together with Redgrove's autobiographical poem) have one clear thing in common: the representations of coma and BI are built around the lived experience of coma. In this regard, these factually rigorous texts chime with Antonio Damasio's own observations of coma survivors who 'can recall the descent into the nothingness of coma' but 'nothing at all' of the coma itself, coming to the conclusion that, 'It is legitimate to assume, given all the evidence, that little or nothing was in fact going on in the mind' of the coma patient (2000: 95).

Revisiting Jean-Dominique Bauby's memoir, *The Diving Bell and the Butterfly*, while this primarily focuses upon his traumatic experience of locked-in syndrome, he, too, is at pains to distinguish this paralysed state of awareness from the void of unconsciousness (and the lack of awareness) of coma, writing, 'I myself had twenty days of deep coma and several weeks of grogginess and somnolence before I fully appreciated the extent of the damage' (2004: 12). In writing about his emergence from coma, he describes how he 'surfaced', an image that is similarly deployed by Hollyman in his fictional portrayal of coma, influenced by his interviews with coma survivors. Later, Bauby extends his discussion of the coma void, describing the comatose patients as, 'Poor devils at death's door, plunged into endless night' (39). In writing of her own experiences, Kate Allatt, too, draws the distinction between coma and locked-in syndrome in her memoir *Running Free*. After suffering a catastrophic brainstem stroke, Allatt describes 'slip[ping] in and out of consciousness like someone is pressing the pause button on my life', after which she 'regained consciousness' having 'been in a coma for three days' (2011: 3, 5). She later explains that, 'The doctors had been keeping me in a coma to give my brain a rest and the chance to recover', thereafter writing, 'When I came round, I had been left "locked in"' (6), once more describing the dividing line between the blankness of coma, and the awareness of the locked-in state.

James Cracknell, in his autobiography *Touching Distance* (written with his former wife Beverley Turner, to provide an alternative account of her ex-husband's recovery from coma and BI), similarly focuses upon the void of coma. At the very start of the memoir, at the moment of his catastrophic biking accident, he writes: 'I sit back in the saddle; take a deep breath. I've never felt so alive. And then . . . there is nothing' (2013: 2). It is some 225 pages later when Cracknell returns to describing what happened post-accident and he opens this section of his memoir with: 'My next memory is of lying down in a strange room. But I can see Bev, and there's Mark. That's all. One weird disassociated image and then it fades. They call these "islands", sudden breakthroughs of conscious memory, in what is otherwise a total blank' (227). In the case of one of the members of The Write Way, Steph Grant, the blankness of his coma continues to 'haunt' his consciousness throughout his post-coma recovery. In 'Blue Polystyrene Shoes', for example, Grant paints another picture of these post-coma 'islands' between which he must confusedly navigate, a void in consciousness sitting between each island and signalled by Grant's repetition of a two-word phrase appearing throughout the story: 'Then nothing'. He describes a sequence of disconnected, jarring scenarios, from 'waking up' in hospital and seeing 'a tube running from the middle of his right arm' (2011: 5) to being 'sat in an armchair' at home with a 'crying-smiling woman' whose name eludes him, but whom he knows 'loves him, and he her' (6) The end of each disjunct memory, and the passage into the next, is heralded by, 'Then nothing' – again, an extension of the void of his coma over-spilling into his post-coma rehabilitation. And Stephen Hattenstone, in describing writer Michael Rosen's coma that was induced by medical staff to try and combat a Covid-19 infection, writes, 'After he [Rosen] came out of the induced coma, it was all a blank. He didn't even know he had been in one', going on to describe the coma itself as a 'seven-week vacuum'. Rosen, himself, describes his coma as 'a pre-death, because it's a nothingness' (Hattenstone 2020), once more drawing on the image of the void (and the void's relationship with death) to try and give voice to his experience of coma.

However, despite this plethora of narratives of lived experience describing the void of coma (and works of fiction that draw on this lived experience), we also find narratives and autobiographical writings that posit an altogether different view of the interiority of coma: memoirs that are more akin to those works of fiction that employ the dream C-Met. In the cases of most members of The Write Way, such complex and detailed memories of the coma are absent, yet one writer, Caroline Waugh, does possess snap-shots of dream-like memory. In her story of post-coma recovery, 'Lager and Black', she describes her physiotherapists feeding her 'frozen cubes of blackcurrant ice [to] stimulate the muscles' of her mouth. She goes on to describe the frequent visits she received from her local vicar because 'staff believed she was going to die'. These two events of the ice cubes and receiving the Last Rites intersect to form her coma 'dream': 'Receiving Holy Communion, in the form of frozen cubes of wine!' (2014: 29). So how are we to read or comprehend this depiction of a coma-dream in light of the narratives describing the coma void, and in the knowledge that effectively, in coma, brain functions are flattened with no sleep/wake cycle? After all, as Ben Platts-Mills writes, 'A stroke or other injury switches a person off the way a computer is switched off if you pull the plug or drop it from a first-floor window' (2019: 56). The key to answering this may lie in Waugh's acknowledgement of her doubt surrounding the timeline of her recovery in which this dream-memory occurred, using non-traditional form to emphasize her cognitive confusion. In trying to pinpoint exactly when this 'dream' occurred, she writes, '?Probably about the same time as this?' using question marks as parentheses to illustrate her uncertainty. When writing of the memory itself, she describes it as 'a very vivid dream(?)', again emphasizing her vacillating opinion on whether this was a genuine memory from coma, or a dream arising from her return to consciousness as her brain functions and synapses gradually return: the 'islands' of post-coma confusion about which Cracknell, too, writes.

5.3 Post-coma 'lightening' and the near-death experience

This confusion regarding at which point of coma recovery such 'dreams' occur is itself a fascinating area of debate leading to the common, burning questions: what exactly occurs in coma? And what is remembered? One of the leading British climbers of the 1980s and 1990s, Paul Pritchard, like Cracknell, draws the dividing line between coma and the semi-conscious state of post-coma. In his account of his TBI incurred through a rock-climbing accident, his repetitions and hallucinatory traumatic experiences only occur after emergence from his induced coma. Writing about the occurrences in the world around him, he writes, 'Obviously I wasn't aware of any of these goings on, I was unconscious or hallucinating wildly for the best part of four days' (1999: 52). The 'unconscious' stage, a blankness in experience, Pritchard attributes to the coma itself; his dream-like hallucinations to his traumatic, cognitive confusion post-coma. These post-coma 'islands' are akin to the vivid hallucinations which Cracknell experienced, one of which saw Cracknell imagining 'Gary Linekar . . . living under [his] hospital bed while [he] was sharing it with his wife' (227).

Writing as witness to her son's coma and subsequent TBI, Ruthann Knechel Johansen paints a similar picture to the first-hand experience of Pritchard and Cracknel. Her account deliberately avoids using the designation 'waking' to describe her son's emergence from coma. She discusses her son's coma 'lightening' (62), only using the words 'sleep' and 'napping' to describe the post-coma condition, a confusing, frightening and hallucinogenic experience that is again similar to that described by Pritchard and Cracknell. Importantly, Johansen, herself, uses inverted commas for these designations, almost to emphasize the metaphorical, even ironic nature of her terminology. This term 'lightening' is also used by McCarthy in describing the Enactor's gradual emergence from coma which itself constitutes a hallucinatory state – when the Enactor's 'mind was still asleep but getting restless and inventing spaces and scenes for [him] to inhabit' (51). As discussed earlier, Damasio, too, makes reference to this transitional phase of coma, going on to describe how this can lead to the PVS (continuing or chronic VS) in which the sleep/wake cycle, crucial for the generation of dreams, is reinstated (2000: 237). Moreover, Plum and Posner's pioneering work *The Diagnosis of Stupor and Coma*, from the outset, makes it abundantly clear that, 'Between the extreme states of consciousness and coma stand a variety of altered states of consciousness' (1980: 3), qualifying this with the fact that, 'The limits of consciousness are hard to define satisfactorily and quantitatively' and going on to assert that, 'We can only infer the self-awareness of others by their appearance and by their acts' (2). The slippages between states of consciousness discussed in *The Diagnosis* are also referred to by Johansen, commenting that, 'Coma was not simply a clearly demarcated state of unconsciousness. In many patients coma does not end suddenly, as if turning on a light switch' (61), thereby questioning this immediate 'light-switch moment' of recovery prevalent in much of coma fiction discussed herein.

Yet despite this blurring of boundaries between coma and other low-awareness states, many writers of the lived experience of coma still attribute their dreams to the coma itself and not to this 'lightening' period of post-cognitive recovery and confusion. Most puzzling is Swedish poet Artur Lundkvist's memoir, *Journeys In Dream and Imagination*. The tagline to this book is, 'The hallucinatory memoir of a poet in a coma', yet in his foreword to the book, David Ingvar, writes, 'After two months [in coma], miraculously, Artur Lundkvist woke up' (1991: 8). Ingvar goes on to describe how, 'As both Maria [Artur's wife] and Artur tell it, the moments of wakefulness, and clarity, grew longer and longer' while, 'At the same time, Artur Lundkvist began dreaming, richly and strangely' (8). In essence, the strange hallucinations of Lundkvist's 'dream journey' (23) that he describes throughout the book are not dreams occurring within his coma at all, but, as is the case with Waugh and Cracknell, within the cognitive confusion of his 'lightening' of coma. Moreover, the fact that Lundkvist was unconscious for two months would suggest his coma had progressed to a continuing VS.

In a similar vein, in the foreword to Sandra Lyman's autobiography, *Waking Up: Memoirs Of A Coma Recoverer*, she writes: 'I dedicate this book primarily to my God. He gave me [. . .] the memories of coma' (2007: 3), yet peculiarly, she relates very few memories of the deep coma which she inhabited. What soon becomes clear is that those 'memories' of coma that she attests to are rather thought processes which come into consciousness, not within deep-coma, but again within the semi-conscious state that she reaches through her lightening of and emergence from coma. In narrating her story, she fluctuates between relating factual detail of the occurrences in the hospital room ('The nurses just changed the tube to a smaller one and left me in bed') and internalized, frustrated utterances, marked by her use of italics ('*There is nothing to do. Maybe I can pick up that box with my foot. I can!*' (60)). Because these interiorized thoughts and narration of physical actions are separate from the events of the hospital room, there becomes a blurring between what is real and what is not. This sense of cognitive confusion is heightened through Lyman's description of her locked-in (yet physically active) state as her 'nightmare' (55) from which she wakes up, yet it soon becomes clear that what she claims to remember about her coma are actually the confused memories of the 'lightening' coma as she transitions through other DoC or liminal states. Couser postulates that, 'The relation between bodily dysfunction and personal narrative is a complex one; the former may both impel and impede the latter' (1997: 5). This recoding of the interiority of coma and the blanks in consciousness it has left as a remembered experience, I propose, seems to embody perfectly this impulse to narrate the dysfunction of coma/BI while simultaneously revealing the impediments of this process.

But Lyman's dedication to God in the foreword of her memoir also raises another important, and controversial, topic of debate when discussing autobiographical narratives of coma 'dreams' – the coma as near-death experience (NDE) or outer-body experience (OBE) during which the patient sees him or herself travelling to Heaven and communing with God. Richard Selzer's memoir of the comatose state which he entered after contracting *Legionella pneumophila* is one such example of an autopathography depicting an OBE and NDE. Adopting the third-person pronoun, Selzer purports an ability to reveal the secrets of his coma: 'Even to death and beyond, he will be the teller of tales, collecting impressions, defying forgetfulness, and meeting gods all along the road, the way you do when reading Homer or Virgil. He can do all that? In coma? Oh, yes he can. Dream, imagination – these are the chariots that the comatose body rides' (1993: 28). This declaratory preface to his coma memoir seems to contradict many of the autobiographical coma-texts discussed earlier and in terms of linguistic styling has more in common with some of the fiction I have cited to-date, not least Garland's *The Coma* through Selzer's comparison of coma to 'dream'. Unlike Garland's protagonist, though, Selzer's comatose self is not daunted by the loss of story and of selfhood as he confronts and apparently overcomes the 'forgetfulness' of post-coma. Furthermore, Selzer's final line in this passage seems to suggest, through the use of the indefinite article, that every 'comatose body' is able to narrate their own experience of coma in a rather presumptuous and inaccurate generalization. This assumption is further called into question as, adopting third-person narration, he develops a narrative of OBE, focusing on the objective external perspective of his degenerating body, looking down upon himself through the imagined eyes of the medical staff. He writes, 'He has been in coma for almost three weeks. What is it like?' (30), yet what follows, in spite of flurries of figurative language, are simply descriptions of straightforward medical processes and details that struggle to inhabit the two realms of 'dream, imagination'. He writes that, 'It is like being encased in a layer of wax that separates him from the rest of mankind', a simile that merely reinforces the inert physical condition of all coma victims. He goes on to describe the 'immense weight' that 'holds down his thin bluish eyes', again a figurative utterance that brings textual colour to an otherwise medical description of coma that is retrospectively narrativized – the fact that he cannot open his eyes.

However, as the coma extends over the weeks, Selzer appears to describe more vividly the interior state of his unconsciousness. Again using the third-person pronoun, Selzer describes himself as 'like a gardener digging in the earth who makes a decision to lower himself to the underworld', exploiting the metaphor of katabasis used by such writers of fiction discussed extensively in Chapter 3 – a narrative of NDE. Similar to Redgrove, he describes the underworld of coma in organic terms, 'Swinging from root to root' among the 'worms, gulches, darkness' and describing 'the mushroom scent of hell' (31), once more aligning his descent into coma with a chthonic katabatic quest. At one point, Selzer describes how 'silt has settled in his veins' (33), in a startling echo of Redgrove's retrospective image of the 'soil' in his 'limbs' (1999: 7). Prior to this vision of the underworld of coma, Selzer makes yet another allusion to that archetypal katabatic adventurer of Christian teachings, Lazarus:

> This morning he even made a gesture as if to reach up and claw from him the skin of wax that is his coma. It is the same gesture made by Lazarus in the painting (School of Rembrandt) when he sits up in the tomb and begins to unwrap his cerements. But unlike Lazarus, the man in bed cannot manage it. (30–1)

Yet in this admission, and later revelations that include one moment whereby Selzer turns his head and stares at one of his nurses before ripping out his breathing tubes, we find a possible explanation for why the visions of his interiority of coma have become more vivid – these physical actions that Selzer perform reveals the fact that, by now, he has left coma and is now inhabiting a low-awareness state. The veracity of Selzer's memoir of coma is also called into question through his own summary of his literary agenda, rejecting 'facts' for 'impressions' (26). We may therefore return to his assertion that 'dream, imagination' are what allows him to narrate his coma – the dreams that arise from his lightening of coma, and his imagination which allows him to fill in the gaps. Selzer calls his memoir a 'chronicle of an illness told afterward' (26), this adverb 'afterward' being most pertinent to our discussions. Between the traumatic event of coma and the 'afterwardsness' (nachträglichkeit) of narrating this event, Selzer is still unable to write, in detail, of the experience within the coma itself, and, like Redgrove, develops the language with which he can figuratively and retrospectively describe the void of coma. This autopathographical process is emblematic of what Couser refers to as 'one generic convention that crops up in various forms of disability autobiography [namely] the conversion narrative' (185). Closely aligned to Arthur Frank's 'restitution' narrative, the conversion narrative sees 'the redemptive shifting of emphasis from the body to the mind', an act of 'self-rehabilitation' which 'involves in large part redefining the self as more a function of mind and spirit than of the flesh' (1997: 185). For Selzer, this conversion narrative becomes a means for the reclamation of control that was lost in coma.

Mark Sherry, in his own 'insider research' (or 'emancipatory disability research'), working with coma and BI survivors, discusses at length the 'embodied' experience of coma, and the memories of the interiority of coma held by some of the people he has worked with and interviewed. One particular member of his research group, Rick, talks about remembering one of his friends coming to visit him while he was in coma, the friend putting his new born baby in Rick's arms who 'felt it lying there' (2006: 185). Sherry goes on to discuss how, while in coma, Rick's wife read to him and after emerging from coma, Rick 'began reading from the exact page where she had been reading to him' (185–6). Crucially, though, in describing what appears to be a 'light-switch' moment of emergence from coma, Sherry does not state how long after emergence Rick was able to do this. Sherry also describes how Rick 'still retained an embodied sense of self and some awareness of the environment around him' even 'when he was in his least responsive state', with Rick himself describing some of his 'very vivid dreams' (186). Sherry goes on to pinpoint several other cases of coma embodiment within members of his research group that tip over into the realm of the NDE. One member, Reg, describes being 'engulfed by the light' that is 'beautiful' and which 'really feels great', before he 'was brought back to life' (186). Madonna, too, describes an NDE while in coma: 'When I died a couple of times, I went up top and saw Peter, Saint Peter' (187). Sherry also discusses how she reported a vision of the Virgin Mary: 'Mary came down and seen me [. . .] She told me to walk and I did it in front of her' (187). In evaluating the veracity of these stories, Sherry discusses his own NDE, himself a BI survivor: 'Like Reg, I was transformed from one place where I was in enormous pain to another where I was surrounded by light and was completely pain free'. He discusses how he was 'immersed in this light', surrounded by other 'beings of some sort, almost shaped like clouds' that spoke to him (187). He also makes reference to the archetypal 'tunnel' of the NDE, down which he travelled before he 'came back to this life' (188).

Now compare these narratives and experiences of the NDE (and those of Selzer's) with those of Dr Eben Alexander outlined in his coma memoir, *Proof Of Heaven*. Alexander's autobiographical account of his bacterial meningitis-induced coma describes multiple places to which he travels, all of which he views as indicative of an NDE. In the initial stages of his katabasis (which he describes in a chapter titled 'Underworld') he refers to 'objects around [him] . . . a little like roots, and a little like blood vessels in a vast, muddy womb' (2012: 30), drawing on the kind of chthonic language and imagery employed by Selzer and Redgrove, alongside the image of the womb and rebirth so common across works of coma literature. Zasetsky, for example, Luria's Second World War TBI patient introduced in Chapter 1, encapsulates his own 'second birth' (to refer to Johansen's description of her son's post-coma identity) by describing himself as 'a kind of newborn creature' (1975: 88). This level of coma-underworld (in which a 'kind of rebirth' can occur) Alexander refers to as 'the Realm of the Earthworm's-Eye View', a place where he 'wasn't human [. . .] wasn't even animal' (30–1). Later, Alexander hears the 'most complex, most beautiful piece of music' that heralds a 'pure white light' (38) that descends upon him, transporting him to 'a place of clouds' where 'flocks of transparent orbs, shimmering beings [arc] across the sky'. These are 'simply different from anything I had known on this planet. They were more advanced. *Higher*' (45). In this place, Alexander feels 'an explosion of light, color, love, and beauty' (46), leading to a state of transcendental euphoria – a religious experience.

Seemingly predicting the cynicism and doubt with which his account of his NDE will be met, Alexander, in the book's coda, outlines and argues against a sequence of more logical, pragmatic explanations for his NDE, yet despite this defence, his account is still not without its detractors. Mark Shermer, in his attempts to explain NDEs and OBEs, argues that Alexander's account is, like many reports of NDEs, 'Indistinguishable from those of people who have had drug-induced hallucinatory trips' (2018: 91). Moreover, Shermer makes the significant point that the 'near-death' experience isn't actually death (though points out that often, writers of the NDE are at pains to emphasize that they were 'dead' or 'absolutely' or 'clinically' dead). He observes that those within the near-death condition 'may undergo stress, be deprived of oxygen, release neurochemicals that can mimic the hallucinatory trips of drug users, or experience any one of the dozens of anomalous neurological anomalies, abnormalities or disorders that have been documented by neurologists and neuroscientists' (90). One such scientist was the late Oliver Sacks, who himself conducted experiments upon himself using hallucinogens to mimic religious epiphanies or states akin to NDEs[1]. Sacks, himself, takes issue with Alexander's account of his NDE, and his presumptuous statement that this provided him with 'proof of Heaven'. Writing in *The Atlantic*, Sacks observes that, 'When one hallucinates voices, the auditory pathways are activated; when one hallucinates a face, the fusiform face area, normally used to perceive and identify faces in the environment, is stimulated' (2012b) – in short, hallucinations *feel* real because they exploit the same areas of the brain used for standard perception. Sacks points out the fact that Alexander describes his emergence from coma as a sudden 'awakening', going on to assert, however, that, 'One almost always emerges gradually from coma;

there are intermediate stages of consciousness'. It is these stages of coma 'lightening' to which Sacks attributes the experience of the NDE, concluding that, in Alexander's case, 'His NDE occurred not during his coma, but as he was surfacing from the coma and his cortex was returning to full function' (another significant use of the verb 'surfacing', here). This could similarly be an explanation for the experiences of NDEs of some of the members of Mark Sherry's research group. It is significant that, in discussing both his participants and his own NDE, Sherry neglects to mention the stage of unconsciousness they inhabited and fails to reference coma lightening or other DoC despite, earlier in the book, defining the vegetative state as distinct from coma. In Alexander's case, he is convinced that his travails in the underworld of coma constituted a genuine religious encounter due to the fact that, as he asserts throughout his memoir, 'His cortex was off' (184). He maintains that his brain *'hadn't been working at all'*, concluding, 'The part of my brain that years of medical school had taught me was responsible for creating the world I lived and moved in [. . .] was down and out' (129–30). Alexander even predicts and argues against the brain-hallucination explanation that Sacks would go on to posit, although his reasoning is less than convincing, arguing that he had previously experimented with hallucinogens and the effects that were induced were 'most chaotic and unpleasant, and bore no resemblance whatsoever to my experience in coma' (184), an explanation that Sacks sees not just as unscientific but 'antiscientific'. But as Anne Hunsaker Hawkins posits, 'Even if science has tended to replace religion as the official mythology of a secular culture, religious ways of thinking and imagining still persist, as if from a deeper instinctive level and an earlier age' (1999: 49). Yet the controversy surrounding Alexander's memoir runs even deeper. Shermer challenges Alexander's assertion that his cortex had completely shut down, and his insistence that there was 'no way' he 'could have experienced even a dim and limited consciousness' during his time in coma. Shermer points out that Dr Laura Potter, the attending physician at the moment Alexander was taken to ER, induced his coma in order to keep him alive and that whenever they reduced his medication keeping him within coma, he 'thrashed about, pulling at his tubes' and tried 'to scream', revealing the reality that 'his brain was not completely shut down'. Moreover, Shermer explains, when Potter later challenged Alexander about this factual distortion, 'Alexander told her his account was "artistic licence" and "dramatised, so it may not be exactly how it went, but it's supposed to be interesting for readers"' (93). While within his coma, and by his own admission, Alexander writes that, 'I had no memory of prior existence, my time in this realm stretched way, way out. Months? Years? Eternity?' (31). So if he had no concept of time, how did he know exactly when his NDE began? These experiences could equally have occurred within minutes, as often dreams do, and within those moments when he was being brought out of induced coma – when he entered the 'lightening' period of the post-coma condition.

Astonishingly, this is not the most contentious example of the reporting of the interiority of coma as an NDE. In the bestselling coma memoir, *The Boy Who Came Back From Heaven*, Kevin Malarkey describes the events surrounding his son's two-month coma and brain and spinal injury after a catastrophic car accident that left him quadriplegic. The memoir also includes eight-year-old Alex's memories of the coma itself, memories that constitute both the OBE and NDE. After being admitted to hospital, Alex writes, 'When we got to the hospital, I was watching everything that happened from the corner of the emergency room, near the ceiling. Jesus was standing there beside me' (2011: 29). What follows is an affirmatory depiction of a religious epiphany that allowed young Alex to survive. Yet when Alex reached the age of sixteen, he recanted his alleged true story, revealing on his blog that he had made it all up. He writes, 'I did not die. I did not go to heaven. When I made the claims, I had never read the Bible. People have profited from lies, and continue to. They should read the Bible, which is enough'. Suing the specialist Christian publisher, Tyndale House, for damages, Alex's lawsuit states that he 'remembers absolutely nothing from the time he was in a coma' (Flood 2018) – the NDE, ceded to the void once more.

5.4 After brain injury; against sleeping beauty

As discussed, for the victim of trauma, the initiating traumatic event, while not being fully comprehended or confronted at the time it occurred, may be recovered and 'mastered' through therapy, or through a process of repetition and working through; for the survivors of coma, this event may never be recovered, as all memory of it may have been obliterated completely through organic damage to the brain. For the coma survivor, the traumatic event may forever remain as a void and beyond the borders of consciousness, an eventuality that is no less traumatic than if the memory and cognition of the trauma had remained intact. This transformation that has occurred, as Catherine Malabou posits, 'through destruction', will 'not allow patients to return to a previous state, to seek refuge in a past of any kind' (48). And while Malabou concedes that for both the victim of 'sociopolitical trauma' and of 'organic trauma' there exists the 'same relation between the psyche and catastrophe' (11), the victims of organic trauma undergo 'an *unprecedented metamorphosis* [. . .] of identity' [original italics], as if they become 'separated from themselves' (15). However, for the coma and BI survivor (one victim of 'organic' trauma), despite this unprecedented metamorphosis alongside the gap in consciousness that the coma, itself, has created, he may still repeatedly return to snap-shots of memory from the pre-coma mind of his 'separated' self, memories that, while not traumatic per se, become traumatic through their incoherence, temporal rupture and detachment from all frames of reference that may allow him to make sense of them, thus constituting the 'shredded' psyche to which Malabou makes reference (48). Despite these differences, however, both the trauma survivor and the coma survivor are linked by these doomed repetitions of fractured memories (Freud's traumatic 'hauntings') that are, themselves, symptomatic of a process of survival that has taken place. As Caruth concludes when discussing Freud's constantly shifting approaches to trauma, 'What Freud encounters in the traumatic neurosis is not the reaction to any horrible event but, rather, the peculiar and perplexing experience of survival' (1996: 60). Whether or not the coma victim ever recovers memory of the traumatic, initiating event, or whether this forever remains a void in consciousness, he is still confronted with the problematic condition of all survivors of trauma: survival itself. And while Malabou calls for 'new forms of treatment that would no longer be based on the investigation of the past, the exploration of memory, or the reactivation of traces' (48), the coma and BI survivor will inevitably be drawn back into this traumatic repetition in the desperate hope and need to recover and reunite with their old 'self', but also to appease the desperation of their loved ones who hope for such a recovery to take place.

One such example of post-recovery hope appears in Johansen's narrative of her son's recovery from coma when, writing figuratively, she describes the coma itself as 'a lost "realm" we could not enter' (63), but it is a lost realm that can neither be recalled by her son, through the irreparable brain damage he has sustained. Erik's recovery seems to hinge upon his loved ones' attempts to fill in the void of consciousness and selfhood through the telling of stories: 'We tried to present stories that linked his former, healthy self with his present, recovering self and that projected a future of restored well-being' (131). But this proves difficult due to the fact that TBI 'breaks all familiar coherence to smithereens' (131), an image which resonates with Malabou's 'shredded' psyche and which embodies Erik's 'unspeakable grief' – the unexperienced disaster, to return to Blanchot, which 'escapes the very possibility of experience [. . .] the limit of writing' (1995: 7) or, in Erik's case, the limit of self-narrative.

This traumatic confrontation with the fractured past self that existed prior to BI is similarly explored by Steph Grant in his story 'Blue Polystyrene Shoes' when he writes:

> *Who knows when later? A few hours? A few days? A week? Five weeks? It matters not. The man who has a crying-smiling woman that loves him, and he her, is sat in an armchair, apparently reading an edition of J.S. Mill's* Utilitarianism. *Nothing goes into his head out of the book for the man is unable to understand written language. But he looks the part.* (2011: 6–7)

Grant's meta-narration reflects the temporal rupture that the coma has created. What is also noticeable is the use of third-person narration, signifying the detachment between the narrator, Steph, and the Steph that emerged from coma, inextricably altered from his identity pre-coma. It is a technique similarly deployed by Richard Selzer, who, writing of his decision to use the third-person pronoun, explains that the use of '*he* gives a blessed bit of distance between myself and a too fresh ordeal in which the use of *I* would be rather like picking off a scab only to find that the wound had not completely healed' (1993: 26). Interestingly, in discussing his narrative technique, Selzer uses a most apposite metaphor to describe his attempt to distance himself from the trauma of his coma experience, the image of the unhealing wound/trauma. The premature picking of a scab is indicative of a traumatic repetition during which one is both repulsed by the action of picking and compelled to continue until the scab is removed and the wound reopened.

This dichotomy of repulsion/compulsion of the reopening of the wound/trauma is similarly expressed by Grant when describing the need to inhabit his pre-traumatized self. The comment, 'But he looks the part' reflects this idea of the ruptured, post-traumatic identity, as though he is playing a role in his attempt to return to his pre-traumatized self, a goal that is rendered impossible due to the reality and permanence of his BI. The role he attempts to play is that of his old 'self' as he tries to belong to this new world into which he has been 'reborn'. Despite the futility of this post-coma role-play, Grant persists with it in a pattern of behaviour that reflects Freud's repetition compulsion of traumatic neurosis: attempting to re-read Mill, for example, despite not understanding a single word. In his preface to the story, Grant refers to his attempts to reunify the 'ripped apart remnants' of his identity and this is conveyed through his struggle to attempt to play the 'role' of his pre-coma self. These ripped apart remnants again exemplify Catherine Malabou's notion of the 'shredded psyche', both in the linguistic violence of the two phrases, but also in their conceptual construction, both referring to the idea of a shattered, fragmented post-BI identity. It is a designation similarly drawn upon by Luria in describing Zasetsky, referring to his 'fragmented' world – a world in which, as Zasetsky himself says, he has become 'a completely different person, precisely the reverse of what I was before this terrible injury' (87).

Grant, in discussing publicly his decision to use third-person narration, still speaks of the emotional difficulty of facing his accident and subsequent coma and BI, an experience that, by his own admission, he had never been able to voice fully prior to the writing of 'Blue Polystyrene Shoes' due to its traumatic nature. In his biographical note in the second edition of *Head-lines*, Grant writes, 'Experiences became dismembered from my sense of self. Those things which I was able to recall clearly were memories of someone else. Those memories that I create have an alien quality for me' (Grant 2014: 38). Again, the image of a violent severing of one identity and one set of memories from the other is conjured, exacerbating the concept of the permanent alienation of selfhood that occurs within the coma and/or BI survivor. Luria, again in a similar manner, describes Zasetsky's post-TBI relationship to the world as 'alien, colourless' (87). Mark Sherry similarly reports such experiences of detachment from selfhood among the members of his research group. One member, Reg, reflects upon how,

> One day I was a human being, and I've got twenty years of experience in everything I've ever learnt from the age of birth . . . The next day I woke up after the head injury, I didn't remember any of that', going on to discuss how he had to 'come to terms with where I was and what I was. (183)

The use of the word 'what' is particularly powerful, especially when juxtaposed with his initial observation of one day being a 'human being', the implication being that a little of his humanity has been lost. Similarly, Sherry also refers to one participant, Kirsten, who 'experienced a significant period of confusion after her traumatic brain injury' (178). Kirsten draws attention both to the void of coma and to the voids of post-coma cognitive confusion, commenting: 'Okay, the actual hospital part after I came out of the coma, I have no idea! I can't remember that at all' (179). Sherry reflects upon the information delivered bluntly to him by his own neurosurgeon: 'Get it into your head you're brain damaged. You'll never be the same again. You can't recover from brain damage' (182). Sherry even refers to his recovery diary, in which he laments, 'I feel like so much of "me" has been killed in the accident' (182), employing the kind of violence of language drawn on by Grant and Malabou when describing brain damage and its impact upon selfhood. Sherry refers to another participant, 'J', who reflects, 'You have to reinvent yourself' (185). But in the case of Grant attempting to re-read Mill, he is trying not to reinvent himself, but to recover his old self, a pursuit that becomes inherently traumatic as we see in Grant's follow-up to 'Blue Polystyrene Shoes', 'Unremembered Memoirs'. In this story, set a number of months after his emergence from coma, Grant writes about his 'disturbing behaviours' (2014: 4). After one particular unremembered, violent incident, Grant's wife observes: 'There's still something wrong with you' (8), both acknowledging the change in her husband but simultaneously implying that at some point in an unknown future this 'wrong' will right itself, allowing Grant to become his 'old' self again, or at least a simulation of this old self. Grant's second story narrates multiple instances during which he tries to recapture his lost self by simulating the habits and behaviours of that pre-coma self. Moreover, friends and loved ones are, likewise, keen for Grant to perform such simulations: to get back to 'normal' or, to use McCarthy's language, to go 'through the zero' (2010: 110). However, all of these attempts to recapture the lost self (like the Enactor's simulacra) ultimately end in failure. For Grant, even going to the local pub with his friends Bass and Neil ends in disaster, their trademark larking about ending in an 'eruption of violent behaviour' (4). The invitation of an old school friend to visit the house ends in Grant chasing him and his family to his car, yelling 'scabs' and 'blacklegs' (8): in an attempt to simulate a friendship of his lost self, all that is remembered (all that remains) is the fact that his friend broke the picket line during the miners' strike of the 1980s. This trace is the only remainder in Grant's memory of their relationship, meaning that the simulation of a *healed* friendship, post-strike, is impossible. There is also an attempt to take Grant to hear one of his heroes, Arthur Scargill, speak at Ollerton Miners Welfare Club: 'Steph can remember having a front seat to hear Arthur speak. He can remember seeing Arthur and hearing him speak – but he also remembers 'that it was as if Arthur was speaking a completely alien language not one word of which he had been able to understand. *Not a solitary single word*' (Grant 2014: 9). Again in an 'alien' environment, and just as in 'Blue Polystyrene Shoes', Grant attempts to simulate his former self (he is again playing a part) but the simulation fails due to his BI and post-coma cognitive confusion that have created a schism between who he is post-coma and who he was prior to his accident.

But what Grant also writes of is another emotional problem arising from long-term neurological conditions: inflexibility and obsessionality, known as 'perseverations' and sometimes referred to as 'target fixation'. Trevor Powell notes that, 'This type of rigid behaviour is rather like 'tunnel vision'', most often caused by 'direct neurological injury to the frontal lobes' and leading to the patient having 'difficulty 'switching' from one line of thought to another' (1994 132). Beverley Turner, too, writes of James Cracknell's perseverations post-injury, noting that, 'James "perseverates" on trying to get somewhere but he doesn't know where' (196), James's sister describing it 'as like seeing an old LP stuck on repeat' (197) – an evocation of McCarthy's 'feedback loop' and the Enactor's own perseverations that become increasingly extreme, alongside Umberto Eco's overt allusion to Yambo being 'like a stuck record'. Another member of the writing group, Gwynfa Grant, who sustained a hypoxic BI after an anaesthetic mishap while in hospital, captures the realities of post-BI perseveration and behavioural feedback in one of her 'Whacky Rhymes': 'There was a young fellow called Ted | Who had suffered a blow to the head | From that day onwards | He went backwards and forwards |Then started all over again' (2014: 37). Superficially whimsical, this limerick succinctly embodies the trauma of post-TBI repetition compulsion and perseverations, but also the permanence of these behaviours – 'from that day onwards', every day since the initial injury, these behaviours are exhibited. The 'backwardsness' of Grant's description also evokes Zasetsky's allusion to becoming the 'reverse' of his former self – a subversion or inversion of identity. Grant, in her use of 'Whacky Rhymes', shrewdly probes the word 'whacky' itself, drawing attention to the derogatory nineteenth-century lexical origin, a *'whacky'*, referring to 'a person who behaves as if he had been whacked on the head' (*Collins English Dictionary*). But in the seemingly simplistic, child-like form of these whacky rhymes, Grant also satirizes and subverts nursery rhymes which often pivot around comical images of BI: 'Jack and Jill' and 'Humpty Dumpty', for example, alongside the snoring old man who 'went to bed | and bumped his head | and couldn't get up in the morning'.

Laurence Cox, another member of The Write Way and TBI survivor of a motorcycle accident, similarly draws attention to his own perseverations in his story, 'Going Out and Hating Myself':

> Going out and hating myself god knows I don't need to be feeling this way but I am so there's nothing to do but to persevere and write something to try and put my mind at rest and maybe I could so something about the size of the page or the fact that the cursor keeps jumping around to random spots on the screen like it's done at least five times since I started writing this. (2014: 34)

Cox overtly refers to the need to 'persevere' and what follows is a snapshot of repeated behaviours, feedback loops and cognitive confusion: the computer cursor that repeatedly interrupts his narrative flow, leading him back to the beginning of his attempts to write; meeting a 'wheelbarrow-pushing lad' at the local chapel whom Cox recognises yet whose name he 'keep[s] forgetting' (34); being outside the chapel 'with an odd sense of *déjà vu*', feeling as though he must have been inside the chapel at some point but not quite remembering it (34); carrying on his journey through the city and immediately 'feeling anxious' at 'the image of the busy pedestrian crossing on Eccleshall Road flashing' in his mind (35). Even the form of Cox's stream-of-consciousness reflects his perseverations, the lack of punctuation and paragraphing in the opening sequence of the story evoking a sense of determination, frenzied and frustrated obsessionality. Zasetsky, too, refers to his 'morbid writing' (77), the narrative of his illness that he writes 'again and again' (78) in order to try and recover his lost self, and to try and forge a new self in the face of devastating injury.

This indelible impact of BI upon the identity of survivors is explored across a range of texts detailing lived experience of long-term neurological conditions. Beverley Turner, in reflecting upon James Cracknell's condition immediately after his accident and while he was still in coma, notes, 'He will henceforth be known as a TBI survivor' (180), underscoring the permanent redevelopment and reframing of selfhood post-accident. Later, Cracknell himself questions, 'Who was I? I looked the same (in the mirror at least) but *was* I the same person? The honest answer was no' (238). Like McCarthy's Enactor, Cracknell has become *the-same-but-different*, the trace of a former self staring back at him from the mirror – an 'inexact replica', to once more call upon Platts-Mills's designation. Steph Grant similarly expands upon this disconnection between selves caused by TBI: 'Rehab helps people re-remember their selves but their *sense* of self can never be the same organism as before the accident' (2014: 38). Grant uses the term 're-remember', evoking Nicola King's label of 'rememory' within trauma studies, that is, 'remembering again . . . after a period of forgetting' (2000: 151) and the 'point of intersection between individual memory of personal experience and cultural or collective memory' (150). In Grant's case (as in the case, also, of Erik Johansen), the self that existed prior to the organic trauma of BI is reconfronted through rehab and evoked through the collective memory of loved ones – but it is also permanently lost and only exists within these memories, thus his sense of self can never be the same post-accident. This loss of the old self, for the BI survivor, is also coupled with the often arduous, frustrating process of creating a new self, superimposed over the *trace* of the old – again, there is rarely the 'light-switch' moment of 'awakening'. As Platts-Mills succinctly states, '[T]o recover from coma is nothing like waking from sleep' (56). Cracknell consistently draws attention to this struggle to find a new self, discussing one step of his recovery which involved 'making a plan and following it through logically', observing that this is often 'something that victims of frontal lobe injury lose the ability to do', as supported by Powell who notes that such loss of executive functioning caused by damage to the frontal lobes 'often produces [. . .] subtle deficits recently labelled "Dysexecutive Syndrome"' (85). To counter this syndrome, Cracknell relates how he tried to follow recipes for lasagne and a Victoria sponge and recreate a meal. He writes, 'I was convinced I'd always made a mean Victoria sponge. Months later I asked my mum about my legendary sponges and she said to her knowledge I'd never made one in my life' (235). Cracknell exhibits the propensity for the BI survivor for confabulation, the 'verbalizations about people, places or events with no basis in reality – usually after memory impairments' (Powell 1994: 210). As discussed in the previous chapter in the case of McCarthy's Enactor, gaps in memory and a loss of selfhood can lead to confabulations, attempts to rediscover or recreate a sense of self; to fill in gaps in consciousness in order to find (or re-find) one's place in the world. In this sense, Cracknell lucidly highlights the complexity of the term 'recovery' in the case of BI survivors. Recovery implies a regaining of something that has been lost – but what we really see in Cracknell's case, and in the case of many of the other narratives of lived experience discussed herein, is that what survivors really experience is not the *recovery* of an old self, but the *discovery* of a new one.

Another member of The Write Way, Joel Wilde, approaches this concept of injury and selfhood from a slightly different direction, largely due to the fact that he sustained his injury 'at the age of three'. He writes, 'Apparently, I had a brain tumour. Apparently it was aggressive' (2011: 14). This use of 'apparently' is an interesting one, suggesting doubt in the reports given to him (King's 'collective memory') regarding his injury. This doubt is manifested in Wilde's observation, 'It's not that I don't believe them but I think they're making it up for some reason' (14). While much of this doubt seems to stem from the fact that Wilde was so young when he sustained his injury and therefore completely eludes memory and lived experience, the denial of his injury echoes the denials of disability voiced by some of the participants in Sherry's research group, with one particular member, Rick, asserting, 'I see myself as a recycled man. I had a brain injury but I see that it's in the past. I don't see it as going to affect me in the future [. . .] I have some difficulties but they're not permanent. Therefore I don't see myself as disabled' (174). This sense of identity seems to be in stark contrast to Sherry's own conception of his post-injury self, as framed by his consultant with the blunt declaration: 'You'll never be the same again'. Rick's sense of self, too, conflicts with the permanent sense of detachment from the pre-injured self explored by The Write Way authors, Steph and Gwynfa Grant and Cox. Wilde, though, similar to Rick, writes, '*I'm not aware that I have any difficulties or what they are*' (15), utilizing italics to emphasize this evasive self-awareness, embodying Luckhurst's concept of the 'emergency phase' of traumatic memoirs. In the end, Wilde concludes rhetorically, 'Am I me because of me or am I me because of what has happened to me?' (15), underlining the concept of a new self born out of injury and the dichotomy of destructive plasticity – a *'creation through the destruction of form'* (Malabou 2012: 17, original emphasis).

Such narratives of lived experience do not only counter the mythologies of the post-coma, brain injured condition, they also examine the condition of coma itself, dispelling the particularly prevalent C-Met of the sleeping beauty. Caroline Waugh, for example, writes of the 'demi-jars filled with black tar syphoned directly from her lungs' and satirises the 'sexy' language of the 'Tilt Table' used to exercise her body. The 'pale shit-brown padded plastic' sharply diverges from the language of the equipment description in a medical catalogue, a description that intrudes on Waugh's own writing in the form of a facsimile of this advertisement and which describes the Tilt Table as having a 'foam padded top' with 'oven baked finish', providing 'silent and smooth lifting action' (2014: 27). Similar to other writers discussed, Waugh refers to her 'new life' that 'had become her own', while admitting she had no idea how this transition had come about. Both Bev Turner and Paul Pritchard similarly describe the degradation of the body of the coma patient. Turner describes graphically the 'IV' that 'courses' through her ex-husband's veins, 'Removing excess fluid from his cranial cavity'. She goes on to write of how the 'ventilator breathes for him'; of the 'feeding tube' that 'pumps in nutrients that emerge pale yellow into a bag attached to a catheter' (179). And Pritchard, as he enters the stage of post-coma lightening, describes his 'dribbling saliva', the tubes that emerge from his 'neck and nose and cock' and the 'waste' that comes out 'in a steady trickle down the tube emanating from my bladder' (55). He also writes of the 'grinding pain' (55) in his abdomen, later recalling, 'Try as I might, I couldn't get a crap out' – his long-term immobility meaning that he couldn't excrete for a week, and not without frequent enemas (57).

The Chilean novelist Isabel Allende, in writing of her daughter's coma after developing the rare metabolic disorder porphyria, also draws attention to the alienating, uncanny relationship between the body and the machines that sustain it: 'I look at you in that bed, connected to a half dozen tubes and wires, unable to even breathe without help. I scarcely recognize you; your body has changed and your mind is in the shadows' (1996: 34). Allende's description implies the onset of muscle atrophy and her daughter's wasting body and so once more, there is a sustained focus on the degradation of the body. Allende later refers to the 'spine-chilling vomit of blood followed by convulsions' (20) that were the prelude to the coma, and then later, the 'ghostly' colour of Paula's complexion and her 'glassy, dilated eyes', observing ultimately that, 'You were still as death, not breathing' (21). Allende evokes the fine dividing line between images of coma and images of death, but she complicates matters further when she writes, 'You have been sleeping for a month now' (9), channelling the triangular conflation of the coma-sleep-death metaphor. Earlier, Allende reflects on the words spoken to her by a young woman and survivor of porphyria who 'assures' Allende that 'being in a coma is like a sleep without dreams, a mysterious parenthesis' (7), a description that implies that the coma constitutes a void, for what exactly is sleep without dreams? Allende, too, uses the image of birth and the womb, musing, 'Have you returned to the place of total innocence, to the waters of my womb, like the fish you were before you were born?' (35). Again, the coma is imagined to be a form of womb but unlike other authors discussed (Johansen; Hollyman), there is no rebirth – Paula is not 'unwombed' (to again refer to Hollyman's fictional account of coma lightening), never to emerge from coma. Nevertheless, Allende often deploys, as Alice Hall notes, 'The dominant cultural myths and discourses around coma in her narration' (2014: 138). At one point, the author refers to her daughter's 'mysterious state', imbuing the coma with a kind of romantic ideal, while drawing upon mythologies of rebirth, metamorphosis and transfiguration, going on to describe the coma as a 'cocoon' and musing, 'I ask myself what kind of butterfly will emerge when you awake' (162). This language of hope and transformation is similar to that of Jean-Dominique Bauby's description of his own mind trapped within his inert, locked-in state: the animation and beauty of the butterfly, trapped within the dead weight of the diving bell of the paralyzed body. Yet, as Hall notes, 'These myths coexist with a focus on the intricacies of physical care' (138), and while Allende at one points writes of Paula, 'You looked as beautiful as a sleeping bride' (94), seemingly playing into the hands of the sleeping beauty phenomenon, Allende consistently uses contrapuntal imagery of critical care and the degradation of the body. Moments prior to the sleeping beauty image, for example, Allende describes the 'humming of the respirator' and Paula's 'bandaged' feet, her 'arms bruised purple' (79), alongside the 'harsh hole' in her throat, her blocked 'lungs' and the 'deformation' of her body through muscle atrophy (156).

We also see a slippage between coma and the chronic VS, as Allende writes, 'It has been exactly one hundred days since you fell into your coma' (128), providing us with a timeline which suggests that Paula has actually left coma and entered a chronic VS (having been unconscious for over three months following an Acquired Brain Injury (ABI)). This is made clear, later, when Allende actually takes her daughter home to care for her and writes of how, 'Sometimes, she is frightened, trembling, her eyes wide and staring, as if she were seeing visions from Hell' (271), Paula clearly having wakefulness but *without detectable awareness*. This description also highlights another key trope found within coma fiction – the image of Hell, suggesting Paula's PDoC is a katabatic ordeal. But it is an attribution coming from the external perspective of her mother-carer.

Allende's memoir is an interesting one as it oscillates between the language, metaphor and mythologies of hope and medical prognosis, caught between the realities of her daughter's situation and the need for optimism in the face of critical care for Paula. In the final chapter, I will explore further this language of hope alongside the use of the C-Met and B-Met in the depiction and reporting of coma and BI, examining how these conditions are used as a means of 'narrative prosthesis' (to refer to Mitchell and Snyder's concept which describes how literature employs representations of disability as a convenient means for telling stories). I will draw this investigation to a close by discussing exactly how such narratives might affect our collective understanding of these conditions, and the potential real-world impact this might have.

6

Metaphor and narrative prosthesis

Throughout this volume, I have discussed a range of representations of coma and BI in both fiction and non-fiction, eliciting various iterations of the C-Met and B-Met. As discussed in Chapter 1, Susan Sontag sees such metaphorical conversion of illness as 'harmful and destructive', ultimately arguing that illness itself 'can and should be experienced without recourse to metaphoric thinking' (Hawkins 1999: 22). And yet, paradoxically, Sontag opens her second treatise on the subject, *AIDS and Its Metaphors*, with the following admission: 'Of course, one cannot think without metaphors. But that does not mean there aren't some metaphors we might well abstain from or try to retire' (1991: 91). So what are we to make of this seeming inconsistency?

6.1 Revisiting Sontag

Anne Hunsaker Hawkins quite rightly points out the fact that despite Sontag's call for resistance to illness metaphor, she herself pivots her argument *around* a geographical metaphor: separating those who are born into 'the kingdom of the well' from those inhabiting 'the kingdom of the sick' (Hawkins 1999: 23). Furthermore, and in line with Sontag's ambiguity, Hawkins posits that thinking about illness without metaphor is 'an expectation that few of us could live up to. Metaphoric thinking is built into our very mental faculties' (23). This is a position seemingly in support of Lakoff and Johnson in their development of conceptual metaphor theory (CMT) whereby 'conventional patterns of metaphorical expressions in language (e.g. "He *shot down* all of my arguments") are seen as evidence of conventional patterns of metaphoric thought, or conceptual metaphors (e.g. ARGUMENT IS WAR)' (Potts and Semino 2019: 82). As Lakoff and Johnson propose, 'Metaphor is pervasive in everyday life, not just in language, but in thought and action' (1980: 3), arguing that 'human *thought processes* are largely metaphorical' (6). They draw attention to orientational metaphors that associate *up/down* designations with particular feelings, for example (and pertinent to this discussion), 'Get up. Wake up [. . .] He *fell* asleep [. . .] He *sank* into a coma' (15). The latter example is closely linked to the image of 'surfacing' that we find in a lot of coma fiction to describe the emergence from coma

– the *up/down* orientations of *sinking/surfacing* also epitomized by Alex Garland's principle of 'waking is rising and dreaming is sinking'. We might also think about the katabatic C-Met: coma 'is hell' and hell, certainly in Western thought, 'is down'. These orientational metaphors of consciousness, Lakoff and Johnson go on to argue, have a 'physical basis': the fact that 'humans and most other animals sleep lying down and stand up when they awaken' (15).

Barbara Clow similarly calls into question Sontag's argument against illness metaphor. In her ethnographic study of cancer patients and their narratives throughout the last century, Clow explicates the brutal, intrusive nature of early medical cancer care and treatment that was 'frequently disabling as well as disfiguring'. She concludes that 'it is hardly surprising [. . .] that cancer has served as an extraordinarily evocative metaphor in the twentieth century' (2001: 307). Moreover, Clow posits that Sontag's writings 'obscured or ignored the fact that cancer metaphors were rooted in the lived experience of the disease' (307–8). And in an argument that runs in opposition to Couser's assertion that, 'Sontag has brilliantly illustrated how cancer discourse has tended to stigmatize and marginalize the ill' (1997: 45), Clow postulates that the nature of the disease and its treatment was inherently stigmatic, and that, 'Rituals and euphemisms did not necessarily render sufferers mute or helpless: in many cases, they helped patients, families, friends, and physicians to cope with a devastating disease' (311). This is a position supported by Hawkins in her appraisal of myth-making in illness narratives when she notes how 'a fair number of cancer patients, particularly those who use visualization therapy, find undermining the "reality" of their disease to be helpful, and Sontag's assumption that sick people have no control over their illness is one that many pathographers would challenge' (40). Furthermore, in analysing the use of the "battle" myth in describing the treatment of disease (and of which Sontag is so critical), Hawkins argues that its use is 'not at all surprising', even 'predetermined' as, 'We often understand disease as the consequence of a breach of the body's "defense system", a concept that seems very much a function of our habit of thinking militarily' (63-64).

So how are we now to view the use of the C-Met and B-Met in light of this reappraisal of Sontag's central tenet of her argument against illness metaphor? Phillip Lopate contends that while Sontag 'was well aware that her call to reject interpretation made no sense on practical levels' she still 'maintained the zealot's posture while calling for impossibilities that she knew to be impossible. She simply put forward in deadpan her extremist demands' (2009: 32). In this regard, Sontag knowingly disseminated a polemic which, by her own admission, was acutely controversial and contradictory which nevertheless, in Clow's words, 'has had a profound influence on our understanding of the discourse of disease'. As Clow concludes, despite some of the questionable reasoning within her arguments, 'Without Sontag's vision, without her impassioned prose, we might have been much slower to appreciate the importance of language in the illness experience' (311).

Despite the criticism of Sontag's polemic, most recently Potts and Semino, in analysing this dimension of the cancer metaphor, have again highlighted how it is most often utilized in deeply negative discourse, for example, in describing the 'cancer' of political corruption and the need to 'cut out' the disease; or in describing 'violent extremism' which is '*metastasizing* to neighbouring regions' (2019: 92). In their very different conclusions to Hawkins and Clow, they postulate that, 'Overall, the choice of an extremely common illness as a metaphor for a wide range of alleged evils can therefore be described not just as generally insensitive for people affected by cancer but also as reinforcing a view of the disease that may exacerbate anxiety, distress, pessimism, even stigma' (93). It is such an attribution of illness metaphor to wider socio-political discourses that is most germane to our discussions of the C-Met and B-Met.

Yet there is an even more complex dynamic to the C-Met and B-Met. Both Sontag and those theorists revisiting her work are examining illness metaphor when describing the lived experience of illness. This volume has been chiefly discussing illness metaphor when describing fictional experiences of illness whereby the subtext and associations of the C-Met and B-Met have become detached from the realities of lived experience. We might return to the 'coma is hell' C-Met to exemplify this dilemma. Lived experience tells us that coma is not 'hell', at any rate, a conceptual hell based upon mythological archetypes or religious teachings, but is in fact a void. Nevertheless, authors adopt the 'hell' C-Met in its literal biblical or mythological form, depicting complex grand narratives of katabasis that eclipse lived experience. Ben Platts-Mills, in describing his step-mother's coma, demonstrates how myth-making can be employed to more accurately represent the lived experience of illness. He writes, 'Sitting with a person in coma, we feel that there is a separation at play, that their consciousness is not destroyed but elsewhere . . . They have [. . .] gone down, telescoping somehow into a distance that can't be described by normal relations. They are in a place of dream or shadow' (171). Using the Orpheus myth as an example, Platts-Mills describes wanting 'to go down into the shadows and find the person, reach out, guide them back to the light', a quest that, like Orpheus's, is a failure. After all, 'Who could pass this ridiculous trial, this arbitrary test of faith?' (171). The author uses myth-making as a means for encapsulating the realities of coma survival, and the negative prognosis for his step-mother. The failure of the myth of Orpheus correlates quite closely with the failure of Platts-Mills to rescue his step-mother and contrasts with the fictional narratives of katabasis which suggest an easy road out of hell, with a full and immediate recovery.

The fictional C-Met and B-Met, it seems, are products of what Mitchell and Snyder term 'narrative prosthesis', a 'perpetual discursive dependency upon disability' which 'pervades literary narrative'. Its function is twofold: '[F]irst, as a stock feature of characterization and, second, as an opportunistic metaphorical device' (2000: 47). The authors go on to explain how their hypothesis is 'a paradoxical one: disabled people's social invisibility has occurred in the wake of their perpetual circulation throughout print history' (52), a contradiction further supported, they write, by Paul Longmore who has 'perceptively formulated this paradox, asking why we screen so many images of disability and simultaneously screen them out of our minds' (51). Most germane to our discussions, and in particular those arising out of the examination of the katabic C-Met in Chapter 3, Mitchell and Snyder draw attention to what they term 'supplementing the void'. They write, 'The very need for a story is called into being when something has gone amiss with the known world, and, thus, the language of a tale seeks to comprehend that which has stepped out of line. In this sense, stories compensate for an unknown or unnatural deviance that begs an explanation' (53).

The rest of this chapter will examine works of fiction that use coma and BI as narrative prosthesis and the manifestations of the C-Met and B-Met to which this leads – 'opportunistic metaphorical devices'. But it will also look at how such metaphors have filtered into media reportage, prostheticizing news stories of DoC recovery in order to create engaging narratives and an overly simplistic understanding (and conflation) of the conditions. I will conclude by examining the real-world impact this has upon the public understanding of DoC, and the affect this has, in turn, on coma and BI survivors.

6.2 Coma, the neomort and narrative prosthesis

Robin Cook's 1977 novel, *Coma*, follows the investigations of a medical student, Susan Wheeler, as she tries to uncover the mysteries surrounding a number of patients who have inexplicably fallen into coma following otherwise routine operations within Boston Memorial Hospital. Throughout the novel, Cook employs the level of medical detail that one would expect from a writer who, himself, is a trained medical doctor. Central to the novel is the deconstruction of the image of the coma patient as 'sleeping beauty' and consequently, of the sleep C-Met. This is evidenced in the descriptions of Nancy Greenly, the young coma victim who instigates Susan's investigations. Focalizing the confrontation with the comatose patient through Susan, Cook depicts the steady, almost immediate degradation and corruption of Nancy's body and, moreover, of her humanity. Susan, along with her fellow students, notices that there is 'no sign of life save for the rhythmical hiss of the breathing machine' (2008: 51). Like Isabel Allende's descriptions of her daughter, Paula, the organic body has become mechanized and this dehumanizing of the patient is not just a physical process. Nancy is also dehumanized through the attitudes shared by the experienced physicians as they cease to recognize her humanity. Dr Bellows views Nancy purely in terms of medical process, needing to keep 'the ions at the right level', 'the urine output up', 'the bacteria at bay', the absence of the personal pronoun 'her' in Cook's writing indicative of Bellows's determination to obliterate 'the human element' for which he simply doesn't 'have time for' (53). Later, another physician, Stark, sees the 'comatose patient' as being, ultimately, enormously 'rewarding' due largely to the fact that 'the teaching aspect alone is priceless' (75). This process of depersonalizing and dehumanizing the comatose patient is best summed up by Susan who, reflecting upon this dilemma of the body and of personhood, concludes that, 'Nancy Greenly had become a technical challenge, a game to be played' (92).

In his physical description of Nancy, Cook initially seems to conjure the 'sleeping beauty' trope, describing her face as 'marble white' in direct correlation with the aestheticizing of Louis Drax in Liz Jensen's novel. As Cook proceeds to depict the beauty of Nancy's 'sable brown' hair, this process of glorification of the body of the comatose patient seems to be heightening, reflecting the 'elegance' of Lauren's post-accident corporeality in Levy's *If Only It Were True*. However, almost as soon as this sleeping beauty aesthetic is created, Cook begins to depict the degradation of the body. He describes her 'dried and cracked' lips, her 'mouth held open with a plastic mouthpiece' and the 'brownish material' that has 'crusted and hardened on her front teeth'. A similar register of language appears in Richard Dooling's *Critical Care*, discussed earlier, again a novel written by an author who has lived experience of working with patients within DoC. He similarly writes in terms of abjection, the 'swirling mass of vomit, snot, drugs, clotted blood, and whatever else was being siphoned out' alongside the 'cloudy dark brown urine' of the patient (1992: 39) who exhibits a 'death mask of dry skin' (38). It is a description translated to screen by Sidney Lumet, focusing on the grey, leathery complexion and long white hair of Bed Five who looks little more than a withered corpse. In this cinematic representation, Lumet flawlessly renders Dooling's description in the novel: 'Gray, gray, gray. Bed Five's skin color was gray. His hair was gray. His brain was gray. He was gray-faced. He was not alive or dead; he was gray' (1992: 238). Robin Cook, however, continues to intersperse glamorized, figurative language in his description of the comatose patient, as Susan holds one of Nancy's hands 'as if reaching for a delicate piece of porcelain' (54). Again, like Allende, Cook vacillates between imagery of organic degradation and a bodily aesthetic (the image of porcelain used also by Liz Jensen to describe her eponymous comatose hero). Notably, though, this is focalized through Susan herself, conveying her increasingly horrified attitude at the dehumanizing of the coma patient, something to which she is already succumbing in viewing Nancy as a piece of 'porcelain': inanimate and breakable. It is an attitude that is stressed, a short time later, when Bellows declares, in relation to Nancy's prognosis, 'If her squash is gone, I mean wiped out, then we might as well get the kidneys for someone else' (56). This objectification of the comatose patient indirectly references the origins of the vegetative state coined by Jennet and Plum in 1972 in order to designate 'the contrast between the severe mental loss and the subject's preserved autonomic or vegetative functions' (1980: 6). It is a dehumanizing image and sentiment similarly evoked in *Critical Care*, though even more bluntly and cruelly as Werner muses relentlessly: 'Your father is an acorn squash, a turnip, a Mr. Potato, gomerland, a gork, a chunk on a slab, a veg, a stiff, lunch meat, a carcass, a hamburger, fertilizer, a box lunch for worms' (194). For Susan in *Coma*, there is a huge disparity between this kind of attitude and her more humane (and somewhat naïve) approach. At the same time, it serves as a narrative prosthesis for the novel, foreshadowing the events to come and the object of Susan's investigations. Gradually, she begins to uncover a hospital conspiracy whereby patients are deliberately forced into irreversible coma on the operating table, following which they are housed in the sinister Jefferson Institute where their lives are sustained until the last moment when their bodies are 'harvested' for organ donations.

Cook's novel explores debates surrounding medical ethics and black market organ donation, focusing on the comatose patient as a paradigm of what has been termed the *neomort*: the 'new dead', a term coined by the psychiatrist and bioethicist Willard Gaylin in 1974 in his controversial article for *Harper's*, 'Harvesting the Dead'. In this think-piece, Gaylin addresses the issue of the increasing number of vegetative patients whose lives are being sustained in hospitals and care-facilities consuming valuable space. He proposes that such 'neomorts' can be housed in vast '*bioemporia*' or 'farms of cadavers' where they can be 'harvested' for organ transplantation, drug studies and medical teaching and education (1974: 26). Cook's novel, therefore, arises out of such a vision of future medical praxis, although despite including an 'Author's Note' at the end of the novel that contains his own reflections on the inspiration for *Coma*, there is actually no reference to Gaylin's article. Nevertheless, Cook's Jefferson Institute is the archetypal embodiment of a Gaylinian *bioemporium*, with swathes of comatose patients suspended in mid-air by cables within vast hangars or 'barns' (to extend Gaylin's metaphor of farming), their vitals constantly monitored and adjusted by cyber-technology. Even before Susan realizes that these neomorts have been deliberately forced into coma, she finds it difficult, ethically, to accept this situation, struggling to see the comatose patient as anything other than 'a sleeping human being' and not simply 'a brainless shell' (109). In this, Susan voices the opinions and misconceptions of the wider, lay population: that coma is little more than a deep sleep, a concept arising from the proliferation of the C-Met. As her initial investigations lead to a tour of the institute, she gets the 'impression of grotesque, horizontal, sleeping marionettes' (287) hanging above her. Cook again uses dehumanizing imagery to convey Susan's dilemma over exactly what existential state the comatose patient occupies, at one point his protagonist saying, 'It's like some science fiction setting. A machine taking care of a host of mindless people. It's almost as if these patients aren't people' (289). However, Michelle, the Head of Operations at the Institute, is under no illusion as to where on the spectrum of consciousness and, moreover, of humanity these neomorts lie: 'They aren't people [. . .] They *were* people; now they're brain stem preparations', before extolling the virtues the bioemporium offers in a 'cost-effectiveness crisis' (289). This reference to the economic 'value' of the comatose patient reflects Gaylin's own discussion of the 'cost-benefit analysis' of the bioemporium (28), a financial dimension of the neomort that is further exemplified in Michael Crichton's 1978 film adaptation of the novel, with a scene in the Jefferson Institute in which shadowy individuals bid by tele-link on the sale of organs.

In Mikael Salomon's TV mini-series adaptation, Michelle's unwavering perception of the neomort is complicated further through her equivalent character Mrs Emerson (Ellen Burstyn), who, when prompted by Susan, describes the comatose patients thus: 'You see, they're not really alive, but they're not dead either' (2012) in an echo of Dooling's description of Bed Five. Exploring the preoccupations and concerns of the current climate, this adaptation sees the neomort as the perfect subject for the advancement of the Human Genome Programme. By triggering coma in those patients pre-disposed to certain medical conditions (Alzheimer's Disease being of particular concern to this adaptation) the neomorts are used for experimentation and research in the pursuit of finding a cure for such genetic disorders. The bodies are also, as is revealed in one particularly graphic sequence, used as receptacles for surrogate babies, while providing valuable stem cells from umbilical cords. The neomorts are referred to as a herd that must be culled in order to create a eugenics programme for the betterment of mankind, once more conveying Gaylin's use of agricultural metaphor in relation to his cadaver farms. This most recent adaptation uses narrative prosthesis to develop the concept of cyber-phobia (at which Cook hinted in the original source material), with a vast computer-driven bioemporium transporting bodies to 'visiting chambers' where the neomorts, meticulously arranged and groomed, are deposited into beds, ready for their families to visit.

Coma, and its various adaptations, raises some important questions surrounding the identity of the comatose patient. Cook's novel attempts to address some of the misrepresentations and mythologies surrounding this DoC, deconstructing the sleeping beauty C-Met, for example, or presenting the long-term physical effects. It also explores a key and controversial philosophical and bioethical debate regarding the existential positioning of the neomort who can be seen as neither fully alive, nor not quite dead which, by implication, means that they occupy both of these polar existential states. Similarly, it examines the prognosis of continuing or chronic VS and raises difficult ethical questions, introduced by Gaylin's work, with regard to how the neomort might be utilized. Simultaneously, coma is used as a wider metaphor and narrative prosthesis that pivots towards an exploration of a host of more global themes: the sale of black market organs; cyber and techno-phobia; patient depersonalization; medical ethics and sexual politics in the workplace. Throughout the novel, for example, Susan's authority as a physician is persistently undermined by her male colleagues because of her gender. In her analysis of Crichton's adaptation of *Coma* as a 'progressive' text in its representation of a female protagonist, Elizabeth Cowie asserts that, aside from the conspiracy of the bioemporium within the central thrust of the narrative, there exists another dominant conspiracy: 'A kind of male conspiracy, of a collective male prejudice against the idea that a woman could be right – that if a woman is saying something disagreeable she must be neurotic' (1988: 122). In this regard, we might view Susan's career as metaphorically comatose and at the mercy of a controlling, paternalistic profession. In the era of post-Watergate conspiracy dramas, Cook's novel (and film adaptation) seamlessly 'transplanted' the culture of fear and paranoia into the medical thriller, using coma as narrative prosthesis and metaphor for wider thematic and bioethical concerns.

A more problematic example of the use of coma as narrative prosthesis, and one which will help to exemplify the complexities and controversies of the use of the C-Met, is Douglas Coupland's 1998 novel, *Girlfriend in a Coma*. This work of coma fiction is centred upon the fate of Karen McNeil who, after consuming a dangerous concoction of alcohol and a small amount of her mother's downers one night at a party, subsequently collapses into coma.

In his descriptions of Karen, Coupland, similar to Cook, Dooling and Powers, focuses upon the degradation of the body. In descriptions focalized through Richard (who holds vigil by his lover's bed), Coupland describes Karen's 'ever-shrinking hands reduced to talons' (1998: 25), an image similarly evoked in *Critical Care* with the description of 'Bed Five's' 'yellow claw foot' (39). Karen's eyes are likened to those of 'a *photo* of an aquarium fish' (46): not even a *real* fish but a simulacrum of a fish. Karen's stomach bulges 'like a goiter on a crone's neck', her body is 'withered and shrunk to skin and bones, [appearing] more like a yellow leather hide stretched over bone drums' (46, 62). Coupland continues to use animal metaphor to illustrate the ongoing dehumanizing effects of coma, but where before Karen's hands were described as the talons of a living creature, now her body is likened to the skin of a dead animal: she becomes an incarnation of the living dead, again like Dooling's Bed Five. The ethical dilemma over the existential state of the neomort is also addressed with Karen's mother immediately asking, 'Is she *alive*? Is she dead?' (26). And later, over ten years after Karen entered coma, Richard muses, 'And what of Karen? Neither alive nor dead after all these years, ever dimming from the world's mind – rasping, blinded, and pretzeled in a wheelchair'

(74), a description that also emphasizes Karen's gradual physical wastage, her muscle atrophy causing her limbs to desiccate and curl in on themselves.

The novel clearly recodes the sleeping beauty C-Met, representing Richard's unending love for Karen, regardless of her physical decline: she does not need to be physically beautiful for Richard to have feelings for her still. However, we soon discover that the novel's title may be a misnomer: that Karen is not, after all, a 'girlfriend in a coma' but a 'girlfriend in a vegetative state'. This is implied very early on in the novel when her physician explains to her parents that, 'Karen will have sleep and wake cycles and may even *dream*' (26). Later in the novel, Richard describes Karen thus: 'She moves her head, her eyes flicker, and for three seconds she sees the sky and the clouds' (74). It becomes clear that Karen actually inhabits PVS, that disorder of consciousness 'characterized by the complete absence of behavioural evidence for self or environmental awareness' yet with the 'preserved capacity for spontaneous or stimulus-induced arousal, evidenced by sleep-wake cycles' (Giacino et al. 2002: 349). Moreover, Coupland is quite overt about the PDoC into which his heroine slips, with the character Dr Menger announcing to her friends, 'It doesn't give me any pleasure to tell you, kids, but your friend, Karen, is in what's known as a persistent vegetative state'. Coupland, in a literary move that seems to lift information directly from the medical literature on PVS, develops this announcement with Menger asserting that Karen 'is completely unaware of either herself or her environment', despite having 'sleep cycles and awake cycles', lacking any 'high brain function' (41). At the heart of this novel lies a puzzling dilemma whereby Coupland knowingly conflates coma with the persistent vegetative state (in this case, a chronic VS): two markedly different DoC.

Coupland's primary use of the C-Met lies within his characterization of Karen herself, and the narrative prosthesis she performs. Prior to becoming comatose, she warns Richard of a dream she had, a 'dark . . . Future' where 'everybody looks so old' (28), 'meaningless' and '*electronic*' (10). Insisting this is not just a dream but a prophetic vision, she speaks of Richard's (and her friends') future selves, all seeming normal but with 'eyes . . . without souls' (11), what Andrew Tate terms as 'images of a ruined future' that predict 'the prospect of an epoch of debris and an end to originality' (2007: 89). She also predicts her own departure, and even her return from 'wherever it is' she has gone (28). As predicted, Karen emerges from her chronic VS to find that the world has changed, dominated by new technologies, greed and social dysfunction – the dystopia of capitalist postmodernity. Her friends live a collectively vapid existence based upon the bogus 'phenomenon of self-fashioning supposedly afforded by capitalism' (Tate 2007: 78). Richard, her once-teenage lover, is an alcoholic; her friends, Pam and Hamilton, are successful yet vacuous, hooked on heroin, which they treat as a recreational drug of the middle classes; and Linus remains unchanged from high school but stagnating, unable to translate the intellectual promise he exhibited as a teenager into a career that is worthy of his talents. Coupland, therefore, uses the C-Met and narrative prosthesis as a means for critiquing postmodern capitalist society and what Tate refers to as 'desire culture' and an 'economy that relies on a ceaseless flow of images' (53–4) and which impacts upon identity politics of Coupland's 'Generation X', a 'generation 'purposefully hiding itself' as it searched, in a distracted, leisurely fashion, for an identity of its own' (Tate 2007: 8). Mark Forshaw views *Girlfriend in a Coma* as a contemporary satire which adopts 'an Irving-derived device' in order to critique 'a world of dehumanizing and, ultimately, pointless accelerated capitalism' (2000: 46). Forshaw name checks Washington Irving, referring to his story of 1819, *The Tale of Rip Van Winkle*, which itself, nearly two-hundred years before *Girlfriend in a Coma*, used the 'deep sleep' metaphor to satirize the hardships of the American Revolution through which Rip had the good fortune to sleep. In Coupland's novel, the C-Met is used to target his Generation X. Prior to going into coma, for example, Karen speaks of her need to consistently fit into her 'size-five bikini' (18) and the Valium she ingests prior to falling unconscious seems to be at least one method to suppress her appetite. While in coma, and as Jefferson Faye observes, Karen is finally able to achieve her 'supermodel physique' (2001: 507), Coupland simultaneously presenting the physical implications of PDoC while satirizing postmodern society and the existential crisis of self-image of those who inhabit it. There is also an explicit reference to Irving's protagonist with Karen, in a reluctant post-'coma' interview with a cable news channel that is desperate to report on her 'miracle' recovery, being asked by a reporter: 'How does it *feel* to be a modern Rip Van Winkle?' (166). It is a motif that is similarly utilized in Wolfgang Becher's tragi-comedy *Good Bye, Lenin!* (2003) in which an East German woman and proud supporter of the Communist regime, Christiane, suffers a near-fatal heart attack and falls into coma during an anti-government demonstration in which her son is arrested. During her eight-month 'coma' (in reality, a chronic VS), she missed the fall of the Berlin Wall and the gradual Westernization of East Germany, her daughter, for example, abandoning her economics studies for a job in Burger King. Christiane, herself, is depicted as a sleeping beauty figure, with a high colour in her tranquil face and no degradation of the body, frequently referred to, by her son who narrates the film, as inhabiting a deep sleep. Her emergence from coma, like sleeping beauty, is triggered by a kiss – but in an interesting subversion of the fairy tale, it is a kiss between her son and his lover, a nurse in charge of Christiane's care. Speaking of her emergence from coma, her doctor says, 'That she woke up is a miracle but she might not be the same as she was', primarily referring to her amnesia. Because of this, her son is told she's still in danger and should be protected from any potential shocks that might worsen her condition and so her son, fearing a confrontation with such political upheaval might bring on another heart attack, sets about maintaining the illusion that reunification has never occurred. The coma is a perfect narrative prosthesis for exploring and satirizing socio-political issues in 1990s Germany.

In a moment of life imitating art, this version of the Van Winkle C-Met used to satirize socio-political upheaval can be seen in the reportage of a real-life modern 'Rip Van Winkle', Jan Grzebski. Grzebski emerged, in 2006, from a nineteen-year chronic VS to find that Poland was no longer under the rule of the Soviet Union or a communist president, that the Berlin Wall had fallen, and that the world had become a slave to unrecognizable technologies and consumer culture, dominated by mobile phones and ipods (Parfitt, *The Guardian* 2007).

In Coupland's novel, Karen, as a Van Winkle figure, provides another narrative prosthesis to explore the changed world on the brink of the millennium with Coupland further deploying the C-Met in the representation of Karen trapped within a stuttering loop of a past existence. Her body 'retains memories long after [her] mind' (135) has forgotten them: an organic, corporeal databank. And Coupland emphasizes this image, writing, 'Karen is a time capsule – a creature from another era reborn' (137). It is these reborn memories, this yearning, nostalgic invocation of the 1970s that makes Karen the ideal subject through which her friends (and the reader) can view the world with a fresh pair of eyes: the eyes of the resurrected neomort.

Coupland's use of the C-Met intensifies when Karen's post-coma prophetic predictions of an apocalypse turn out to be not just satirical representations of postmodern society, but of a literal, global apocalypse. The world's population (with the exception of Karen and her friends) succumbs to a sleeping sickness pandemic which causes the victim to drift into a somnolent state, shortly after which they die. This cataclysmic disaster is described, significantly, as the 'whole world [going] into coma' (229). Coupland simultaneously uses the coma-as-sleep and coma-as-death versions of the C-Met with similar undertones of the socio-political metaphor, for example, employed by Senator Lloyd Bentsen and throughout Chuck Palahniuk's *Diary*, discussed earlier, in which protagonist Misty Wilmot sees her husband's coma as a metaphor of her own life, trapped as she is within a loveless, joyless and ambitionless limbo. It is also deployed, perhaps somewhat ironically given the realist depiction of coma within the novel, in the paratextual review quote by Joe Stretch on the cover of Hollyman's *Lairies*: 'A bedtime story for a country in a coma'. It is a quote that at once uses the socio-political C-Met to describe a stunned, affectless society while simultaneously using the sleep C-Met to convey the fact that this is a bedtime story for this somnolent, comatose population.

Despite facing the apocalypse, Karen's friends still fail to change their selfish and materialistic lives, and it is within the final denouement of the novel that Coupland's use of the C-Met and narrative prosthesis is amplified. The novel takes a fantastical direction, with Karen, together with the ghost of a former high-school friend, Jared (through whom this last section of the novel is focalized) proclaiming to her friends that it is within their power to restore the world to its former pre-apocalyptic state. All they have to do is to alter their shallow existence and promise to do everything in their power to change the ways of the world by forever challenging the iniquities and vagaries of modern society: by 'boiling the carcass of the old order' (271). There is one big catch. In order for this to happen, the ultimate sacrifice has to be made: Karen has to return to her comatose state, positioning the novel as a work of 'fantastic' literature. The fantastic, Todorov asserts, is a literary genre in which a character is confronted by seemingly supernatural events. Both the character and the reader are uncertain whether these events have been artificially created through illusion or trickery (in which case, the laws of nature remain unbroken) or whether these events have truly taken place (in which case, there is an acceptance of extant laws that are unknown to us). It follows that the fantastic occupies this duration of uncertainty (1973: 25). It is usual, Todorov goes on to discuss, that at the end of a story the reader ceases to hesitate and comes to a decision, whether the character does or not. If he decides that 'the laws of reality remain intact and permit an explanation of the phenomena described', then the narrative belongs to the subgenre of the 'uncanny'. However, if he decides that the events truly are of the supernatural order, then the narrative slides into another subgenre: the 'marvellous' (41). On first glance, it would seem that Coupland's novel is an example of what Todorov would term the marvellous in its 'pure state' (52), whereby the reader accepts immediately the events as being of the supernatural order. After all, Coupland, from the outset, suggests that the novel is truly 'marvellous' by creating a first chapter narrated from the point of view of a ghost: Jared. It is also Jared who picks up the narration in the last section of the novel, directly influencing Karen and her friends in what they must do to save mankind from the apocalyptic sleeping sickness plague. In this use of the fantastic and the supernatural, the novel is also paradigmatic of what Tate sees as a 'revival of interest in dreams, altered states of perception and the power of the supernatural' in late twentieth and early twenty-first century narrative (60). This provides a further explanation for the modes of narrative employed in coma novels *Marabou Stork Nightmares* (1996) and Alex Garland's *The Coma* (2004), despite these appearing concurrently with the rise of the neuronovel and a shift towards novels of the brain. In the end, despite Coupland's medical, realist descriptions of Karen's physical wastage while in coma, the coma itself is revealed to be a 'marvellous' phenomenon, a motif of the curse of deep sleep so common in fairy tales that, Todorov posits, occupy 'marvellous' fiction. Moreover, Karen's descent into and return from coma can be likened to mythological tales of the katabatic hero who descends into hell and receives prophetic knowledge. Returning once more to the earlier description of Karen while in coma, Coupland's description of her respirator tube 'hissing sick threats of doom' serves to subvert the sleeping beauty archetype and embodies the 'marvellous' function of her character—her precognitive powers and messianic status that she finally attains. It is a status that is similarly granted to Stephen King's katabatic hero, Johnny Smith, and so both Coupland's novel and King's develop a marvellous embodiment of coma (or, more accurately, chronic VS), set against the backdrop of an impending apocalypse, thereby elevating each protagonist to the position of modern-day messiah, with Karen and Johnny ultimately sacrificing themselves to save mankind. Yet despite Coupland's novel residing within the genre of 'fantastic' fiction, within its use of coma as narrative prosthesis lies a deeply problematic ethical question.

6.3 Narrative prosthesis, metaphor and the hope economy

In an article for the Toronto *Globe and Mail* in 2007, fellow Canadian novelist, Robert Wiersema, discusses his own work of coma fiction, *Before I Wake* (2006), a literary fantasy that similarly exploits the motif of the coma patient as a 'miraculous' being. The novel follows three-year-old Sherry Barrett who, while in coma after a hit-and-run incident, has the power to cure the illnesses of those who come in contact with her. In his article 'Wake Up, Wake Up, You Sleepyhead', Wiersema, writing of the inevitable comparison of Jan Grzebski's recovery to the Rip Van Winkle archetype, asserts that, 'Characters in comas don't lend themselves well to dramatic conflict [. . .] a comatose character perhaps isn't the best vehicle for narrative tension. Awakening from a coma, however, is another matter entirely' (2007). Wiersema, in a similar vein to Alex Garland commenting upon how the condition of coma allowed him to write expansively about wider concerns (in his case, dreams), discusses how the coma trope provides a useful narrative prosthesis and metaphor that allows authors to creatively explore a range of wider existential questions and crises. This comment also resonates with Couser's observation that, 'Disability generally does not impose the sort of narrative scripts or plots that illnesses do' (1997: 185), possibly providing us with a further explanation as to why the C-Met proliferates, and why there is an erasure in fiction of a representation of the permanence of BI. Wiersema refers to Grzebski's 'nineteen-year coma', alongside his potential for, like van Winkle, a 'long, contented life' that appears to be on the 'horizon'. Yet again, we encounter the slipperiness of the language of coma and PDoC and we must remind ourselves, once more, that comas do not tend to last for more than a few weeks, thereafter patients enter the PVS (continuing/chronic VS). But it also erases the potential for BI, applying a 'comic plot' to represent disability, to refer again to Couser's analysis of illness narratives. It is useful therefore to explore the Grzebski case in more detail before examining the coma trope at play within Wiersema's own novel.

Shortly after the report of Grzebski's 'miraculous' and 'fairy tale' recovery, it was revealed that the first time Grzebski, himself, had heard about his likening to Rip Van Winkle was when he read it in the local Polish newspaper that originally broke the story. In truth, he revealed that he was only in a 'coma' for four years, after which he was confined to a wheelchair. However, the editor-in-chief of the newspaper defended the story, contending that, 'There are different kinds of coma. There is a kind of coma where people are unconscious and others where they wake up from time to time, and then fall back into coma' (Leidig, *Media Guardian* 2007). Yet such a description seems to reflect the state of 'coma vigil' or 'akinetic mutism' in which there are prolonged 'wakeful periods' during which the patient presents 'silent, alert-appearing immobility ... in which sleep-wake cycles have returned, but externally obtainable evidence for mental activity remains almost entirely absent and spontaneous motor activity is lacking' (Plum and Posner 1980: 7). Most interesting is that both Grzebski's physician and wife maintained that he 'was not in a coma' for all that time, only being comatose for 'the first four years' (Leidig), although even this four-year coma seems contentious, given what we know about the transition from coma to the vegetative state. Again, this discrepancy in the perception and reportage of Grzebski's PDoC lies in the slippage of language used to describe such disorders, similarly seen in many of the works of fiction discussed herein, and openly acknowledged by Coupland in his fictional physician's diagnosis of Karen's PVS/chronic VS. Thus, what the editor-in-chief of Grzebski's local newspaper denotes as being a 'coma' was, more than likely, a chronic VS. Grzebski's recovery, therefore, was not a 'miracle' or an immediate 'awakening' from coma with an effortless transition back to pre-coma personhood, but a painful and protracted transition between traumatic DoC: from coma to the persistent vegetative state to the minimally conscious state to consciousness, and extensive rehabilitation thereafter. As an interesting coda to this case, in the BBC's initial reporting of Grzebski, their news website contains a paragraph (a supposedly factual pull-quote defining coma) that is particularly informative for our discussions: 'Although those in coma do not respond to stimuli in a meaningful way, contrary to popular belief they do not always lie quiet and still – in some cases they can move, open their eyes and even talk' (*BBC News Online*: 2007). Certainly, the comatose patient may respond to pain stimuli, for example, the testing of motor functions being one criterion for determining the depth of coma and an eventuality that is rendered in Cook's novel *Coma*, as Susan pinches Nancy's thigh. Susan '[recoils] in horror' as Nancy's body stiffens in a 'painful contraction', her jaw performing a 'side-to-side chewing motion' (110). However, it is explained that Nancy has had 'a seizure of some kind', contrasting markedly with what the BBC classification purports, a definition that describes the PVS rather than coma.

This slippage between the language of coma and wider PDoC is apparent, too, in Wiersema's novel, a core narrative turning point centred around the moment when Sherry is disconnected from her life-support machine and artificial respirator, a moment which the medical staff expect to be the point of 'Sherry's death' (2006: 52). But what seems to be Sherry's 'breath, her last breath, escaping from her' turns out not to be so: 'There was a wheeze as she breathed against the pressure of the machine, against the tubes in her mouth and nose [. . .] Another breath. And then choking . . . choking' (55). Despite the fact that (as we shall see) spontaneous, autonomous breathing is a key indicator of the PVS/chronic VS, suggesting that this is the existential liminal state which Sherry now occupies, Wiersema exploits the miraculous element of her survival from coma, with even medical staff observing, 'No one could explain why, but her condition didn't deteriorate. Her vital signs were absolutely normal [. . .] None of the things we would normally be on the lookout for, from bedsores to muscle atrophy to infections, ever manifested' (72). Sherry's VS is a state of miraculous (and 'marvellous') *otherness* as we soon discover when she becomes a manifestation of a living Christian relic, with pilgrims flocking to her in order to be cured of their terminal illnesses. Despite his assertion in his *Globe and Mail* article that 'awakening from coma' provides the real fascination for authors of fiction, for Wiersema, awakening plays an insignificant role in his novel and similar to Coupland's Karen, Sherry 'wakes' (albeit briefly) before immediately sacrificing herself in a messianic act akin to that of both Karen and Johnny Smith, curing all the pilgrims surrounding her home.

There are clear similarities between the novels of Wiersema and Coupland regarding the representation of the miracle coma and the slippage between coma and VS, but we also see a similarity in the way Coupland, too, perceives the coma (and the imagined events following an 'awakening' from coma) as a useful narrative prosthesis or metaphor – and this is where the deep controversy lies.

In an article, again for the Toronto *Globe and Mail* from 1998, Coupland, discussing the inspiration for the novel, told interviewer Stephen Smith that, 'I like the notion that comas can allow a person to radically reinvent themselves upon awakening. I think we all want to do that – radically reinvent ourselves – I think it's our deepest need'. Coupland simultaneously employs the language of sleep ('awakening' from coma) while continuing to refer to Karen's PDoC as 'coma', despite overtly acknowledging it to be a chronic VS within the pages of the novel. The tone and subtext of the comment is likewise controversial, implying that the coma is a fantastic 'opportunity' for the redevelopment of a new self, as though the medical condition offers a *choice* for the coma survivor. Just as Welsh and Garland represent a sense of control *within* coma, Coupland speaks of a sense of control *outside* of coma – freedom presented to the resurrected neomort. The potential for permanent BI is erased once more, reflecting Robert Wiersema's implication that the narrative prosthesis of coma has to be manipulated and exploited in some way if an engaging, commercial fiction is to be created. However, the most problematic aspect of Coupland's comment comes to light when considering the real inspiration for the novel: the high-profile case of Karen Quinlan.

In 1975, Karen Ann Quinlan, after accidentally ingesting a combination of alcohol and sedatives, suffered a heart attack which caused massive brain damage, leaving her in a *permanent* vegetative state. In 1976, her father's application to remove his daughter's ventilator was granted by the New Jersey Supreme Court. However, once removed, Quinlan survived for another nine years in a vegetative state, therefore drawing to the attention of the public the fact that 'VS patients breathe spontaneously' (Latronico et al. 2011: 6), a revelation described in Wiersema's depiction of Sherry's removal from life-support apparatus. The parallels between this case and Coupland's novel are immediately clear: both patient and fictional counterpart enter coma after ingesting a cocktail of alcohol and Valium; both were in the habit of taking prescription drugs as part of an extreme dietary regime; both enter coma, and shortly thereafter, a chronic VS, maintaining and sustaining autonomous aspiration; the full name of Coupland's character is Karen Ann McNeil, the fictional equivalent of Karen Ann Quinlan. This is complicated by the fact that Coupland's novel is clearly a work of marvellous fiction and one might argue that the author does not purport to represent realistically a medical condition since Karen's coma, in the end, is revealed to be a supernatural phenomenon and not a biomedical reality. This being said, the circumstances leading up to the coma, alongside the description of the ensuing chronic VS, are entirely based upon a biomedical reality: on the medical history of Karen Quinlan. Even Jared himself, when explaining to Karen why she was 'chosen' as apocalyptic prophetess, admits that the cause of her coma was a biomedical inevitability when he says, 'You were taking all those diet pills and starving yourself' (212), further indicating mimetic detail within a work of marvellous fiction. Indeed, on closer inspection of the novel's structure, I would argue that there is nothing to overtly suggest that her coma has been supernaturally induced, up until the point whereby Jared re-emerges in the final section of the novel and explains what her function has been (and will be) in the salvation of mankind. This leads us to re-evaluate the subgenre of fantastic literature into which *Girlfriend in a Coma* can be placed. Granted, Jared's initial narration immediately signifies to the reader that the text is a work of marvellous fiction in its 'pure state' (in accordance with Todorov's theory) yet for the characters, it is only really their direct encounter with Jared towards the end of the novel that confirms this. It follows, therefore, that up until this point they are caught within the 'fantastic-marvellous', a class of narrative, as defined by Todorov, that presents itself as fantastic but which ends with an acceptance of the supernatural (Todorov 1973: 52). Thus, the characters (and, by implication, the reader) encounter fantastic events (Karen's coma; the miracle birth of her child while in coma; her miracle 'awakening' with cognition intact; her prophetic visions) that could have rational explanations, but in the end are revealed to be truly marvellous. Despite Jared's initial narration from the grave, Karen's coma could still be real, and this illusion of reality is generated and sustained precisely because of Coupland's use of mimetic techniques (descriptions of medical processes; definitions of PDoC; evocation of real-life patient case studies), an element of the author's style that Robert McGill has referred to as his 'trademark slacker realism' (2000: 252). *Girlfriend in a Coma* therefore embodies Mitchell and Snyder's concept of narrative prosthesis in its fullest sense in both revealing disability in the form of vegetative states and then simultaneously erasing disability through its depiction of total, immediate recovery, eclipsing the inevitable BI of chronic vegetative states.

The socio-political fallout of such cultural representations and conflations of DoC, together with an erasure of representations of BI and long-term neurological conditions, has a palpable impact not only upon the public understanding of coma and other DoC, generating widespread confusion and misinformation, but also upon the public's recognition of and empathy with BI and its survivors. If the public receive representations of coma that largely belie the possibility of BI, or even (in the case of a film like *Trance*) representations of brain injury that propagate the belief that the neurological, organic damage is 'curable', then the public are poorly equipped with the knowledge that would allow them to recognize survivors of BI in the world at large. This has the potential for real-world stigmatization of survivors. Frequently, those survivors I have worked with have alluded to experiences which speak of their stigmatization in a society where misinformation about BI is abound. Both Steph Grant and Caroline Waugh have discussed how, on numerous occasions, they have been mistaken for being 'drunk' because of slurred speech or impaired motor functions. Caroline even spoke of one occasion when, phoning for an ambulance for her sick son, the emergency operator refused to help, again mistaking Caroline's slurred speech (a consequence of her TBI) for alcohol-impairment. Couser writes that 'one response to marginalization by disabled people (like marginalized groups) has been to challenge the prevailing terminology' (1997: 179). Members of The Write Way thus see their writings as a means of doing this: to challenge the prevailing terminology and ableist dominant narratives proliferated across fiction and the media which have somehow 'invalidated' the group's narratives of lived experience.

This 'invalidation' of lived experience of BI is curiously no more evident than in a film *about* BI: Robert Zemeckis's biopic *Welcome To Marwen*, discussed earlier. In collapsing and reordering the timeline of Hogancamp's life, the narrative follows a conventional structure of triumph over adversity that sees Mark's struggle to face his attackers in court which in turn impacts upon his desire to attend his first photographic show. The animation sequences when his models come to life begin to represent psychoanalytical confrontations with the traumatic past and when these are resolved, Mark is then able to attend court and attend his show, creating narrative closure of resolution and restoring the comic plot, to again refer to Couser's work on disability narratives. As discussed, the film, unlike the documentary, does not end with Mark's model beginning to create his own models in a *mise-en-abyme* of traumatic simulation, yet closes on a very similar shot. In Zemeckis's film, Steve Carrell's Mark, triumphant at overcoming his trauma, walks down the road pulling his model truck; in the documemoir, it is Model Mark who pulls the truck, taking photographs of his scaled models as Hogancamp narrates the need for his model to create a system to help him deal with the trauma of the attack. In short, Zemeckis's film seems to erase the permanence of organic BI, even seeming to imply that Mark's hallucinations as the models come to life are purely the product of psychological trauma. In fact, when we first see Mark pulling his model truck to his place of work, Patsy Cline's 'Crazy' plays, this use of non-diegetic sound again depicting Mark's condition as purely functional and negating the permanence of organic damage. *Welcome To Marwen*, then, is another example of erasure of disability through narrative prosthesis that can have a profound effect upon how BI is understood.

John McClure writes extensively on the misunderstanding of BI, examining the role of causal attributions in public misconceptions. Because, largely speaking, 'brain injury is invisible' (2011: 85), the general public, when confronted with the behaviours of a BI survivor (disinhibited or aggressive behaviour, for example), will 'misattribute' these as being facets of the individual's inherent personality or nature. In line with my discussions of the perception of BI being curable, McClure posits that, 'Many of the public believe that . . . a person with even severe brain injury may completely recover apart from some problems with memory' (86), reflecting the preoccupation with memory and amnesia that is common within fictional representations of coma and BI, *Goodbye, Lenin!*, for example. McClure concludes, 'With invisible conditions such as brain injury, people tend to discount the severity of the injury and suggest that the person will fully recover all their normal abilities' (87). This medical perspective reflects Sontag's critique of contemporary culture and, in particular, her notion, discussed earlier, that when a disease becomes a metaphor, the victim of the disease becomes both a victim and a culprit. In the case of the BI survivor, the public extend their sympathy, yet soon lose this when the survivor does not fully recover: when the survivor is perceived to be 'not trying hard enough' to recover. It seems to me that this 'invisibility' that McClure speaks of is perpetuated by the wealth of coma fictions that are in the public domain, highlighting the central findings of the Wijdicks's study of the misrepresentations of coma in motion pictures, and the potential impact and influence that these had, they discovered, on public audiences. Similarly, a study by Hux, Schram and Goeken alongside one by Casarett et al. point towards the proliferation of misinformation surrounding BI in the public consciousness and the links to fictional representations. Hux et al., in their survey replication study that aimed to update information about the public understanding of BI gained in a previous study, discovered that, 'Regarding brain injury recovery, the public has shown increased misperception over the years concerning the feasibility of complete recovery following severe injury' (2006: 550). In assessing possible causes of this misperception, they observe that, 'Speculation about the role of popular forms of media entertainment – such as magazines, newspapers, books, television shows and movies – seems feasible', noting how, 'Many respondents in the current study made comments such as, "I saw that once in a movie" or, "It happened in my soap opera"'. They conclude that because 'many accounts in the popular media portray survivors of brain injury as recovering completely' this does a 'disservice to survivors of brain injury' and 'encourages people to believe that recovery from acquired brain damage is totally within the control of an individual survivor' (552). Casarett et al.'s own study into the representation of prognosis of coma in daytime television dramas come to similar conclusions, observing that, 'Patients in soap operas who experience coma [. . .] are very likely to regain full function' (2005: 1538) and that representations of 'coma and PVS [. . .] is overly optimistic in two key respects': first, in survival rate depicted and second, with the regaining of full function; both outcomes at dramatic odds with medical statistics and prognoses. They conclude that, 'It is reasonable to infer that regular viewers of soap operas may be more likely to hold implausibly favourable views of the prognosis of coma' (1539), an evaluation similar to that of Eelco and Cohen Wijdicks' survey of motion picture representations.

Returning to the potential impact (mis)representations have on the BI survivor, McClure postulates that because of an absence of 'a [physical] marker of injury', the survivor 'does not suffer automatic stigmatization', the 'appearance of normality and wellbeing lead[ing] people who do not understand BI to overlook any disability'. This, McClure suggests, causes 'misconceptions [that] can lead to accusations of malingering and [which] may impede survivors' re-integration into society and fuel discriminatory practices' (88). The survivor, because of the invisibility of the injury, therefore experiences deferred stigmatization through the misattribution of behavioural stigmatizing 'labels' circulating in society ('drunk' or 'benefits cheat', for example, or McClure's own label, 'malingerer'), as well as broader medico-social misattributions of 'mental illness' or 'learning disability'.[1]

This level of stigma and shame and lack of public understanding regarding BI is perhaps most poignantly depicted in Richard Lowenstein's documentary, *Mystify* (2019), about Michael Hutchence, the late-lead singer of Australian band INXS. This film reveals the ongoing trauma Hutchence underwent after he was brutally attacked, leading to organic brain injury: an area of contusion of the interior right and left medial frontal lobes with severed nerves. This led to a total loss of taste and smell alongside erratic, violent behaviours; target fixation and perseverations; loss of higher executive functioning; emotional lability and amnesia. Crucially, Hutchence insisted that this was kept secret indicating a level of shame and stigma and which, in turn, led to his erratic behaviours being stigmatized, his frequent violent outbursts earning him the moniker 'Mad Dingo' in the press. His friend, U2 singer Bono, informatively reflects that Hutchence was traumatized and had 'lost his way', as though there was some way back to the person he once was, again viewing the injury as purely psychological and erasing the possibility of traumatic brain plasticity. The film also shines a light on the multiple functional/organic pathologies of BI, Hutchence's depression born out of physical injury – the trauma of having to cope, privately, with this indelible change to personhood and with the lack of taste and smell. As one neuroscientist observes, such chronic anosmia and ageusia gets worse over time leading to a loss of a sense of self – 'a hole in one's being'. The film concludes by revealing that during Hutchence's autopsy, two large areas of brain damage were found.

In the work of coma and BI survivors I have published, much of the writing focuses upon the trauma, hardship and permanence of post-BI living, and the depression to which this leads. Laurence Cox writes of his 'fear of seeing the world permanently broken into shards, with people wildly out of focus' (2014: 35), evoking the cognitive confusion that he still has many years after the accident and his emergence from coma, alongside the panic that is so often triggered, for him, in crowded social situations. He overtly makes reference to the 'permanence' of his neurological disability which leads to fluctuations in energy, concentration and mood. In communicating these sporadic subjective experiences, Cox employs sparsely-punctuated streams of consciousness, his need to be 'energised exercised worked' often hampered by apathy and emotional flattening, coupled with emotional lability, symptoms of his BI and condition that often make him feel as though he is physically 'ill' (34).

Similarly, in his story 'Unremembered Memoirs', Steph Grant, as discussed in the previous chapter, recounts his post-coma 'fugue-states'. In trying to communicate the cognitive rupture during which he violently assaults his two best friends, Grant exploits *mise-en-page* (Figure 6.1), physically jolting the reader and inviting them into the fearful jumble of snapshot memories that, like those of McCarthy's Enactor in *Remainder*, gradually come back to him, fragmented and out of synch, and that are '*in some sense . . . not real*' (2014: 9) (original emphasis).

[...]

THUMPING BASS HARDER AND MORE FREQUENTLY THAN BASS WAS ABLE TO RETURN

Crossing the footbridge across the dyke and over the style into the bull's field

sitting

on a

kerbside

Catching Neil
And
HITTING
          Him
     repeatedly

with

Rozanne.

Rolling over and over with **Bass**

in the field

trading punches

runningacrosstherailwaylevelcrossingthat
separatedsouthfromnorthlevertoninpursuitofneil

vOiCeS in ALARM trying to ARREST steph's
BEHAVIOUR

(Neil furious with fear)

sCrEaMs

of

distress from Rozanne
and Bass

[...]

- 7 -

Figure 6.1 Facsimile of a page from Steph Grant's 'Unremembered Memoirs'. Copyright © 2014. Courtesy Waggledance Press.

These behaviours that both Grant and Cox describe might be confusing and difficult to comprehend for a general public whose misconceptions of BI are constantly sustained by fictional (mis)representations of the condition. Grant's sporadic violence would possibly demonize him as an individual in the eyes of the public because of the invisibility of his injury and the misinformation they are fed. Interestingly, in McClure's research and social experimentations, when the public were presented with a set of such behaviours and given a photograph of the 'perpetrator' sporting a physical scar or injury, the public were much more forgiving and understanding and more likely to put this behaviour down to some form of perceived BI. However, it is important to reiterate that the prevalence of the C-Met alongside the misleading conflation of PDoC (that have led to this crisis of misunderstanding of BI in society) have not arisen from fiction alone. As touched upon, there are frequently slippages of language and examples of misreporting in media coverage when attempting to describe coma and other DoC, as I will now further illustrate.

In 1984, an Arkansas teenager, Terry Wallis, went into a coma after a serious car crash. Nineteen years later, he emerged from coma (apparently with cognition and speech functions largely and quickly intact) to find himself a middle-aged man with a teenage daughter. In the *Mail Online*'s reportage, the 'miracle recovery' is invoked, describing how the first word he uttered was 'Mom', exploiting the emotive weight of the story (Ryan 2003). The article refers to the 'experts' who point out that, 'Cases like Wallis's, where the patient is able to talk freely after a long period of unconsciousness, are extremely rare'. However, *The Guardian Online* presents an entirely different picture. Here it is revealed that 'a few years' before his dramatic 'calling out for his mother', Wallis had 'begun responding to questions by blinking his eyes' (Goldenberg 2003). As Joseph J. Fins notes, Wallis's 'course was fairly typical. He opened his eyes and moved out of the coma and into the vegetative state about three weeks after his injury' (2015: 59). His utterance of 'Mom', then, nineteen years after entering VS was not a 'miracle awakening' from coma – it was the culmination of a slow, painful, frustrating and traumatic road to recovery, moving between PDoC to finally achieve consciousness. Fins further notes, 'Although media accounts described him as awaking from a coma after nineteen years, or being vegetative up to when he began to speak, in actuality, he was responsive at times within the first year of injury', going on to point out how his mother had noted that, 'Within three to five months he seemed to be following things happening in his room' (65-66). Fins naturally concludes that, 'In retrospect, it seems quite likely that Terry had been aware, lying there in a minimally conscious state since late 1984' (67). Despite the more accurate (and less emotively-charged) reporting of *The Guardian*, however, the headline still reads: 'Crash Victim Wakes Up After 20 Years In Coma', utilizing a non-fictional narrative prosthesis to fulfil a news agenda that not only conflates and confuses DoC but also draws upon the sleep C-Met. As Fins asserts when analysing the ethical and policy implications of late recovery from the minimally conscious state, 'The conflation of these brain states is understandable but never excusable' (2007: 305).

The case of Terry Wallis becomes even more complex when the finer details are examined more closely. Slipping into coma in 1984, eighteen years before the minimally conscious state (MCS) was recognized in 2002, the protestations of Wallis's family that he could '[follow] a command or purposefully [track] an object in his visual field' fell on deaf ears, the physicians putting these observations down to 'wishful thinking rather than useful clinical evidence' (Goldenberg 2003). This exemplifies the confusions that occur with PDoC, even within the medical profession, testified to with the identification of MCS- and MCS+. As Derick Wade points out in his discussion of the ever-changing boundaries of what constitutes death in the light of the rise of the neomort and PDoC, 'There is no absolute boundary, and as medical practice and capabilities advance, so once clear boundaries become increasingly ill-defined, especially so for death' (2002: 425). This ambiguity surrounding states of consciousness is similarly explored through ideas more rooted in philosophy, most notably in Giorgio Agamben's notion of the multiple 'thresholds' between life and death. Reflecting upon the ethical and existential positioning of the comatose patient, Agamben posits, 'The concept "death", far from having become more exact, now oscillates from one pole to the other with the greatest indeterminacy' (1998: 93), an uncertainty that has stemmed, in line with Wade's argument, from increasing discoveries of complex and barely-delineated levels and divisions of consciousness. In one particularly startling research study conducted by Gray, Knickman and Wegner, it was even discovered that participants consistently viewed patients in PVS as 'more dead than dead', ascribing less capacity of mind to such patients than the actual dead (2011). Mike McCormack draws on these ethical dilemmas in his novel of coma-exile, *Notes On A Coma*. At one point, reflecting upon the existential state of the coma 'guinea pigs' housed on the prison ship, the *Somnos*, he muses, 'The present perfect continuous is unable to encompass the exact parameters of the phenomena. What's needed, among other things, is a new tense' (2005: 83). Such ambiguity and confusion was addressed, a quarter of a century earlier, by Robin Cook in *Coma*, communicated at the point at which Susan begins her research into coma: 'The more she read about coma, the less she felt she knew . . . it was not known what determined consciousness, other than saying that the individual was not unconscious . . . In fact, being fully conscious and being totally unconscious (coma) seemed to represent opposite ends of a continuous spectrum' (125). As Wade further explicates, 'The vegetative state is simply one end of a spectrum of awareness, and there is no obvious cut-off between the vegetative state and the low-awareness state' (2001: 353).

The Wallis case is just one example of many that illustrates how the degree of media misreporting and the slippage in language to describe PDoC is rife. In Latronico's study of the quality of reporting on the vegetative state of the Italian woman Eluana Englaro, it was found that, 'The majority of articles (88%) [of 967 articles] were dedicated to non-medical aspects of VS' with the inadequacy of the reporting being 'mostly the result of missing information'. This study also draws attention to the case of Theresa (Terri) Schiavo and the US media coverage of her VS, revealing that, 'Only 1.4% of articles [of 1,141 studied] provided an explanation of VS, with a high number of incorrect or equivocal descriptions' (2011: 3). Latronico exemplifies the dangers of such misrepresentations and the effect these can have upon the public understanding of these conditions: '[A] videotape showing that Ms Schiavo was able to open and move her eyes ignited the public skepticism [sic] over her diagnosis of VS because most viewers had no idea that VS patients can have periods of [sleep-wake] periods in which eyes are open and may move about' (1). In Eric Racine's analysis of the media coverage of the Schiavo case to which Latronico also refers, it is observed that, 'The most frequently used terms to describe Schiavo's neurological condition and diagnosis were "persistent vegetative state", "brain damage", "vegetative state", "severe brain damage", and "coma"' (2008: 1029). This once more evidences the conflation of terminology to describe PDoC, leading to escalating public misinformation and confusion. In this instance, this confusion had a profound impact, most notably, upon Schiavo's 'right-to-die' decision due to the fact that the press, through misreporting of the PVS/chronic VS, suggested that Schiavo's instinctive behaviours represented deeper cognitive functioning, thus influencing a huge public and moral backlash against Schiavo's husband's case to withdraw Artificial Nutrition and Hydration (ANH) to allow his wife to die. Moreover, as Fins observes, such conflations and misinformation provided an opportunity for 'politicians and others' to 'deliberately misus[e] medical terms for ideological purposes' (2015: 26). This left a 'residue of confusion in the public sphere that is amplified by physicians who either do not adequately distinguish between brain states or conflate diagnostic categories putting informed decisions at risk' (26–7) – what Fins refers to as the 'conflation error', present also, as evidenced, within literature and reportage.

Gabrielle Samuel and Jenny Kitzinger's extensive analysis of reporting consciousness in coma explores such case studies, while also examining the rush to report so-called 'miracle recovery' stories, as in the case of Terry Wallis. These do occasionally occur, as Samuel and Kitzinger acknowledge, although they are enormously rare, but what they are primarily concerned with is how even the more routine recoveries (like that of Wallis) are reported in terms of the miraculous event, sometimes 'presenting scientific inaccuracies and confusing use of terminology' (2013: 2). This can be seen, for example, in the case of Vicki Allen, a young girl who failed to come out of her induced coma, administered in order to stem leukaemia cell production. The headline in the *Daily Mail*, 'SAVED . . . BY SUMS', carries all of the emotive weight of a miracle recovery story, with a redemptive undertone, as the article focuses on how she was apparently brought out of coma by her father posing arithmetical puzzles to her, maths being her 'favourite subject' (Dolan 2009: 33). 'It was magical', her father is reported as saying, once more reflecting the obsession the media has with so-called miraculous recoveries from coma. Whether it was the simple sums her father asked her that triggered Vicki Allen's emergence from coma or the possibility that she was already coincidentally entering the lightening stage of coma is unclear, with her doctors asserting initially that it was 'just a coincidence'. This proliferation of miracle recover stories in the media is further supported by Eelco Wijdicks and Marilou Wijdicks's study into the coverage of 'coma' in the headlines of American newspapers from 2001 to 2005. They note that the most popular reporting on coma was constituted by so-called 'miracle awakenings' that were covered by multiple newspapers (2006: 1335). They go on to discuss how, from the details of recovery described in the reports (all involving 'emergence of speech after no communication for decades', as in the Wallis case), 'None of these patients appeared in a persistent vegetative state, and patients were far more likely to be in a minimally conscious state or other severely disabled neurological state' (1334). Furthermore, 'Persistent vegetative state was rarely a subject of interest' (1335), with continual use of 'coma' as a catch-all term, again contributing to Fins' 'conflation error' and therefore public misinformation. Press inaccuracies are clear to see but what is critical about Samuel and Kitzinger's study is that it also examines the role of scientific reporting in creating confusion and misinformation surrounding PDoC. In particular, they refer to a pair of studies that received widespread coverage in popular media, including an edition of BBC One's *Panorama* (November 2012), that experimented with fMRI of the brains of patients within VS in order to ascertain whether lines of communication could be established, and whether such patients could understand simple questions being asked – in other words, to try to ascertain whether the patient in VS was conscious. The first study of 2005, led by Dr Adrian Owen, looked into whether a 23-year-old woman who had sustained a TBI through a car-crash, and who now inhabited a PVS, could retain the ability to understand spoken commands and to respond to them through her brain activity. To test this, the research team conducted an fMRI study during which the patient was given spoken instructions to perform two mental imagery tasks at specific points during the scan: to imagine playing tennis and to imagine visiting the rooms in her house. During the tennis periods, 'Significant activity was observed in the supplementary motor area' (Owen et al. 2006: 1402). In contrast, during the 'house-tour' periods, noticeable activity was observed in the areas responsible for spatial awareness. These reactions were no different, it was noted, to test subjects not in PVS. Owen concluded that these moments represented a 'clear act of intention which confirmed beyond any doubt that she was consciously aware of her surroundings' (2006: 1402). Owen was then involved in a wider study, led by Martin M. Monti, between 2005 and 2009 involving fifty-four subjects and sixteen control subjects. This time, motor and spatial imagery tasks were employed but these were now linked to yes/no answers. Participants were asked if they had any brothers; for "yes", they would imagine the motor-image; for "no" the spatial image. Again, it was found that some participants could wilfully modulate their brain activity, but what is most fascinating, as Samuel and Kitzinger point out, is the markedly hyperbolic response in the mainstream press with headlines such as: The Unconscious Patient Who Can Hear What the Doctors Tell Her (*Daily Mail*, 2006); Woman in Vegetative State Responds to Commands (*Independent* 2006); Patient in Vegetative State Communicates with Scientists Using Power of Thought (*The Times*, 2010); Coma Victim 'Speaks' with His Thoughts (*Mirror* 2010).

Exploring the level of 'hope' that both scientific and media reportage generates, Gabriel and Kitzinger also point towards how 'two senior figures' within the field of medicine 'made public statements' that suggested that the initial fMRI studies revealed the patient's 'rich' or 'complex' inner mental life. However, as Samuel and Kitzinger assert, 'Reports rarely mentioned that only a minority of the patients had responded to the fMRI task and did not discuss the implications for 'non-responders' and their families' (2). Referring to the second study of Monti et al., this limited success is clear with only five subjects out of fifty-four tested being able to 'wilfully modulate their brain activity', and all five of them having a *traumatic* brain injury, not an ABI (stroke, tumour etc.) (Monti et al. 2010: 583). The results and success rate are further called into question when it is revealed that when four out of five patients who were able to respond through fMRI imaging were retested at the bedside, 'Some behavioural indicators of awareness could be detected in two of them' (2010: 585) which suggests that they were entering the lightening stage of VS, or on the cusp of this or of the MCS at the time of fMRI testing, once more echoing Wade's cautiousness and misgivings over the divisions within a spectrum of consciousness and the inexactitude of this alongside diagnostical accuracy. The other two 'remained behaviourally unresponsive at the bedside', despite what fMRI had potentially revealed. Thus, as the research paper itself concludes, 'In a minority of cases, patients who meet the behavioural criteria for a vegetative state have residual cognitive function and even conscious awareness' (585). In addition, Monti's team conducted additional tests in one of the five patients with evidence of awareness through fMRI testing, finding he had the ability to answer simple yes/no questions while applying the imagery/visualization technique. Yet despite undergoing repeated evaluations that indicated he was in a VS, at the time of scanning, 'Thorough retesting at the bedside showed reproducible but highly fluctuating and inconsistent signs of awareness [. . .], findings that are consistent with the diagnosis of a minimally conscious state' (585). Again, we see the precariousness of diagnosis of PDoC, and the palpable sense of flux between levels of awareness on the spectrum of consciousness. Despite the nuanced findings of the report, Samuel and Kitzinger emphasize how much of the press reportage and the subsequent scientific papers 'presented no caveats about the level of cognitive function such patients might possess' (3). They point toward the use of such hyperbole as 'Astonishing Breakthrough Medical Miracle' (*The Sun*, 4 February, 2010) and the *Sunday's Times*' less hysterical yet nevertheless fantastical, 'Telepathic Leap' (7 February 2010) (7). Even the *Panorama* documentary exploited this hyperbolic hysteria with the use of the title: 'The Mind Reader'. These latter examples of media embellishment, in the science fiction infused references to 'telepathy' or 'mind-reading', have their counterparts in science fiction itself, most notably in Tarsem Singh's *The Cell* (2000) and in Kristina Buožytė's psycho-erotic *Vanishing Waves* (2012), both texts depicting the central protagonist being projected into the psyche of a victim of a particular DoC. In *The Cell*, child psychologist Catherine Deane is plugged into the hellish subconscious of serial killer Carl Stargher in order to find the location of his latest would-be victim; in *Vanishing Waves*, neurologist Lukas is inserted into the mind of the comatose Aurora with a view to discovering the inner trauma that is preventing her from emerging from coma: the neomort as virtual-reality pod. Significantly, in both texts, the interiority of coma is akin to a purely psychological (functional) trauma. When Lukas reveals to a scientist friend that nothing on Aurora's medical record explains why she is still in coma, his friend explains that the coma could be caused 'by psychological reasons'. In both films, the 'telepathic leap' into the coma consciousness is likened to a descent into the underworld of the mind, borrowing imagery of the katabatic archetype and exploiting the coma-as-death trope. Lukas, in order to reach Aurora, when first entering her mind, has to traverse vast expanses of water, just as Odysseus had to cross the ocean to commune with the dead. And in *The Cell*, the technology used to connect the minds of Catherine and Stargher (a 'neurological synaptic transfer system', as it is described in a 'here comes the science bit' moment) resembles a death-shroud (the kind of shroud that is stuck to the rotting face of Kazantzakis's Lazarus). It is technology that is both futuristic and archaic: a fine, silken cloth laced with electrodes and receptors that are draped over the faces of both participants. In *Vanishing Waves*, the coma patient, Auroroa, shares the moniker given by Disney to its version of Sleeping Beauty, though despite this similarity, Buožytė goes to great lengths to deconstruct the sleeping beauty C-Met. Her Auroroa is shaven-headed, with a sallow complexion, sunken eyes and decubital ulcers; her airways are blocked by breathing tubes, lips dry and encrusted. It is a physical depiction of coma that is at odds, for example, with Almodovar's Alicia in *Hable con Ella*. In a reversal of this narrative model of the 'external' protagonist 'inserting' themselves into the telepathic mind of the coma patient, the 1978 film *Patrick* (and Mark Hartley's 2013 reboot, *Patrick: Evil Awakens*) sees the murderous eponymous anti-hero, while in coma, telekinetically controlling the overworld to defend himself against those who wish to do him harm, once more representing the fictional 'telepathic leap' of the coma protagonist.

This 'telepathic leap' is one such example of fictional portrayals of medical miracles. Other manifestations are rife, the messianic C-Met, for example. Robert Wiersema's novel *Before I Wake* has an interesting spin on this, the novel interspersed with imagined articles from extant Toronto newspapers that satirize real-world reportage: 'Miracle Vigil for Sherry' (140); 'Miracles? Can Injured Girl Cure the Dying?' (117); and, as the inevitable press and public backlash against the Burnetts gathers pace, 'Miracle Fraud? Investigation Reveals False Healings, Fraud' (189). What is notable in this, though, is how Wiersema's medical miracle with which the fictional press is so fascinated isn't a hyperbolic survival from coma itself, but a *literal* miracle with Sherry possessing healing powers. In John Niven's dark comedy novel *The Amateurs*, we find that other staple of coma fiction – the coma survivor who has developed a special ability and comparable with *I Feel Pretty* in which a brain injury constitutes a positive transformative experience. After a golfing accident, protagonist Gary Irvine emerges from coma and suddenly in the possession of uncannily good golf-skills that proves to be 'a constant process of discovery and amazement' (2010: 175). Prior to his accident, he was woefully inept at the game. In coma, Gary is described as having a 'relatively mild' score on the Glasgow Coma Scale (105) with Niven depicting the interiority of the coma as a 'lightening' process. Gary is described as 'rising very fast from deep black water' and 'exploding through the surface' (123), using linguistic tropes of water and surfacing used in other texts previously discussed. His emergence from coma is immediate with him exclaiming, '*Ya Fucken Beauty!*' coinciding with him hitting a perfect shot in his coma-dream, triggering his light-switch 'awakening'. The sudden post-coma skillset that Gary finds he possesses has its equivalence in those coma recovery stories so popular within the mainstream media that obsess over survivors who suddenly and inexplicably appear to have acquired another language: 'Barber woke from coma speaking fluent French and thinking he was Matthew McConnaughey' (the *Telegraph* 2014); 'Before his coma he spoke English; after waking up he's fluent in Spanish' (*CNN* 2016); 'Aussie man who woke from a coma speaking fluent *Chinese*' (*Mail Online* 2014), narratives of miraculous transformation that are again fictionally rendered in *I Feel Pretty*.

In the conclusion to their study, Samuel and Kitzinger assert that scientific and media misrepresentations and 'hype' contribute to what has been termed the 'political economy of hope'. Coined by Mary-Jo Delvecchio Good in her examination of the discourse of hope in American oncology, the 'political economy of hope', Good posits, sustains 'specialist-research oncology' through maintaining the belief that cancer is 'curable'. This allows 'society's cultural interpretation of "hope" to be perpetuated' and as Good asserts, 'The funding of cancer research both depends on and promotes' the hope that cancer can be cured (1990: 60). This constant drive to sustain hope, a 'dynamics of expectations' to refer to Nik Brown's exploration of this topic (2003: 6), inevitably leads to 'hype': a magnification of the potential of new technologies and scientific developments designed both to sustain hope and to ensure medical funding will continue. Brown is fully aware of the dangers of such build-up of hope through hype, particularly through the over-reporting of new technologies (as seen in the case of the fMRI research). He proposes that, '[As] once distant futures advance towards the present, comparisons are made between past promises and present realities' (9). Of course, there is nothing more damaging than a scientific breakthrough that is suddenly found to be a failure, yet conversely, in order for the breakthrough to be funded and advanced, the language of scientific reportage has to overly 'hype' the breakthrough in order to continue to interest the public and maintain funding and investment.

But we might find this political economy of hope operating within all levels of society and certainly within literary and fictional representations of coma and the use of the C-Met. As discussed in Chapter 3, the C-Met (and coma as narrative prosthesis) allows authors to confront fears over this DoC and what it can be seen to represent: the void in consciousness that may come with death. In this sense, the prevalence of the C-Met not only helps to sustain this political economy of hope, but also reveals the need for a personal and cultural economy of hope. As Zygmunt Bauman further discusses in his analysis of the deconstruction of mortality by modern societies, there is a constant 'drive to mastery' over death which, pertinent to our discussions, is a 'mode of being shot through with hope' (1992: 132). Moreover, Bauman posits, 'The very act of thinking death is already its denial', proposing that, 'Our thoughts of death, to be at all thinkable, must already be processed, artificed, tinkered with' (15). The proliferation of the C-Met and narrative prosthesis within literature and media reportage alike can be seen as a manifestation of the human desire to 'process' death, therefore contributing to a 'mode of hope' and to an overall ethical dilemma. We only need to return to the examples of misleading and confusing reporting on Michael Schumacher's condition, discussed at the beginning of this investigation, to see this mode in operation. All of this overly 'hopeful' reporting conveys the very real need not to conceive of a giant of motor-sport as anything other than 'heroic' and flawless, thus consistently failing to address the possibility of long-term neurological damage. Most recently, we have seen this economy of hope in media reportage of Derek Draper, the husband of TV presenter Kate Garraway, who was put into an induced coma after his health deteriorated due to Covid-19 infection. However, he failed to come out of coma for three months. When he eventually did come out of coma, reportage was again overly positive and hopeful. Garraway herself was quick to address this coverage with a press statement detailing the fact that her husband was in the MCS, stating, 'These headlines are a sign of a level of optimism that might not be justified', describing the 'very slow and uncertain path' to recovery (Capon 2020).

This hope culture and the mythologizing of difficult and traumatic experiences can be further explicated by returning to Ricoeur and his concepts of sedimentation and 'narrative identity'. In his discussions concerning our 'demand' for narrative and storytelling, Ricoeur explores how the self begins to 'know itself' through the 'cultural signs' and 'symbolic mediations' which constitute 'the narratives of everyday life' (1991b: 198). Furthermore, he argues, 'Human lives become more regularly intelligible when they are interpreted in the light of the stories that people tell about them', going on to suggest that these 'life stories' are even more 'intelligible' when 'narrative models' or 'plots' from 'history or fiction' are applied to them (188). Ricoeur therefore suggests that humans consistently use and 'innovate' the sediment of historical and fictional narratives in order to try and understand and explicate their own lives, thereby meaning that we 'never cease to reinterpret the narrative identity that constitutes us, in the light of the narratives proposed to us by our culture' (37). Writing of the function of fiction in 'shaping' reality, Ricoeur proposes that, '[M]imesis is not simply reduplication but creative reconstruction by means of the mediation of fiction' (1991c: 134). Across the works of fiction discussed throughout this book, we see this level of creative reconstruction, to lesser and greater extents – and also, with varying degrees of controversy, as exemplified by, for example, *Girlfriend in a Coma*. For while Coupland's creative agenda is a highly complex and problematic one, it is complicated further by the fact that the author, clearly taking inspiration from the Quinlan case, still discusses the 'potential' that 'coma' has to offer for the shaping of a new identity while fully aware that Quinlan had no such opportunity, raising an ethical question over how authors appropriate illness narratives of patients for their fiction, even if that fiction is 'fantastic' in its form. Yet it is within the complexity of Coupland's agenda that we may find the clues to understanding, further, our relationship with and attitudes towards the (prolonged) disorders of consciousness that challenge our notions of life and death. Coupland's 'deepest need' is not so much the need to radically change ourselves, and the opportunity for this that coma 'offers' us, but the need to *think* that this is what is offered us.

6.4 Controversies

This book has not been a call-to-arms for more accurate, medically-precise and ethical fictional portrayals of coma and BI. Or at least, that has not been my intention. Nor should all works of fiction be treated, viewed or judged as scientifically rigorous narratives. It is important to always acknowledge that the image of coma is most often taken purely as a means for narrative prosthesis which enables creative forays into the imagination and the fantastic. Yet this does not mean that we cannot or should not explore the profound effect that such representations have upon a public understanding or awareness of the condition of coma, wider PDoC and BI. In analysing the ethical dilemmas arising from the proliferation of myths about brain disorders and illnesses, Christian Jarrett rightly observes that the public's belief 'about coma recovery and their understanding of a coma or vegetative patient's levels of awareness are important because of the difficult decisions that often have to be made about a patient's treatment' (2015: 277). He goes on to discuss the controversial case of Terri Schiavo and the impact that misleading portrayals of PDoC in the media and fiction had upon her right-to-die appeal. We may return once more to Eric Racine's report on the media coverage of the case in assessing this impact. Racine and his team found extensive scientifically inaccurate, inconsistent or incorrect prognoses, erratic diagnostic terminology (the conflation of different PDoC), and highly emotively and politically charged language designed to mislead audiences in their conception of Schiavo's end-of-life care. Descriptions of the withdrawal of life support were abound, including references to 'murder' or 'death by starvation', and 'explanations of the basic concept of PVS and other CDCs [chronic disorders of consciousness] were rare' (2008: 1030). It was found that, 'Statements conveying *false hopes for recovery* were disseminated in a general absence of adequate critical examination and background information about PVS and CDCs' (1032) (my emphasis). 'This is where relatives' religious beliefs', Jarrett discusses, 'Their understanding of a coma patient's levels of awareness and suffering, their beliefs about recovery chances – potentially skewed by fictional portrayals – can influence decision making' (277) – the Schiavo case being an exemplar of this dilemma. It is this kind of misinformation and bioethical crisis that has led Eric J. Cassell to describe the case as a 'shocking, clamouring, and very public intrusion into the life and death of Terri Schiavo' (2005: 22). As he sums up, 'People who think that they know what diagnosis is or the treatment should be or what the morally appropriate response is just because they know the name of the disease or have seen a videotape of the patient are often wrong or foolish or both' (23).

We may return to *Just Like Heaven*, the film adaptation of Marc Levy's novel *If Only It Were True*, to exemplify the potentially problematic nature of fictional portrayals of PDoC. As Elizabeth's physicians, at her sister's behest, prepare to take her off life support, David 'kidnaps' her from the ICU and a chase ensues as he tries to navigate her gurney towards escape from the hospital. In the process, her breathing tube becomes tangled, wrenched out and she flatlines. It only takes the kiss of David's Prince Charming to rouse Elizabeth's Sleeping Beauty. But at the point at which she 'wakes', with cognition immediately intact (apart from her memories of David), her sister laments the fact that she came very close to letting Elizabeth die. In this single comment, in conjunction with the representation of a 'light bulb' moment of 'awakening', we see the ethical dilemma of the film as it begins to pivot towards a right-to-die question, but with a fundamentally misleading depiction of a patient within PVS/chronic VS at its heart. It is a portrayal again in contrast, for example, with *Critical Care*'s darkly comic pessimism. At one point, Werner reflects on a comment his colleague has made 'in a voice so loud that any one of four comatose patients might have heard her every word, if they could have only risen from the dead' (Dooling 1992: 22). It is a view of the neomort underscored by the term Werner uses for his patients: 'stiffs' (12), thus negating any chance of complex inner mental life.

Casarett et al. conclude in their review of misrepresentations of coma (and prognosis of survival) in daytime television dramas, 'Soap operas are not designed with the goal of educating the public about the realities of health and illness or even about the realities of interpersonal relationships, but they may contribute to public misperceptions in these areas' (2006: 1539). Just because we shouldn't be overly critical of both fictional and factual misrepresentations of coma and BI, it doesn't mean that we can't look at the socio-political impact of these, or the human cost, a cost that

Nik Brown lucidly outlines. In discussing the circulation of overly positive sickness narratives and medical reportage, he notes there is also often a negative impact upon the patients and loved ones at the centre of such narratives. Stories such as the skewed, overly optimistic reportage of Wallis, Grzebski and Schiavo, alongside the fMRI studies, have 'enormous potency because they tell of the precarious futures of individuals who are desperate for treatment' (2003: 8). In these PDoC cases, the desperation for a 'miracle recovery' so common in fiction or media reportage is shared by the loved ones of the patient, leading to the 'costs of inflated promise', an over-hyped assurance that is further communicated and perpetuated in the press. Samuel and Kitzinger, for example, examine the impact that such reporting of the fMRI studies had on the loved ones of PVS/chronic VS patients. What promised to be a 'telepathic leap' had profoundly negative effects upon loved ones who found themselves suddenly caught in a double-bind. On the one hand, it built hope that they could now communicate to their loved ones (if they did not already have that hope and belief) but on the other hand, with this 'proof' that they could communicate, they now did not know how they could translate hope into a practical means that could help their loved ones to recover. For some, knowing that their loved one did have autonomous awareness of his or her self and surroundings made the situation even more painful. Samuel and Kitzinger also describe, for example, how one particular family member of a patient in PVS was 'bitterly disappointed' when she discovered that 'it would be difficult to access fMRI because – contrary to the expectations raised in her by media reporting – the imaging was only available as part of scientific studies' (2013: 6).

Maybe even more disturbing is the wilful manipulation of linguistic terminology of PDoC in the mainstream press, even in the face of censure. Fins refers to his and his colleagues' pleas to 'avoid diagnostic conflation' of PVS/chronic VS and MCS (2015: 127), warning against 'diagnostic creep' (126) that has the potential to attribute, for example, indicators of awareness found in MCS to the PVS, where there is no detectable awareness. Fins goes on to relate a startling and deliberate case of diagnostic creep when he and colleagues were interviewed by the *The New York Times* for a feature on their work with MCS patients, identifying the small levels of awareness that may be present. Fins notes that despite the award-winning journalist, Carl Zimmer, being 'precise in his descriptions and careful in getting the science right', the ensuing article entitled, 'What if there is something going on in there?' had 'been mangled by editorial staff who conflated the vegetative and minimally conscious states'. Fins points towards one 'memorable header', which had nothing to do with what he and his colleagues had said, that crudely asserted: 'New research suggests that many vegetative patients are more conscious than previously supposed – and might eventually be curable. A whole new way of thinking about pulling the plug' (127). Even more worrying, when challenged about these conflations between PVS and MCS by the eminent professor of neurology and expert on PDoC, Fred Plum, the editor of the *Times* defended his decisions, claiming that, 'The distinction between the vegetative and minimally conscious states was semantic' (128). Such an offhand dismissal, as we have seen, can have critical, real-world impacts upon victims of PDoC, as testified to by Fins himself who notes that shortly after a scientific paper regarding MCS was published, lawyers working on behalf of Terri Schiavo's parents contacted the authors of the paper asking them to support their case in applying these behaviours of low-awareness to Schiavo and to diagnose her as being in MCS, not PVS.

Such ethical dilemmas regarding diagnostic creep and the language and imagery of coma, PDoC and BI in the media and fiction may only become more complex and problematic, particularly as right-to-die and 'best interest' decision-making cases increasingly gain traction as seen in the case of police officer Paul Briggs. In 2015, Briggs suffered a BI in a crash on his way to work and was subsequently diagnosed as being in MCS. In a Court of Protection case of 2016, Briggs' wife won her appeal to withdraw ANH (in spite of his doctor's wishes) citing that this was in his best interests and in-line with his 'previously expressed wishes' (*BBC News Online* 2016). In the absence of a 'living will', this was a landmark case.

In light of such cases, what impact does diagnostic creep have in public perception of PDoC? And how might overly hopeful narratives of prognosis and recovery, coupled with an exaggeration of what degree of awareness and consciousness exists within certain behaviours of different PDoC, affect both how we view such right-to-die cases and our ethical position? Eelco Wijdicks is under no illusion as to what the answers to these questions might be. Concluding his discussions of the impact of misrepresentations of coma and BI in the media and fiction within his seminal book *The Comatose Patient*, he writes,

> Coma is a consequence of a BI that often leads to a severe disability and agony to family members. There should be a sensible depiction in media outlets and an attempt to frame it correctly. Journalists, screenwriters, TV commentators, and correspondents all have a responsibility to be cautious. They ought to. The audience may be quite perceptive but is unable to draw the line. (2008: 226)

Yet even scientists and clinicians familiar with the ambiguities, conflations and diagnostic and linguistic slippage or creep of different PDoC can also exploit the political economy of hope. Dr Adrian Owen, in the very first pages of *The Grey Zone*, his book detailing his pioneering work in fMRI studies in VS patients, asserts, 'We have discovered that *15 to 20 per cent* of people in the VS state who are assumed to have no more awareness than a head of broccoli are fully conscious, although they never respond to any form of external stimulation' (2017: 3). This is a contentious claim, not least because one element of the evidence he gives for this finding, cited in an endnote, is the research paper he co-authored with Martin Monti in which only five out of fifty-four patients responded to the fMRI visualization test. That figure amounts to a mere 9 per cent success rate and this is even before we get into the technicalities, discussed at length in the previous chapter, of whether they were in PVS or MCS, or whether they *were* in PVS but had now *progressed* to MCS. This overtly optimistic, hopeful and 'hyped' scientific position contrasts greatly with the conclusion of the original paper which Owen himself references: that fMRI imaging is only successful in a 'minority of cases'. And even taking into account a separate, apparently more successful EEG study to test awareness to which Owen refers (and in which he was again involved), the figures of success rate still appear to be questionable. While three out of sixteen VS patients did appear to 'generate appropriate EEG responses to two distinct commands' (which does amount to 19 per cent success), only one 'of 11 non-traumatic patients were able to successfully complete this task' (Cruse et al. 2011: 2088). This only amounts to a mere 9 per cent success rate in ABI patients, a finding roughly in line with the Monti study. In fact, I would argue that the very title of Owen's book, *The Grey Zone*, is linguistically contentious. Despite writing extensively about the differences between coma, PVS and MCS, and charting the history of the development of diagnostic criteria to distinguish between them, he continually places all of these patients under this singular umbrella term. In short, the patients to which he refers (whether in PVS or MCS) all inhabit this 'grey zone', a linguistic tic that in itself embodies conflation error and diagnostic creep.

inews, in 2019, ran a feature that is once more paradigmatic of this conflation error. In an article entitled, 'What makes people in comas wake up – from Lynx to Rolling Stones' Satisfaction', we are immediately confronted with the notion of 'sleep-like' coma, an idea from which Plum and Posner were quick to distance themselves in the fourth edition of *The Diagnosis*. Despite acknowledging the fact that patients can progress to PVS or MCS, the article still writes of these as if they are still within the category of coma – testified to by the very title of the article: a catch-all 'grey zone'. And again, despite referring to patients who have inhabited prolonged vegetative states (nineteen years; twenty-seven years), there is no mention of the traumatic consequences of this – no mention of BI, merely, 'The potential for [a] kind of long-term recovery' (Feinmann 2019).

This erasure of the possibility of BI throughout coma narratives consistently contributes to the invisibility of the condition: a condition that is often physically invisible. Christopher Priest, in his coma-novel *The Glamour*, depicts this invisibility in a unique way. Recovering from a coma caused by a terrorist bomb attack, the aptronymous Richard Grey struggles to cope with the BI this has left him: 'A silence of memory inside him, a period of his life irretrievably lost' (2005: 5). Significantly, evoking the kind of language deployed by Redgrove and McCarthy, Grey observes that, 'There was a profound blankness in his mind' (10). Reflecting the two opposing arguments arising between the two world wars regarding the causes of shell shock, and similar to *The Echo Maker*, competing physicians argue over whether Grey's retrograde amnesia is 'an organic loss of memory' or 'psychologically based' (16). Later, it is revealed that Grey might have 'paramnesia' – the propensity to confabulate 'a whole sequence of invented memories' (25). The novel takes a trip into the fantastic when it is revealed that this trauma has reawakened in Grey his natural ability to make himself invisible from the world – to be 'glamorous', Priest therefore invoking the plight of the post-coma BI survivor. In this way, and as Paul Kincaid notes, Priest insightfully comments upon the 'idea of a kind of social invisibility' (Kincaid 1991: 52), exemplified by survivors of coma and BI or long-term neurological conditions, metaphorically portrayed in a work of fantastic fiction that uses narrative prosthesis to explore both coma and BI alongside a range of wider existential questions.

Two more recent examples of fictional works that have brought the portrayal of BI to the forefront of their narratives are Tom Robb Smith's mini-series *MotherFatherSon* (2019) and Paddy Considine's feature film *Journeyman* (2017). At the heart of *MotherFatherSon* is a narrative of brain-trauma and rehabilitation after the vapid newspaper editor, Caden Finch, suffers a massive ABI after a drug overdose. Recovering from coma and his drug-induced stroke, Smith portrays the trauma of Finch's organic BI: loss of motor functions and faculty of speech; emotional lability; disinhibited behaviour and, in one particularly visceral scene, nihilist self-violence, attempting to tear open the deep scar of surgery that runs across his scalp – the scar that, like the Enactor's scar, remains and reminds Finch of who he was and who he now is. In an interesting twist, his wealthy parents place him in a military rehab centre, alongside amputees, soldiers with PTSD . . . and those exhibiting symptoms and behaviours of shell shock, caused by both psychological and organic trauma, and a combination of the two.

But it is Paddy Considine's *Journeyman* that perhaps provides us with the most vivid portrayal of BI recovery. Boxer Matty Burton, after narrowly winning his last fight against a much-younger opponent, suddenly suffers a catastrophic BI – an ABI, in the form of a stroke, it is suggested, but brought on by the TBI of his fight. In this moment, there is no high-drama of the initiating injury: instead, we just see the deferred, slow violence of the trauma that causes Matty to be 'changed' indelibly and irrevocably. Considine meticulously portrays Matty's oscillations between uncontrollable, violent emotion (his emotional lability) and the cool, apathetic flattening to which injury has led. The film is unflinching in its depiction of the trauma of BI and rehab – having to painfully 're-learn' to walk, like McCarthy's Enactor; his disinhibited behaviour; his memory loss; his impassive violence, at one point unpredictably bloodying his wife, Emma's, nose after she refuses to have sex with him – even sealing their baby into the washing machine, her screams unbearable for him to hear. But it also portrays the social isolation of both the BI survivor and his loved ones – Matty and Emma's friends abandoning them, unable to cope with or process Matty's shredded identity; and Emma, left alone, terrified and confused by this person she no longer recognizes: 'Where are you, baby – I need you to come back now', she whispers to her sleeping husband, a narrative of hopeful reinstatement of a lost, former self that is not available to either of them. This sense of a split, post-injury Subject is embodied with the post-injury Matthew consistently coming face-to-face with the pre-injury pugilist Matty – at one point, punching the glass of framed photographs of his previous boxing successes. Once more, the motif of the scar is present: in his severe hair-cut, the sides of his head shaved to the bone, the scar is clear to see: a rem(a)inder. But as the film progresses, so Matty's hair grows back – as he slowly improves, the invisibility of his condition increases, the scar eventually hidden. Considine, in this brutally accurate portrayal of BI, even subverts the conventions of the sporting drama in having, and inherent in the *Rocky* franchise, a 'training montage' – except Matty is not training for a fight, but honing his new self in order to win back his wife and baby: the biggest fight of his life.

It is only when viewing or reading such texts as *MotherFatherSon*, *Journeyman*, *Remainder*, *The Echo Maker* and *Lairies* that painstakingly depict the aetiology and sequelae of coma and BI that we begin to fully realize that we rarely encounter such narratives – and, moreover, that we actually begin to understand that we know very little about these conditions because of the dominant narratives that we do receive. Caspermeyer et al., in the conclusion to their study of stigmatizing language and medical inconsistencies in neurology coverage by American newspapers, posit, 'Public perceptions and attitudes are the foundation of the stigmatizing process' (2006). So while many of the texts, discussed throughout this book, do teach us about wider existential questions and our relationship to these, it is mindful to remember that these are, to return to Fins, 'metaphorically powerful', yet at the same time they propagate what might be deemed to be dominant, ableist ideologies. It is therefore incumbent upon us, as viewers and readers, to continually interrogate such texts and perhaps to seek out narratives that will enable an understanding of such medical conditions, thereby aiding our empathic relationships with both survivors of disorders of consciousness living with long-term neurological conditions and those still occupying DoC who we may encounter in our everyday lives.

Notes

Chapter 2

1. Due to the fact that Garland's novel does not use pagination, I have used my own system of page numbering so that references can be easily located, denoted by the number surrounded with square brackets.
2. Coma as a narrative motif, in fact, features heavily in the world of videogames. See also: *The Coma: Cutting Class* (Devespresso Games, 2019); *Bad Dream Coma* (Desert Fox, 2017); and *Neversong*, formerly *Once Upon a Coma* (Serenity Forge/Atmos Games), the very title of which combines 'Coma' with the linguistic register of the fairy tale with its use of 'Once Upon a'.

Chapter 3

1. Throughout this chapter, I will use 'underworld' and uncapitalized 'hell' as general terms to describe the subterranean place to which all katabatic heroes descend. The capitalized designation 'Hell' will be reserved for the underworld of Christian thought and 'Hades' for the underworld of Greco-Roman tradition. 'Hellish' will be used as an adjectival umbrella term for the underworld.
2. A thorough analysis of the use of homophones and rhyme within the novel should be treated a little with caution, considering the variation of pronunciation across regional dialects within Standard Scottish English.

Chapter 5

1. For further discussion of Sacks's experiments, see *Hallucinations* (2012a).

Chapter 6

1. Similarly, in a recent study conducted by Parkinson's UK, it was found that sufferers of Parkinson's Disease (itself, a neurological, 'invisible' injury) were found to have experienced widespread 'abuse and accusations of being drunk or not disabled enough because of a lack of understanding about their condition' (Matthews-King 2019, the *Independent*).

Bibliography

Adams, T. (2004), 'Coma Chameleon', *The Guardian*, 27 June. Available online: http://www.guardian.co.uk/books/2004/jun/27/fiction.features2 (accessed 30 January 2011).
Adams, Z. M. and J. J. Fins (2017), 'Penfield's Ceiling: Seeing Brain Injury through Galen's Eyes', *Neurology*, 89: 854–8.
Adorno, T. (1997), *Aesthetic Theory*, London: The Athlone Press.
Agamben, G. (1998), *Homo Sacer*, trans. D. Heller-Roazen, Stanford: Stanford University Press.
Alexander, E. (2012), *Proof Of Heaven*, London: Piatkus.
Alighieri, D. ([1320] 1995), 'Inferno', in *The Divine Comedy*, 59–213, trans. A. Mandelbaum, London: Everyman's Library.
Allatt, K. (2011), *Running Free*, Bedlinog: Accent Press.
Allende, I. (1996), *Paula*, London: Flamingo.
Ashbery, J. (1978), 'And Others, Vaguer Presences', in *Houseboat Days*, 48, New York: Penguin.
Bad Dream Coma (2017), [Video Game], Poland: Desert Fox.
Bailly, L. (2009), *Lacan*, Oxford: Oneworld.
Ball, E. (2013), *The Inventor and the Tycoon*, New York: Doubleday.
Banks, I. (1986), *The Bridge*, London: Little, Brown and Company.
'Barber woke from coma speaking fluent French and thinking he was Matthew McConaughey' (2014), *The Telegraph*, 22 December. Available online: https://www.telegraph.co.uk/news/picturegalleries/howaboutthat/11307568/Barber-woke-from-coma-speaking-fluent-French-and-thinking-he-was-Matthew-McConaughey.html (accessed 27 June 2019).
Bates, D. (2001), 'The Prognosis of Medical Coma', *Journal of Neurology, Neurosurgery and Psychiatry*, 71 (Suppl. 1 - 'Neurology In Practice'): 1–29.
Bauby, J.-D. (2004), *The Diving Bell and the Butterfly*, trans. Jeremy Leggatt, London: Harper Perennial.
Baudrillard, J. (1983a), 'The Precession of Simulacra', in *Simulations*, 1–79, trans. P. Foss and P. Putton, New York: Semiotext[e].
Baudrillard, J. (1983b), 'The Orders of Simulacra', in *Simulations*, 83–159, trans. P. Beitchman, New York: Semiotext[e].
Baudrillard, J. (1994), *Simulacra and Simulation*, trans. S. F. Glaser, Ann Arbor: The University of Michigan Press.
Baudrillard, J. (1997), *The Evil Demon of Images*, Sydney: The Power Institute of Fine Arts.
Bauman, Z. (1992), *Mortality, Immortality and Other Life Strategies*, Cambridge: Polity Press.
Baxendale, S. (2004), 'Memories Aren't Made of This: Amnesia at the Movies', *BMJ*, 329 (18–25 December): 1480–83.
Bell, V., S. Wilkinson, M. Greco, C. Hendrie, B. Mills and Q. Deeley (2020), 'What Is the Functional/Organic Distinction Actually doing in Psychiatry and Neurology?', *Wellcome Open Research*. Available online: https://wellcomeopenresearch.org/articles/5-138 (accessed 25 June 2020).

Bernat, J. L. (2008), 'Theresa Schiavo's Tragedy and Ours, Too', *Neurology*, 71: 964–5.
Bevan, D. (1990), 'Introduction', in David Bevan (ed.), *Literature and Exile*, 3–4, Amsterdam: Rodopi.
Biderman, D., E. Daniels-Zide, A. Reyes and B. Marks (2006), 'Ego-Identity: Can It Be Reconstructed After a Brain Injury?', *International Journal of Psychology*, 41 (5): 355–61.
Bigley, K. (2019), *Comaville*, Troy, NY: Clash Books.
Bishop, R. (2009), 'Baudrillard, Death and Cold War Theory', in Ryan Bishop (ed.), *Baudrillard Now*, 47–71, Cambridge: Polity Press.
Blanchot, M. (1995), *The Writing of Disaster*, trans. A. Smock, Lincoln and London: University of Nebraska Press.
Brison, S. (2002), *Aftermath: Violence and the Remaking of a Self*, Princeton, NJ: Princeton University Press.
Brooks, P. (1977), 'Freud's Master Plot', *Yale French Studies, Literature and Psychoanalysis. The Question of Reading*, 55/56: 280–300.
Brown, N. (2003), 'Hope Against Hype – Accountability in Biopasts, Presents and Futures', *Science Studies*, 16 (2): 3–21.
Bruno, M., S. Majerus, M. Boly, A. Vanhaudenhuyse, C. Schnakers, O. Gosseries, P. Boveroux, M. Kirsch, A. Demertzi, C. Bernard, R. Hustinx, G. Moonen and S. Laureys (2011), 'Functional Neuroanatomy Underlying the Clinical Subcategorization of Minimally Conscious State Patients', *Journal of Neurology*, 259: 1087–98.
Burn, S. J. (2015), 'Neuroscience and Modern Fiction', *Modern Fiction Studies*, 61 (2): 209–25.
Bush, S. (2019), 'Unity Government Is Cloud Cuckoo Land', *i*, 16 August.
The Cabinet of Dr Caligari (Das Cabinet Des Dr Caligari) (1919), [Film] Dir. Robert Weine, Germany: Friedrich-Wilhelm-Murnau-Stiftung.
Canguilhem, G. (1991), *The Normal and the Pathological*, trans. C. A. Fawcett, New York: Zone Books.
Campbell, J. (1968), *The Hero with a Thousand Faces*, New York: Bollingen.
Capon, T. (2020), '"Very Slow Path" Piers Morgan Warns Kate Garraway's Husband Derek Waking from Coma "is not all positive" and Recovery is "uncertain"', *The Sun*, 6 July. Available online: https://www.thesun.co.uk/tvandshowbiz/12041136/piers-morgan-kate-garraway-derek-coma/ (accessed 24 July 2020).
Cartlidge, N. (2001), 'States Related to or Confused With Coma', *Journal of Neurology, Neurosurgery and Psychiatry*, 71 (suppl I): i18–i19.
Caruth, C. (1995), *Trauma: Explorations in Memory*, Baltimore, MD: The Johns Hopkins University Press.
Caruth, C. (1996), *Unclaimed Experience*, Baltimore, MD: The Johns Hopkins Press.
Casarett, D., J. M Fishman, H. J. MacMoran, A. Pickard and D. A. Asch (2006), 'Epidemiology and Prognosis of Coma in Daytime Television Dramas', *BMJ*, 331: 1537–9.
Caspermeyer, J. J., E. J. Sylvester, J. F. Drazkowski, G. L. Watson and J. I. Sirven (2006), 'Evaluation of Stigmatizing Language and Medical Errors in Neurology Coverage by US Newspapers', *Mayo Clinical Proceedings*, 81 (3): 300–6.
Cassell, E. J., (2005), 'The Schiavo Case: A Medical Perspective', *The Hastings Centre Report*, 35 (3): 22–3.
The Cell (2000), [Film] Dir. Tarsem Singh, USA: New Line Cinema.
The Centers for Disease Control and Prevention, *Injury Prevention & Control: Traumatic Brain Injury*, 'What are the Leading Causes of TBI?'. Available online: http://www.cdc.gov/traumaticbraininjury/causes.html (accessed 26 November 2013).

Charter, D. (2014), 'Michael Schumacher "an invalid for life" Says Coma Specialist', *The Times*, 20 June. Available online: http://www.thetimes.co.uk/tto/news/world/europe/article4125140.ece (accessed 14 October 2014).

Cheer, L. (2014), 'The Australian Man Who Woke from a Coma Speaking Fluent Chinese (but couldn't remember English) . . . and Went on to Host a Chinese Game Show and Study in Shanghai', *Mail Online*, 2 September. Available online: https://www.dailymail.co.uk/news/article-2740708/Aussie-man-wakes-coma-car-crash-speaking-MANDARIN.html (accessed 27 June 2019).

Cheyne, J. (1812), *Cases of Apoplexy and Lethargy*, London: Thomas Underwood.

Clandfield, P. and C. Lloyd (2007), 'Redevelopment Fiction: Architecture, Town-Planning and "Unhomeliness"', in Berthold Schoene (ed.), *The Edinburgh Companion to Contemporary Scottish Fiction*, 124–31, Edinburgh: Edinburgh University Press.

Clark, R. J. (1979), *Catabasis: Vergil and the Wisdom-Tradition*, Amsterdam: B.R.Grüner.

Clegg, B. (2007), *The Man Who Stopped Time*, Stroud: Sutton Publishing.

Clevenger, C. (2007), *Dermaphoria*, London: Harper Perennial.

Clow, B. (2001), 'Who's Afraid of Susan Sontag? or, the Myths and Metaphors of Cancer Reconsidered', *Social History of Medicine*, 14 (2): 293–312.

Cohn, D. (1978), *Transparent Minds*, Princeton, NJ: Princeton University Press.

Cold Lazarus (1996), [Television drama] Dir. Renny Rye, UK: Channel 4, April.

Colebrook, M. (2013), '*Lanark* and *The Bridge*: Narrating Scotland as Post-Industrial Space', in M. Colebrook and K. Cox (eds), *The Transgressive Iain Banks*, 28–44, Jefferson, NC: McFarland & Company.

Collier, J (2003), 'Sleeping Beauty', in *Fancies and Goodnights*, 311–26, New York: New York Review Books.

Collins, J. and B. Mayblin (2012), *Introducing Derrida*, London: Icon Books.

Collyer, R. H. (1871), *Mysteries of the Vital Element in Connexion with Dreams, Somnambulism, Trance*, London: Henry Renshaw.

Coma (1978), [Film] Dir. Michael Crichton, USA: United Artists.

Coma (2012), [TV miniseries] Dir. Mikael Salomon, USA: A&E Network.

The Coma: Cutting Class (2019), [Video Game], Seoul: Devespresso Games.

Cook, R. ([1977] 2008), *Coma*, London: Pan Books.

Coupland, D. (1998), *Girlfriend in a Coma*, London: Harper Collins.

Couser, G. T. (1997), *Recovering Bodies*, Madison: The University of Wisconsin Press.

Couser, G. T. (2011), 'Introduction: Disability and Life Writing', *Journal of Literary & Cultural Disability Studies*, 5 (3): 229–42.

Couser, G. T. (2016), 'Body Language: Illness, Disability, and Life Writing', *Life Writing*, 13 (1): 3–10.

Cowie, E. (1988), 'The Popular Film as a Progressive Text – a Discussion of *Coma*', in C. Penley (ed.), *Feminism and Film Theory*, 105–40, London: Routledge.

Cox, L. (2014), 'Going Out and Hating Myself', in M. Colbeck (ed.), *Head-Lines*, 2, 34–6, Blythe Bridge: Waggledance Press.

Cracknell, J. and B. Turner (2013), *Touching Distance*, London: Arrow Books.

Craig, C. (1999), *The Modern Scottish Novel*, Edinburgh: Edinburgh University Press.

Criss, D. (2016), 'Before His Coma He Spoke English; after Waking Up He's Fluent in Spanish', *CNN*, 25 October. Available online: https://edition.cnn.com/2016/10/24/health/teen-spanish-new-language-trnd/index.html (accessed 27 June 2019).

Critical Care (1997), [Film] Dir. Sidney Lumet, USA: Village Roadshow Pictures.

Cruse, D., S. Chennu, C. Chatelle, T. A. Bekinschtein, D. Fernández-Espejo, J. D. Pickard, S. Laureys and A. M. Owen (2011), 'Bedside Detection of Awareness in the Vegetative State: a Cohort Study', *Lancet*, 378: 2088–94.

Culbertson, R. (1995), 'Embodied Memory, Transcendence, and Telling: Recounting Trauma, Re-Establishing the Self', *New Literary History: Narratives of Literature, the Arts, and Memory*, 26 (1): 169–95.
Cullen, W. (1790), *First Lines of the Practice of Physic*, Vol. 2, Worcester, MA: Isaiah Thomas.
Damasio, A. (2000), *The Feeling of What Happens*, London: Vintage.
Damasio, A. (2003), *Looking for Spinoza: Joy, Sorrow, and the Feeling Brain*, Orlando: Harcourt.
Damasio, A. (2005), *Descartes' Error: Emotion, Reason, and the Human Brain*, New York: Penguin.
Davies, S. E. (1910), 'Some Account of a Proposed New College for Women', in *Thoughts on Some Questions Relating to Women*, 85–107, Cambridge: Bowes and Bowes.
Davis, J. P. (1994), *Stephen King's America*, Bowling Green, OH: Bowling Green State University Popular Press.
Davison, K. and C. R. Bagley (1970), 'Schizophrenia-like Psychoses Associated With Organic Disorders of the CNS', *British Journal of Psychiatry*, 4: 113–84
The Dead Zone (1983), [Film] Dir. David Cronenberg, USA: The Dino De Laurentiis Company.
De Bruxelles, S. (2014), 'Schumacher "is being brought out of coma"', *The Times*, 30 January (page unknown).
Delvecchio Good, M. J., B. J. Good, C. Schaffer and S. E. Lind (1990), 'American Oncology and the Discourse on Hope', *Culture, Medicine and Psychiatry*, 14: 59–79.
Derrida, J. (1973), *Speech and Phenomena and Other Essays on Husserl's Theory of Signs*, trans. D. Allison, Evanston, IL: Northwestern University Press.
Derrida, J. (1981), *Positions*, trans. A. Bass, London: The Athlone Press.
Dieguez, S. and J.-M. Annoni (2013), 'Stranger than Fiction: Literary and Clinical Amnesia', *Monographs in Neural Sciences*, 31: 137–68.
The Diving Bell and the Butterfly (2007), [Film] Dir. Julian Schnabel, France: Pathé.
Docherty, T. (2012), *Confessions: The Philosophy of Transparency*, London: Bloomsbury.
Dolan, A. (2009), 'Saved . . . By Sums', *The Daily Mail*, 3 November: 33.
Dooling, R. (1992), *Critical Care*, New York: William Morrow and Company.
Doran, J. M. (1990), 'The Capgras Syndrome: Neurological/Neuropsychological Perspectives', *Neuropsychology*, 4: 29–42.
Driver: San Francisco (2011), [Video game] Dirs. Martin Edmondson and Craig Lawson, UK: Ubisoft.
Eagleman, D. (2016), *The Brain*, Edinburgh: Canongate.
Eco, U. (1987), 'Travels in Hyperreality', in *Travels in Hyperreality*, 1–58, trans. W. Weaver, London: Picador.
Eco, U. (2006), *The Mysterious Flame of Queen Loana*, London: Vintage.
Elliott, J. K. (1993), *The Apocryphal New Testament*, Oxford: Clarendon Press.
Falconer, R. (2007), *Hell in Contemporary Literature*, Edinburgh: Edinburgh University Press.
Faulks on Fiction, 'The Hero' (2011), [TV documentary], UK: BBC Two, 5 November.
Faye, J. (2001), 'Canada in a Coma', *American Review of Canadian Studies*, 31 (3): 501–10.
Feinmann, J. (2019), '"What makes people in comas wake up – from Lynx to Rolling Stones" Satisfaction', *inews*, 18 June. Available online: https://inews.co.uk/news/health/coma-patient-waking-up-rolling-stones-satisfaction/ (accessed 29 June 2019).
Finer, E. (2010), *Turning into Sterne: Viktor Shklovskii and Literary Reception*, Leeds: Legenda.

Fins, J. J. (2007), 'Correspondence', *Neurology*, 68 (1): 79.
Fins, J. J. (2015), *Rights Come to Mind*, New York: Cambridge University Press.
Fins, J. J., N. D. Schiff and K. M. Foley (2007), 'Late Recovery from the Minimally Conscious State', *Neurology*, 68: 304–7.
Flood, A. (2018), 'Boy Who Came Back From Heaven Author Sues Book's Christian Publisher', *The Guardian*, 12 April. Available online: https://www.theguardian.com/books/2018/apr/12/boy-who-came-back-from-heaven-author-sues-books-christian-publisher (accessed 28 June 2019).
Forshaw, M. (2000), 'Douglas Coupland: In and Out of "Ironic Hell"', *Critical Survey*, 12 (3): 39–58.
Frank, A. W. (1997), *The Wounded Storyteller*, Chicago: University of Chicago Press.
Freud, S. (1939), *Moses and Monotheism*, trans. K. Jones, Letchworth and Herts: Hogarth Press.
Freud, S. (1958), 'Remembering, Repeating and Working-Through', in *The Standard Edition of the Complete Psychological Works of Sigmund Freud*, 145–56, trans. J. Strachey, London: Hogarth Press.
Freud, S. ([1930] 2002), *Civilization and Its Discontents*, trans. D. McLintock, London: Penguin.
Freud, S. ([1899] 2003), 'Screen Memories', in *The Uncanny*, 1–22, trans. D. McLintock, London: Penguin.
Freud, S. ([1920] 2003), 'Beyond the Pleasure Principle', in *Beyond the Pleasure Principle and Other Writings*, 43–102, London: Penguin.
Freud, S. ([1919] 2003), 'The Uncanny', in *The Uncanny*, 121–61, trans. D. McLintock, London: Penguin.
Freud, S. ([1918] 2005), 'Timely Reflections on War and Death', in *On Murder, Mourning and Melancholia*, 167–94 trans. S. Whiteside, London: Penguin.
Freud, S. ([1899] 2006), *Interpreting Dreams*, trans. J. A. Underwood, London: Penguin.
Freud, S. ([1925] 2008), 'A Note Upon the Mystic Writing Pad', in P. Rieff (ed.), *General Psychological Theory*, 211–16, London: Simon & Schuster.
Freud, S. and J. Breuer ([1893] 2004), *Studies On Hysteria*, London: Penguin.
Frost, M. (2017), *Twin Peaks: The Final Dossier*, London: Macmillan.
Frye, N. (1963), *Fables of Identity: Studies in Poetic Mythology*, New York: Harbinger.
Frye, N. (1964), *The Educated Imagination*, Bloomington, IN: Indiana University Press.
Frye, N. (1981), *The Great Code*, New York: Harcourt Brace Jovanovich.
Fueshko, T. M. (2016), 'The Intricacies Of Shell Shock: A Chronological History Of The Lancet's Publications By Dr. Charles S. Myers And His Contemporaries', *Peace & Change*, 41 (1): 38–51.
Fulton, J. F. (1942), 'Blast and Concussion in the Present War', *New England Journal of Medicine*, 226 (1): 1–8.
Galen (1962), *On Anatomical Procedures: The Later Books*, trans. W. L. H. Duckworth, Cambridge: Cambridge University Press.
Galen (2006), *Galen: On Diseases and Symptoms*, trans. I. Johnston, Cambridge: Cambridge University Press.
Garland, A. (2004), *The Coma*, London: Faber and Faber.
Gaylin, W. (1974), 'Harvesting the Dead', *Harper's*, 249 (1492): 23–38.
Ghost Stories (2017), [Film], Dir. J. Dyson and A. Nyman, UK: Lionsgate Films.
Giacino, J. T, S. Ashwal, N. Childs, R. Cranford, B. Jennett, D. I. Katz, J. P. Kelly, J. H. Rosenberg, J. Whyte, R. D. Zafonte and N. D. Zasler (2002), 'The Minimally Conscious State: Definition and Diagnostic Criteria', *Neurology*, 58: 349–53

Giacino, J. T., D. I. Katz, N. D. Schiff, J. Whyte, E. J. Ashman, S. Ashwari, R. Barbano, F. M. Hammond, S. Laureys, G. S. F. Ling, R. Nakase-Richardson, R. T. Seel, S. Yablon, T. S. D. Getchius, G. S. Gronseth and M. J. Armstrong (2018), 'Practice Guideline Update Recommendations Summary: Disorders of Consciousness', *Neurology*, 91: 450–60.

Goldenberg, S. (2003), 'Crash Victim Wakes Up After 20 Years', *The Guardian*, 9 July. Available online: http://www.theguardian.com/world/2003/jul/09/usa.suzannegoldenberg (accessed 19 July 2014).

Goldie, D. (2015), *The Cambridge Companion to British Fiction Since 1945*, New York: Cambridge University Press.

Good Bye, Lenin! (2003), [Film] Dir. Wolfgang Becker, Germany: X Verleih AG and Sony Pictures Classics.

'The Gospel of Nicodemus' ([c.4th Century AD] 1993), Latin A text, *The Apocryphal New Testament*, trans. J. K. Elliott, Oxford: Clarendon Press.

Gowers, W. (1893), *A Manual of Diseases of the Nervous System*, Vol. 2, Second edn, London: J. & A. Churchill.

Granacher, R. P. (2008), *Traumatic Brain Injury: Methods for Clinical and Forensic Neuropsychiatric Assessment*, Boca Raton, FL: CRC Press.

Grant, G. (2014), 'Whacky Rhymes', in M. Colbeck (ed.), *Head-Lines*, 2, 37, Blythe Bridge: Waggledance Press.

Grant, S. (2011), 'Blue Polystyrene Shoes', in M. Colbeck (ed.), *Head-Lines*, 1, 5–9, Blythe Bridge: Waggledance Press.

Grant, S. (2014), 'Unremembered Memoirs', in M. Colbeck (ed.), *Head-Lines*, 2, 4–9, Blythe Bridge: Waggledance Press.

Gray, A. (2007), *Lanark*, Edinburgh: Canongate Books.

Gray, A. (2003), *1982 Janine*, Edinburgh: Canongate Books.

Gray, K., T. A. Knickman and D. M. Wegner (2011), 'More Dead Than Dead: Perceptions of Persons in the Persistent Vegetative State', *Cognition*, 121 (2): 275–80.

Greenberg, J. (1998), 'The Echo of Trauma and the Trauma of Echo', *American Imago*, 55 (3): 319–47.

Gronwall, D., P. Wrightson and P. Waddell (1990), *Head Injury: The Facts*, New York: Oxford University Press.

Guignon, C. (2004), *On Being Authentic*, London: Routledge.

Guignon, C. (2008), 'Authenticity', *Philosophy Compass*, 3/2: 277–90.

Hable con Ella (Talk To Her) (2002), [Film] Dir. Pedro Almodóvar, Spain: Sony Pictures Classics.

Halbwachs, M. (1992), *On Collective Memory*, trans. and ed. L. A. Cosler, Chicago and London: The University of Chicago Press.

Hall, Alice (2014a), 'Representing Chronic Disorders of Consciousness: The Problem of Voice in Allende's *Paula*', *Literature and Medicine*, 32 (1): 133–47.

Hall, Allan (2014b), 'Michael Schumacher Moved Out of Intensive Care, Report Claims', *The Express*, 13 June. Available online: http://www.express.co.uk/news/world/482136/Michael-Schumacher-moved-out-of-intensive-care-but-still-in-coma-claim-reports (accessed 26 June 2019).

Hall, C. S. and V. J. Nordby (1973), *A Primer of Jungian Psychology*, New York: Mentor.

Harlow, J. M. (1868), *Recovery from the Passage of an Iron Bar Through the Head*, Boston: David Clapp & Son.

Harrington, A. (1985), 'Nineteenth-Century Ideas on Hemisphere Differences and "duality of mind"', *The Behavioral And Brain Sciences*, 8: 617–60.

Harris, S. L. and G. Platzner (1995), *Classical Mythology: Images and Insights*, Mountain View, CA: Mayfield.

Harrison, R. P. (2003), *The Dominion of the Dead*, Chicago: The University of Chicago Press.
Hattenstone, S. (2020), 'Michael Rosen on His Covid-19 Coma: "It felt like a pre-death, a nothingness"', *The Guardian*, 30 September. Available online: https://www.theguardian.com/books/2020/sep/30/michael-rosen-on-his-covid-19-coma-it-felt-like-a-pre-death-a-nothingness (accessed 2 October 2020).
Hendricks, G. (1975), *Edweard Muybridge: The Father of the Motion Picture*, London: Secker & Warburg.
Herman, J. (1997), *Trauma and Recovery*, New York: Basic Books.
Herman, L. and Bart Vervaeck (2009), 'Capturing Capgras: *The Echo Maker* by Richard Powers', *Style*, 43 (3): 407–28.
Hillman, J. (1979), *The Dream and the Underworld*, New York: Harper and Row.
Hippocrates (1817), *The Aphorisms of Hippocrates*, New York: Collins & Co.
Hippocrates ([430 to 330 BC] 1978), *Hippocratic Writings*, ed. G. E. R. Lloyd, Harmondsworth: Penguin.
Hirsten, W. and V. S. Ramachandran (1997), 'Capgras Syndrome: A Novel Probe for Understanding the Neural Representation of the Identity and Familiarity of Persons', *Proceedings: Biological Sciences*, 264 (1380): 437–44.
Hoffman, K. A. (2006), 'Sleeping Beauties In The Fairground', *Early Popular Visual Culture*, 4 (2): 139–59.
Hogancamp, M. and C. Shellen (2016), *Welcome To Marwencol*, New York: Princeton Architectural Press.
Holland, S. (2003), *Bioethics: A Philosophical Introduction*, Cambridge: Polity Press.
Hollander, J. (2001), 'The Rhetoric of Consciousness', *Social Research*, 68 (3): 589–608.
Hollyman, S. (2013), 'Interview with M. Colbeck', 12 November.
Hollyman, S. (2021), *Lairies*, London: Influx Press.
The Holy Bible, King James Version Homer ([c.8th century BC] 1991), the *Odyssey*, trans. Richmond Lattimore, New York: Harper Perennial.
Horspool, D. (2010), 'A Pioneer and a Murderer: The Man Who Gave Us Moving Pictures', *The Times* (Review), 14 August: 6–7.
Hunsaker Hawkins, A. (1986), 'A. R. Luria and the Art of Clinical Biography', *Literature and Medicine* 5: 1–15.
Hunsaker Hawkins, A. (1992), 'Charting Dante: The *Inferno* and Medical Education', *Literature and Medicine*, 11 (2): 200–15.
Hunsaker Hawkins, A. (1999), *Reconstructing Illness*, 2nd edn, West Lafayette, IN: Purdue University Press.
Hutchinson, R. (2005), *Head/Case*, London: Oberon Books.
Hux, K., C. D. Schram and T. Goeken (2006): 'Misconceptions About Brain Injury: A Survey Replication Study', *Brain Injury*, 20 (5): 547–53.
I Feel Pretty (2018), [Film] Dirs. Abby Kohn and Marc Silverstein, USA: STX Entertainment.
Ibieta, G. (1990), 'Transcending the Culture of Exile' in D. Bevan (ed.), *Literature and Exile*, 67–76, Amsterdam: Rudopi.
Illes, J., M. P. Kirschen and J. D. E. Gabrieli (2003), 'From Neuroimaging to Neuroethics', *Nature Neuroscience*, 6 (3): 205.
Irving, W. ([1819] 2009), 'The Tale of Rip Van Winkle', in *The Tale of Rip Van Winkle and Other Stories*, 9–43, Ware, Herts: Wordsworth.
James, W. (1890), *The Principles of Psychology Vol. 1*, New York: Henry Holt.

Janet, P. (1925), *Psychological Healing: A Historical and Clinical Study*, trans. E. and C. Paul, London: George Allen & Unwin.
Jarrett, C. (2015), *Great Myths of the Brain*, Chichester: Wiley Blackwell.
Jennett, B. (2002), 'The Vegetative State', *Journal of Neurology, Neurosurgery and Psychiatry*, 73: 355–7.
Jennett, B. and G. Teasdale (1976), 'Predicting Outcome in Individual Patients After Severe Brain Injury', *The Lancet*, May 15: 1031–4.
Jensen, L. (2005), *The Ninth Life of Louis Drax*, London: Bloomsbury.
Jian, M. (2008), *Beijing Coma*, trans. F. Drew, London: Vintage.
Jones, B. (2013), 'Imperfect Doubles: The Recasting of Place, Object and Character in the Dream Narratives of *The Bridge*', in M. Colebrook and K. Cox (eds), *The Trangressive Iain Banks*, 76–86, Jefferson, NC: McFarland & Company.
Jones, E., N. T. Fear and S. Wessely (2007), 'Shell Shock and Mild Traumatic Brain Injury: A Historical Review', *Journal of American Psychiatry*, 164: 1641–5.
Journeyman (2017), [Film] Dir. Paddy Considine, UK: Film 4.
Jung, C. (1959), 'The Archetypes of the Collective Unconscious', in Sir H. Read, M. Fordham and G. Adler (eds), *The Collected Works of C.G. Jung*, vol. 9, part 1, trans. R. F. C. Hull, London and Henley: Routledge and Kegan Paul.
Jung, C. (1973), *Psychological Reflections*, ed. Jolande Jacobi and R. F. C. Hull, New York: Princeton/Bollingen.
Jung, C. (1977), *The Collected Works of Carl Jung*, ed. Sir H. Read, M. Fordham and G. Adler, 18, trans. R. F. C. Hull, London and Henley: Routledge and Kegan Paul.
Just Like Heaven (2005), [Film] Dir. Mark Waters, USA: DreamWorks.
Kaplan, F. (1974), '"The Mesmeric Mania": The Early Victorians and Animal Magnetism', *Journal of the History of Ideas*, 35 (4): 691–702.
Kazantzakis, N. (1975), *The Last Temptation*, London: Faber and Faber.
Kellner, D. (2009), 'Jean Baudrillard (1929–2007): A Critical Overview', in R. Bishop (ed.), *Baudrillard Now*, 17–27. Cambridge: Polity Press.
Kill Bill Volume 1 (2003), [Film] Dir. Quentin Tarantino, USA: Miramax.
Kincaid, P. (1991), 'Only Connect: Psychology and Politics in the Work of Christopher Priest', *Foundation*, 0: 42–58.
King, N. (2000) *Memory, Narrative, Identity*, Edinburgh: Edinburgh University Press.
King, S. ([1979] 2007) *The Dead Zone*, London: Hodder and Stoughton.
Kirkman, R. and T. Moore (2013), *The Walking Dead: Volume 1: Days Gone Bye*, Berkeley, CA: Image Comics.
Knechel Johansen, R. (2002), *Listening in the Silence, Seeing in the Dark*, Berkeley and Los Angeles: The University of California Press.
Knirsch, C. (2014), 'Richard Powers's "The Echo Maker": Reassessing the Neuronovel in American Literature', *American Studies*, 59 (1): 47–62.
Koehler, P. J. and E. F. M.Wijdicks (2008), 'Historical Study of Coma: Looking Back through Medical and Neurological texts', *Brain*, 131: 877–89.
Kontinen, J. (2009), 'Modern Day Lazarus: Man Regains Full Consciousness After 23 Years in Coma', *Wryte Stuff*. Available online: http://jkontinen.wrytestuff.com/swa558023-Modern-Day-Lazarus-Man-Regains-Full-Consciousness-After-23-Years-In-Coma.htm (accessed 17 July 2012).
Kristeva, J. ([1941] 1982), *Powers Of Horror*, New York: Columbia University Press.
Lacan, J. (2006), *Écrits*, trans. B. Fink, New York: W. W. Norton & Company.
LaCapra, D. (2001), *Writing History, Writing Trauma*, Baltimore: The Johns Hopkins University Press.

Laing, R .D. (2010), *The Divided Self*, London: Penguin.
Lakoff, G. and M. Johnson (1980), *Metaphors We Live By*, Chicago: The University of Chicago Press.
Laplanche, J. (1999), *Essays On Otherness*, Abingdon: Routledge.
The Last Temptation of Christ (1988), [Film] Dir. M. Scorsese, USA and Canada: Universal.
Latronico, N., O. Manenti, L. Baini and F. A. Rasulo (2011), 'Quality Reporting on the Vegetative State in Italian Newspapers: The Case of Eluana Englaro', *PLoS ONE*, 6 (4): e18706.
Laureys, S., G. G.. Celesia, F. Cohadon, J. Lavrijsen, J. León-Carrión, W. G. Sannita, L. Sazbon, E. Schmutzhard, K. R. von Wild, A. Zeman, G. Dolce and the European Task Force on Disorders of Consciousness (2010), 'Unresponsive Wakefulness Syndrome: a New Name for the Vegetative State or Apallic Syndrome", *BMC Medicine*, 8 (68): 1–4.
Lea, D. (2012), 'The Anxieties of Authenticity in Post-2000 British Fiction', *Modern Fiction Studies*, 58 (3): 459–76.
Leidig, M. (2007), '"The 19-year Coma" Story Rubbished', *The Guardian (Media Supplement)*, 5 June. Available online: http://www.theguardian.com/media/2007/jun/05/pressandpublishing.broadcasting (accessed 18 July 2014).
Levy, M. (2000), *If Only It Were True*, London: Fourth Estate.
Life On Mars (2006–07), [TV series] Dir. Various, UK: BBC One.
Lifton, R. J. (1995), 'An Interview with Robert Jay Lifton', in Cathy Caruth (ed.), *Trauma: Explorations in Memory*, 128–47 Chicago: The Johns Hopkins University Press.
Littell, E. (1847), *The Living Age*, 8, Boston: E. Littell & Company.
Longenecker, R. N. (2003), *The Westminster Theological Wordbook of the Bible*, ed. D. E. Gowan, Louisville: John Knox Press.
Lopate, P. (2009), *Notes On Sontag*, Princeton, NJ: Princeton University Press.
Luckhurst, R. (2008), *The Trauma Question*, London and New York: Routledge.
Lundkvist, A. (1991), *Journeys in Dream and Imagination*, trans. A. B. Weismann and A. Planck, New York: Four Walls Eight Windows.
Luria, A.R. (1970), *Traumatic Aphasia*, The Hague and Paris: Mouton.
Luria, A. R. (1975), *The Man With a Shattered World*, Harmondsworth: Penguin.
Luria, A. R., M. Cole and K. Levitin (2010), *The Autobiography of Anton Luria*, New York: Psychology Press.
Lyman, S. (2007), *Waking Up: Memoirs of a Coma Recoverer*, Baltimore, MD: Publish America.
Mackay, D. and A. Hall (2014), 'F1 Hero Michael Schumacher Can Lead "Relatively Normal Life" Soon, Says Former Ferrari Boss', *The Metro*, 7 October 2014. Available online: http://www.mirror.co.uk/sport/formula-1/f1-hero-michael-schumacher-can-4395046 (accessed 26 June 2019).
Mackay, M. (2003), '*Marabou Stork Nightmares*: Irvine Welsh's Anthropological Vision', *National Identities*, 5 (3): 269–81.
Macmillan, M. (2002), *An Odd Kind of Flame: Stories About Phineas Gage*, Cambridge, MA and London: The MIT Press.
Malabou, C. (2008), *What Should We Do With Our Brain?*, trans. S. Rand, New York: Fordham University Press.
Malabou, C. (2012), *The New Wounded: From Neurosis to Brain Damage*, trans. S. Miller, New York: Fordham University Press.
Malarkey, K. and A. Malarkey (2011), *The Boy Who Came Back From Heaven*, Carol Stream: Tyndale House.
Manea, N. (2012), *The Fifth Impossibility*, New Haven and London: Yale University Press.

Mansfield, N. (2000), *Subjectivity*, New York: New York University Press.
Marwencol (2010), [Film documentary] Dir. Jeff Malmberg, Canada: Kinosmith.
Mason, M. P. (2008), *Head Cases*, New York: Farrar, Straus and Giroux.
Matthews-King, A. (2019), 'Parkinson's Patients Abused and Accused of Being Drunk Or Not Disabled Enough, Survey Reveals', *The Guardian*, 11 April. Available online: https://www.independent.co.uk/news/health/parkinsons-disease-symptoms-stigma-drunk-disabled-abuse-a8863756.html (accessed 20 November 2020).
Mawson, R. (1999), *The Lazarus Child*, London: Bantam Books.
McAleer, P. (2011), 'I Have the Whole World in My Hands . . . Now What? Power, Control, Responsibility and the Baby Boomers in Stephen King's Fiction', *The Journal of Popular Culture*, 44 (6): 1209–27.
McCarthy, T. (2008), 'What's Left Behind: An Interview with Tom McCarthy', conducted by R. Orwell, The London Consortium, London: Static.
McCarthy, T. (2010), *Remainder*, Richmond: Alma Books.
McCarthy, T. (2011), 'Interview with Tom McCarthy', conducted by F. Fernandez Armesto', *The White Review*. Available online: www.thewhitereview.org/interviews/interview-with-tom-mccarthy-2/ (accessed 26 June 2019).
McClure, J. (2011), 'The Role of Causal Attributions in Public Misconceptions About Brain Injury', *Rehabilitation Psychology*, 56 (2): 85–93.
McCormack, M. (2005), *Notes On A Coma*, London: Jonathan Cape.
McGill, R. (2000), 'The Sublime Simulacrum: Vancouver in Douglas Coupland's Geography of Apocalypse', *Essays on Canadian Writing*, Spring, 70: 252–76.
Memento (2000), [Film] Dir. Christopher Nolan, USA: Summit Entertainment.
Middleton, P. M. (2012), 'Practical Use of the Glasgow Coma Scale; a Comprehensive Narrative Review of GCS Methodology', *Australasian Emergency Nursing Journal*, 15: 150–83.
Middleton, T. (1999), 'The Works of Iain. M. Banks: A Critical Introduction', *Foundation*, 76 (Summer): 5–16.
Miller, G. (2007), 'Welsh and Identity Politics', in Berthold Schoene (ed.), *The Edinburgh Companion to Contemporary Scottish Fiction*, Edinburgh: Edinburgh University Press.
Mindell, A. (1989), *Coma: Key to Awakening*, Boston: Shambhala.
Mitchell, D. T. and S. L. Snyder (2000), *Narrative Prosthesis*, Ann Arbor: The University of Michigan Press.
Monti, M. A. Vanhaudenhuyse, M. R. Coleman, M. Boly, J. D. Pickard, L.Tshibanda, A. M. Owen and S. Laureys (2010), 'Wilful Modulation of Brain Activity in Disorders of Consciousness', *New England Journal of Medicine*, 362 (7): 579–89.
MotherFatherSon (2019), [TV mini-series] Dirs. Various, UK: BBC Studios.
The Multi-Society Task Force on PVS (1994), 'Medical Aspects of the Persistent Vegetative State', *The New England Journal of Medicine*, 330 (21): 1499–508.
Myers, C. (1915), 'A Contribution to the Study of Shell Shock', *The Lancet*, February 13: 316–20.
Mystify (2019), [Documentary Film] Dir. Richard Lowenstein, USA: Dogwoof.
Nettleton, S. J., Kitzinger and C. Kitzinger (2014), 'A Diagnostic Illusory? The Case of Distinguishing Between "Vegetative" and "Minimally Conscious" States', *Social Science & Medicine*, 116: 134–41.
Neversong, formerly *Once Upon A Coma* (2020), [Video Game], Boulder, CO: Serenity Forge/Atmos Games.
The Ninth Life of Louis Drax (2016), [Film] Dir. Alexandre Aja, UK, USA, Canada: Miramax.

Niven, J. (2010), *The Amateurs*, London: Random House.
Nochi, M. (2000), 'Reconstructing Self-narratives in Coping with Traumatic Brain Injury', *Social Science & Medicine*, 5: 1795–804.
Nolan, J. (2002), 'Memento Mori', in L. Dark (ed.), *The O. Henry Prize Stories*, New York: Anchor Books.
Novoa, A. (2005), 'Whose Talk Is It? Almodóvar and the Fairy Tale in *Talk to Her*', *Marvels & Tales*, 19 (2): 224–48.
O'Driscoll, K. and J. P. Leach (1998), '"No longer Gage": An Iron Bar through the Head', *BMJ*, 317: 1673–4.
Oltermann, P. (2014), 'Michael Schumacher Being Brought Out of Induced Coma, Says Manager', *The Guardian*, 30 January. Available online: http://www.theguardian.com/sport/2014/jan/30/michael-schumacher-brought-out-induced-coma (accessed 26 June 2019).
Owen, A. (2017), *Into The Grey Zone*, London: Guardian Books.
Owen, A. M., M. R. Coleman, M. Boly, M. H. Davis, S. Laureyst and J. D. Pickard (2006), 'Detecting Awareness in the Vegetative State', *Science*, 313 (5792): 1402.
Pachalska, M., B. D. MacQueen, B. L. J. Kaczmarek, M. Wilk-Franczuk and I. Herman-Sucharska (2011), 'A Case of "Borrowed Identity Syndrome" After Severe Traumatic Brain Injury', *Med Sci Monit*, 17 (2): CS18–CS28.
Page, B. (2011), 'Martin Amis: Only Brain Injury Could Make Me Write for Children', *The Guardian*, 11 February 2011. Available online: http://www.theguardian.com/books/2011/feb/11/martin-amis-brain- injury-write-children (accessed 26 June 2019).
Page, D. L. (1955), *The Homeric Odyssey*, Oxford: Clarendon Press.
Page, R. (2012), *Stories and Social Media*, Abingdon: Routledge.
Palahniuk, C. (2003), *Diary*, London: Jonathan Cape.
Panorama, 'The Mind Reader: Unlocking My Voice' (2012), [TV Documentary], UK: BBC One, 13 November.
Parfitt, T. (2007), 'Fairytale Awakening After 19 Years Leaves Man Astonished at Post-communist Life', *The Guardian*, 9 June. Available online: http://www.theguardian.com/world/2007/jun/09/tomparfitt.international (accessed 26 June 2019).
Paterson, T. (2014), 'Michael Schumacher: Doctors Voice Concerns Over Coma "Recovery" Claims', *The Telegraph*, 17 June. Available online: http://www.telegraph.co.uk/sport/motorsport/formulaone/michael-schumacher/10905287/Michael-Schumacher-Doctors-voice-concerns-over-coma-recovery-claims.html (accessed 26 June 2019).
Patrick (1978), [Film] Dir. Richard Franklin, Australia: Filmways.
Patrick: Evil Awakens (2013), [Film] Dir. Mark Hartley, Australia: Umbrella Entertainment.
Pattie, D. (2013), 'The Lessons of *Lanark*: Iain Banks, Alasdair Gray and the Scottish Political Novel', in M. Colebrook and K. Cox (eds), *The Trangressive Iain Banks*, 9–27, Jefferson, NC: McFarland & Company.
'PC Paul Briggs: Life Support Treatment "should stop"' (2016), *BBC News*, 20 December. Available online: https://www.bbc.co.uk/news/uk-38382771 (accessed 28 June 2019).
Petrie, D. (2004), *Contemporary Scottish Fictions*, Edinburgh: Edinburgh University Press.
Pike, D. L. (1997), *Passage Through Hell*, Ithaca, NY: Cornell University Press.
Pinkerton, N. (Date Unknown), 'Interview with James B. Harris', *Film Comment*. Available online: https://www.filmcomment.com/interview-james-b-harris-part-one/ (accessed 16 July 2020).
Plath, S. (1965), 'Lady Lazarus', in *Ariel*, 16–19, London: Faber and Faber.

Plato ([c.380BC] 1995), 'The Allegory of the Cave' and 'The Myth of Er', in S. L. and G. Platzner (eds), *Classical Mythology: Images and Insights*, 826–38, trans. F. M. Cornford, Mountain View, CA: Mayfield.
Platts-Mills, B. (2019), *Tell Me The Planets*, London: Penguin.
Platts-Mills, B. (2020), 'On Matthew's Mind', *Aeon*, 17 July 2020. Available online: https://aeon.co/essays/matthew-had-a-brain-injury-who-is-he-after-brain-surgery (accessed 20 July 2020).
Plum, F. and J. B. Posner (1980), *The Diagnosis of Stupor and Coma*, 3rd edn, Philadelphia, PA: F. A. Davis Company.
Plum, F., J. B. Posner, C. B. Saper and N. F. Schiff (2007), *The Diagnosis of Stupor and Coma*, 4th edn, New York: Oxford University Press.
'Pole Wakes Up from 19-year Coma' (2007), *BBC News*, 2 June 2007. Available online: http://news.bbc.co.uk/1/hi/6715313.stm (accessed 26 June 2019).
Poster, M. (1996), 'Postmodern Virtualities', in G. Robertson (ed.), *Futurenatural: Nature, Science, Culture*, 183–202, London: Routledge.
Poster, M. (2009), 'Swan's Way: Care of Self in the Hyperreal', in R. Bishop (ed.), *Baudrillard Now*, 72–99, Cambridge: Polity Press.
Potter, D. (1996), *Karaoke and Cold Lazarus*, London: Faber and Faber.
Potts, A. and E. Semino (2019), 'Cancer As a Metaphor', *Metaphor and Symbol*, 34 (2): 81–95.
Powell, T. (1994), *Head Injury: A Practical Guide*, Bicester, Oxon: Winslow Press.
Power, H. and L. W. Sedgwick (1882), *The New Sydenham Society's Lexicon of Medicine and the Allied Sciences*, Vol. 2, London: The New Sydenham Society.
Powers, R. (2006), *The Echo Maker*, New York: Picador.
Priest, C. (2005), *The Glamour*, London: Jonathan Cape.
Pritchard, P. (1999), *The Totem Pole*, London: Constable and Company.
Racine, E., R. Amaram, M. Seidler, M. Karczewska and J. Illes (2008), 'Media Coverage of the Persistent Vegetative State and End-of-Life Decision Making', *Neurology*, 71: 1027–37.
Ramachandran, V. S. and S. Blakeslee (1998), *Phantoms in the Brain*, London: Fourth Estate.
Redgrove, P. (1999), 'Lazarus and the Sea', in *Selected Poems*, 7–8, London: Jonathan Cape.
Redgrove, P. (2006), 'Lazarus and the Visionary Truth', in Neil Roberts (ed.), *The Colour of Radio*, 142–62, Devoran: Stride.
Remainder (2015), [Film] Dir. Omer Fast, UK and Germany: BFI.
Reuben, C. (2003), 'Exile, Identity and Memory: The Boundaries of Perception', in M. Stroińska and V. Cecchetto (eds), *Exile, Language and Identity*, 197–212, Frankfurt: Peter Lang.
The Review Show (2011), [TV Documentary Series], UK: BBC Two, 3 June.
Richards, G. (2020), *The Guardian*, 11 June 2020. Available online: https://www.theguardian.com/sport/2020/jun/11/michael-schumacher-stem-cell-surgery-reports-are-premature-motor-sport (accessed 16 June 2020).
Ricoeur, P. (1985), '*Anatomy of Criticism* or the Order of Paradigms', in E. Cook, C. Hosek, J. MacPherson, P. Parker and J. Patrick (eds), *Centre and Labyrinth*, 1–13, Toronto: University of Toronto Press.
Ricoeur, P. (1991a), 'Life in Quest of Narrative', in D. Wood (ed.), *On Paul Ricoeur*, 20–33, London: Routledge.
Ricoeur, P. (1991b), 'Narrative Identity', in D. Wood (ed.), *On Paul Ricoeur*, 188–99, London: Routledge.

Ricoeur, P. (1991c), 'The Function of Fiction in Shaping Reality', in M. J. Valdés (ed.), *A Ricoeur Reader*, trans. D. Pellauer, 117–36, Hemel Hempstead: Harvester Wheatsheaf.

Ripley's Believe It Or Not Cartoon Of Phineas Gage (1947), St. Paul, MN: Brown and Bigelow.

Roberts, N. (2012), *A Lucid Dreamer: The Life of Peter Redgrove*, London: Jonathan Cape.

Rose, F. D. and D. A. Johnson (1996), *Brain Injury and After*, Chichester: John Wiley & Sons.

Roth, M. (2009), 'The Rise of the Neuronovel', *n+1*, Issue 8: Recessional. Available online: https://nplusonemag.com/issue-8/essays/the-rise-of-the-neuronovel/ (accessed 25 June 2020).

Rothberg, M. (2000), *Traumatic Realism*, Minneapolis: University of Minnesota Press.

Royal College of Physicians (2020), *Prolonged Disorders of Consciousness Following Sudden Onset Brain Injury: National Clinical Guidelines*, RCP: London.

Royle, N. (2011), *Regicide*, Oxford: Solaris.

Ryan, R. (2003), 'Coma Man Wakes After 19 Years', *Mail Online*. Available online: http://www.dailymail.co.uk/health/article-187920/Coma-man-wakes-19-years.html (accessed 26 June 2019).

Sacks, O. (2012a), *Hallucinations*, London: Picador.

Sacks, O. (2012b), 'Seeing God in the Third Millennium', *The Atlantic*, 12 December. Available online: https://www.theatlantic.com/health/archive/2012/12/seeing-god-in-the-third-millennium/266134/ (accessed 26 June 2019).

Said, E. (2000), 'Reflections on Exile', in *Reflections on Exile and Other Literary and Cultural Essays*, 173–86, London: Granta.

Sampson, E. E. (1989), 'The Destruction of the Self', in J. Shotter and K. Gergen (eds), *Texts of Identity*, 1–19, London: Sage.

Samuel, G. and J. Kitzinger (2013), 'Reporting Consciousness in Coma', *JOMEC Journal*. Available online: https://www.researchgate.net/publication/249994415_Reporting_consciousness_in_coma_Media_framing_of_neuro-scientific_research_hope_and_the_response_of_families_with_relatives_in_vegetative_and_minimally_conscious_states (accessed 26 June 2019).

The San Francisco Chronicle (1875), February 6.

Sarup, M. (1992), *Jacques Lacan*, Hemel Hempstead: Harvester Wheatsheaf.

Sarup, M. (1993), *Post-Structuralism and Postmodernism*, 2nd edn, Hemel Hempstead: Harvester Wheatsheaf.

Sayer, N. (1989), 'Atlanta', *Grand Street*, 8 (3): 207–27.

Schlesinger, P. (2004), 'W.G.Sebald and the Condition of Exile', *Theory, Culture and Society*, 21 (2): 43–67.

Schnider, A., C. von Daniken and K. Gutbrod (1996), 'The Mechanisms of Spontaneous and Provoked Confabulations', *Brain*, 119: 1365–75.

Seidel, M., (1986), *Exile and the Narrative Imagination*, New Haven, CT: Yale University Press.

Selzer, R. (1993), *Raising the Dead*, Beckenham: Whittle Direct Books.

Shermer, M. (2018), *Heavens On Earth*, London: Robinson.

Sherry, M. (2006), *If I Only Had a Brain*, New York: Routledge.

Shimamura, A. P. (2002), 'Muybridge in Motion: Travels in Art, Psychology and Neurology', *History of Photography*, 26 (4): 341–50.

Shively, S. B and D. P. Perl (2012), 'Traumatic Brain Injury, Shell Shock, and Posttraumatic Stress Disorder in the Military—Past, Present, and Future', *Journal of Head Trauma Rehabilitation*, 27 (3): 234–9.

Silva, J. A. G., B. Leong, R. Weinstock and C. L. Boyer (1989), 'Capgras Syndrome and Dangerousness', *Bull Am Acad Psychiatry Law*, 17 (1): 5–14.
Smith, S. (1988), 'Dictators and Comas', Toronto *Globe and Mail*, 14 March 1998.
Smith, Z. (2008), 'Two Paths for the Novel', *The New York Review of Books*, 20 November. Available online: http://www.nybooks.com/articles/archives/2008/nov/20/two-paths-for-the-novel/?pagination=false (accessed 26 June 2019).
Some Call It Loving (1973), [Film] Dir. James B. Harris, USA: Two World Film.
Sontag, S. (1966), 'Against Interpretation', in *Against Interpretation and Other Essays*, 3–14, New York: Picador.
Sontag, S. (1991), *Illness as Metaphor and AIDS and Its Metaphors*, London: Penguin.
The Sopranos, 'Mayham' (2006), [TV Series Episode] Dir. Jack Bender, USA: HBO.
Source Code (2011), [Film] Dir. Duncan Jones, USA: Summit.
Stephenson, R. L. ([1886] 1999), *The Strange Case of Dr Jekyll and Mr Hyde*, London: Wordsworth Classics.
Strengell, H. (2005), *Dissecting Stephen King*, Madison: The University of Wisconsin Press.
Stroińska, M. (2003), 'The Role of Language in the Re-construction of Identity in Exile', in M. Stroińska and V. Cecchetto (eds), *Exile, Language and Identity*, 197–212, Frankfurt: Peter Lang.
Tal, K. (1996), *Worlds of Hurt*, Cambridge: Cambridge University Press.
Tate, A. (2007), *Douglas Coupland*, Manchester: Manchester University Press.
Teasdale, G., A. Maas, F. Lecky, G. Manley, N. Stocchetti and G. Murray (2014), 'The Glasgow Coma Scale at 40 years: Standing the Test of Time', *Lancet Neurology*, 13: 844–54.
Tew, P. (2007), *The Contemporary British Novel*, London: Continuum.
Thwaites, T. (2000), 'Miracles: Hot Air and Histories of the Improbable', in N. Lucy (ed.), *Postmodern Theory: An Anthology*, 264–81, Oxford: Blackwell Publishers.
Todorov, T. (1973), *The Fantastic*, Ithaca, NY: Cornell University Press.
Trance (2013), [Film] Dir. Danny Boyle, UK and France: Fox Searchlight.
Trilling, L. (1972), *Sincerity and Authenticity*, London: Oxford University Press.
Trumbo, D. ([1939] 2009), *Johnny Got His Gun*, London: Penguin.
Turner-Stokes, L., J. Kitzinger, H. Gill-Thwaites, E. D. Playford, D. Wade, J. Allanson and J. Pickard (2012), 'fMRI for Vegetative and Minimally Conscious States: A More Balanced Perspective', *BMJ*, 345: e8045.
28 Days Later (2002), [Film] Dir. Danny Boyle, UK: 20th Century Fox.
Twin Peaks: The Return (2017), [TV Series] Dir. David Lynch, USA: Showtime.
Van Der Kolk, B. A. and O. Van Der Hart (1995), 'The Intrusive Past: The Flexibility of Memory and the Engraving of Trauma', in C. Caruth (ed.), *Trauma: Explorations in Memory*, 158–82, Baltimore, MD: The Johns Hopkins University Press.
Vanishing Waves (2012), [Film] Dir. Kristina Buožytė, Lithuania, France, Belgium: Autonomy Pictures.
Vermeulen, P. (2012), 'The Critique of Trauma and the Afterlife of the Novel in Tom McCarthy's *Remainder*', *Modern Fiction Studies*, 58 (3): 549–68.
Vickroy, L. (2002), *Trauma and Survival in Contemporary Fiction*, Charlottesville and London: University of Virginia Press.
Virgil ([29 to 19 BC] 2004), the *Aeneid*, trans. M. Oakley, London: Wordsworth.
Wade, D. (2001), 'Ethical Issues in Diagnosis and Management of Patients in the Permanent Vegetative State', *BMJ*, 322: 352–4.
Wade, D. (2002), 'The Dis-integration of Death', *The Lancet*, 360: 425–6.
The Walking Dead, 'Days Gone Bye' (2010), [TV Series Episode] Dir. Frank Darabont, USA: AMC.

Waugh, C. (2014), 'Lager and Black', in M. Colbeck (ed.), *Head-Lines*, 2, Blythe Bridge: Waggledance Press.
Weatherhead, S. and D. Todd, eds (2002), *Narrative Approaches to Brain Injury*, London: Karnac Books.
Weinstein, E. A. and O. G. Lyerly (1968), 'Confabulation Following Brain Injury: Its Analogues and Sequela', *Archives of General Psychology*, 18: 248–54.
Welcome To Marwen (2018), [Film] Dir. Robert Zemeckis, USA: Universal.
Welsh, I. (1996), *Marabou Stork Nightmares*, London: Vintage.
Whitehead, A. (2004), *Trauma Fiction*, Edinburgh: Edinburgh University Press.
Wiersema, R. (2006), *Before I Wake*, Toronto: Random House Canada.
Wiersema, R. (2007), 'Wake Up, Wake Up, You Sleepyhead', Toronto *Globe and Mail*, June 23. Available online: http://www.theglobeandmail.com/arts/wake-up-wake-up-you-sleepyhead/article723881/ (accessed 26 June 2019).
Wijdicks, E. F. M. (2008), *The Comatose Patient*, New York: Oxford University Press.
Wijdicks, E. F. M. (2017), 'C. Miller Fisher and the Comatose Patient', *Neurocritical Care*, 30 (1): 1–4.
Wijdicks, E. F. M. and A. Coen (2006), 'The Portrayal of Coma in Contemporary Motion Pictures', *Neurology*, 66: 1300–3.
Wijdicks, E. F. M. and A. Coen (2007), 'Correspondence', *Neurology*, 68 (1): 79–80.
Wijdicks, E. F. M. and Marilou F. Wijdicks (2006), 'Coverage of Coma in Headlines of US Newspapers From 2001 Through 2005', *Mayo Clinic Proceedings*, 81 (10): 1332–6.
Wilde, J. (2011), 'Thoughts; Feelings', in M. Colbeck (ed.), *Head-Lines*, 1, Blythe Bridge: Waggledance Press.
Williams, M. (1979), *Brain Damage, Behaviour, and the Mind*, Chichester: John Wiley & Sons.
Williams, R. (1992), *Notes on the Underground*, Cambridge, MA: MIT Press.
Wilson, L. (1990), 'European or Caribbean: Jean Rhys and the Language of Exile', in D. Bevan (ed.), *Literature and Exile*, 77–89, Amsterdam: Rudopi.
Winick, J. (2006), 'Daedalus and Icarus: The Return of Jason Todd', in *Batman Annual*, 25, Burbank, CA: DC Comics.
World Cup Qualifier: Portugal Vs USA (2014), [Sports coverage], UK: BBC One, 22 June.
Yapijakis, C. (2009), 'Hippocrates of Kos, the Father of Clinical Medicine, and Asclepiades of Bithynia, the Father of Molecular Medicine', *In Vivo*, 23: 507–14.
Zeman, A. (2014), 'Neurology Is Psychiatry—and Vice Versa', *Practical Neurology*, 14 (3): 136–44.

Index

abjection 96, 163; *see also* Kristeva, Julia
abreaction 61–3
Achilles 85
Adorno, Theodor 8
afterwardsness 44, 58, 148; *see also* nachträglichkeit
Agamben, Giorgio 178
ageusia 17, 142; *see also* loss of taste
Alexander, Eben 149–50
Aligheri, Dante 86, 90–1, 93–4, 96–7, 102
Allatt, Kate 143
Allende, Isabel 157–8, 162–3
Almodóvar, Pedro 1–2, 9, 43, 105, 182; *see also* Hable con Ella
altered states of consciousness 18, 20, 34, 145
Alzheimer's disease 164
Amateurs, The 182
American new-wave cinema 113–14
Amis, Martin 33, 36
amnesia 3, 7–8, 25–7, 35, 68, 70, 108–9, 116–17, 174–5; *see also* memory
   anterograde amnesia 119–20
   paramnesia 188
ANH; *see* artificial nutrition and hydration
animal experimentation 15–16, 19, 140; *see also* Galen
anosmia 25, 142, 175
apocalypse 35, 78, 168–9
apoplexy 15, 17–19, 28
archetypal psychology 7, 84–5; *see also* depth psychology; psychology
archetypes 70–7, 84–6, 90, 94–103, 161, 169, 181; *see also* Jung, Carl; Hillman, James
Aristotle 98
artificial nutrition and hydration 179, 187
Ashbery, John 34
astral projection 43, 45, 49, 60; *see also* psychic shift

authenticity 105–8, 110–17, 119, 123–5, 131, 134
autopathography 11, 139, 146, 148

Banks, Iain; *see The Bridge*
Batman franchise 69–70
Bauby, Jean-Dominique; *see Diving Bell and the Butterfly, The*
Baudrillard, Jean 113–14, 117–19, 121–6, 131, 133
   The Evil Demon of Images 113–14
   the hyperreal 118, 121, 124–5, 131–3
   hypersimulation 124, 127
   'The Orders of Simulacra' 124
   'The Precession of Simulacra' 117–18
   the real 121, 123–7, 130–1
   reference principle 117–18
   'The Remainder' 125, 133
Bauman, Zygmunt 101, 183
Becher, Wolfgang; *see Good Bye, Lenin*
Before I Wake, 169, 171–2, 182; *see also* Wiersema, Robert
Beijing Coma 37–8, 55
Bentsen, Lloyd (Sen) 33, 168
BI; *see* brain injury
bioemporium 164–5; *see also* Gaylin, Willard
bioethics 5, 9, 31, 100, 163, 165, 185; *see also* ethics
Blanchot, Maurice 122, 152
Blofeld, Henry 126
B-Met 36, 158–9, 160–2
   definition of 33
Borges, Jorge Luis 117, 119
Boyle, Danny
   Trance 35, 173
   28 Days Later 35
Boy Who Came Back From Heaven, The 150–1
brain death 4, 5, 9
   Harvard Brain Death Committee 4
   the Minnesota Criteria 5

brain injury (BI)
    acquired brain injury (ABI)   139, 158, 180, 188–9
    amygdala damage   111
    closed head trauma   25, 137
    confabulations   109–10, 116–17, 122, 136, 156
    Dysexecutive Syndrome   156
    emotional flattening   109, 111, 175, 189
    emotional lability   175, 189
    frontal cortex   111, 140, 142
    frontal lobe damage   27, 114, 140–1, 154, 156, 175
    as functional or organic damage   9, 24–7, 32, 35, 111, 136–7, 173–5, 181
    impaired vision   25, 27, 129, 142
    invisibility of   25, 135, 161, 174–5, 177, 188–9, 191 n.1 (ch.6)
    and the Limbic System   111, 136
    lived experience of   27, 109–10, 139–58, 161, 163, 173
    long-term neurological condition   11, 100, 105, 111, 127, 154–5, 173, 183, 188–9
    misattribution of behaviours   174–7
    non-traumatic brain injury   32, 188 (*see also* brain injury, acquired brain injury)
    perseverations   154–5, 175
    physiotherapy   113, 144
    rehabilitation   27–8, 46–8, 50, 113, 127–9, 136, 141, 148, 188–9
    stigma   36, 140, 160–1, 173, 175, 189
    traumatic brain injury (TBI)   24–9, 35, 50, 105–8, 111–16, 133–4, 141–55, 173, 189
brain plasticity   32, 112–14, 120
    destructive plasticity   114, 123, 128, 135, 157, 175
    impact on the hippocampus   112–13
    lesional plasticity   112
brain tumour   3, 41, 156, 180
breathing machine   162; *see also* ventilator, breathing tubes
breathing tubes   70, 147, 182, 185; *see also* ventilator, breathing machine

Bridge, The   86–97, 102, 108
Brison, Susan   72
Brooks, Peter   66–7

Cabinet of Dr Caligari, The   22; *see also* German expressionism
Campbell, Joseph   87
cancer   32–3, 36, 160–1, 183
Canguilhem, George   12
Capgras syndrome   135–7
car accident   7, 45, 109, 139, 150
Carrell, Steve   129, 131, 173; *see also* Welcome To Marwen
carus   18; *see also* karos
Caruth, Cathy   41–2, 44, 65, 74, 87
catalepsy; *see* katalepsis
causus   14
Cell, The   181
Charcot, Jean-Martin   20
Charon   75–6, 95
Cheyne, John   19–20
Christ   17, 70–1, 73, 78–80, 83–4, 95
chronic vegetative state (VS)   68–70, 77, 80, 100, 145, 158, 165–73, 185–6; *see also* continuing vegetative state; persistent vegetative state
    definition of   32
Circe   81
circuits   115, 121, 131; *see also* patterns
Clevenger, Craig; *see* Dermaphoria
C-Met   33–4, 68, 101, 144, 157, 159–83
    definition of   33
Cohn, Dorrit   58–9
Cold Lazarus   39–40, 69, 73
Collier, John; *see under* sleeping beauty
Collyer, Robert Hanam   21–22
coma
    and comata   18
    control of in fiction   58–60, 86
    death metaphor   16–17, 22–3, 35, 71–8, 83, 100–3, 157, 168, 181–3
    deep coma   4, 20, 31, 34, 74, 80, 86, 143, 146
    definition of   3–4, 6, 29
    as described by Herman Boerhaave   18
    as distinct from prolonged disorders of consciousness   1, 4–5, 12, 29–32

Index

dream metaphor   6–12, 48–50, 60, 68, 78, 87–101, 116, 142–8, 182
false memories   48, 58, 116, 117
Glasgow Coma Scale   19, 28, 30–1, 182 (*see also* Jennett, Bryan; Teasdale, Graham)
induced coma   5, 38, 74–5, 135, 144–5, 149–50, 179, 183
islands (of memory)   144–5
lightening   4, 120, 135, 145–50, 157–8, 179–82
'light-switch' recovery   146, 148, 156, 182
lived experience of   139–58, 161, 163, 173
miracle recoveries
   in fiction   4, 110, 167, 171–2, 182
   in the media   170, 177, 179–82, 186
pseudo-coma fiction   39, 69, 85
rebirth imagery   39, 50–1, 69, 75–89, 134, 143, 149, 158
response to stimuli   3, 28–30, 170–1
as sleep   3–4, 6–9, 13–19, 21–4, 38, 43, 60, 77–8, 156–8, 162–71
socio-political metaphor   33, 90, 161, 167–8, 173
surfacing   51, 135, 143, 150, 159–60, 182
train imagery   40, 44, 46, 49, 91–3, 134
   in videogames   191 n.2 (ch.2) (*see also* Driver: San Francisco)
the womb   39, 51–2, 77–8, 143, 149, 158
Coma (film)   164–5
Coma (novel)   162–5, 170, 178
Coma (TV series)   164
Coma, The   46–54, 56–69, 76–8, 169–71, 191 n.1 (ch.2)
   coma as hellish descent   82, 85, 97
   and language signification   134
   loss of narrative   147
   as metaphor of consciousness   160
Comaville   7, 38, 46, 48, 61, 116
conceptual metaphor theory   159
conflation error   179, 188; *see also* diagnostic creep
Considine, Paddy; *see Journeyman*

continuing vegetative state (VS)   37, 145–6, 165, 170; *see also* chronic vegetative state; persistent vegetative state
   definition of   32
contrapasso; *see* punishment *under* hell
Cook, Robin; *see Coma* (novel)
Coupland, Douglas; *see Girlfriend in a Coma*
Couser, G. Thomas   71, 129, 146–8, 160, 169–70
   the comic plot   8–10, 173
   illness metaphor   33, 36
   physician narratives   27, 100
Covid-19   144, 183
Cox, Laurence   155, 157, 175, 177
Cracknell, James   143–6, 154–6
Craig, Cairns   59–60, 89
Crichton, Michael   164–5; *see also Coma* (film)
Critical Care (film)   101, 163
Critical Care (novel)   100, 163–5, 185
Cronenberg, David; *see The Dead Zone* (film)
Cullen, William   18–19

Daily Mail   177, 179–80, 182
Damasio, Antonio   3–4, 7, 111, 114, 128, 143, 145
   coma as distinct from sleep   3, 18
   the proto self   107
Dead Zone (film), *The*   77, 79
Dead Zone (novel), *The*   76–85, 105, 108, 169–71; *see also* King, Stephen
De Anima Brutorum   18; *see also* Willis, Thomas
decade of the brain   32, 103
deep insulin coma therapy; *see* coma, induced coma
degradation of the body   35, 43–5, 73, 134, 157–8, 162–7
dehumanization   55, 134, 162–5, 167
déjà vu   116, 155
Deleuze, Gilles   107, 129
De Niro, Robert   113–14
depth psychology   86, 102
   and archaeology   58
   excavation imagery   10, 86–7
Dermaphoria   109–10, 113, 120

Derrida, Jacques 114–15, 136; *see also* same-but-different, the; trace, the
Diagnosis of Stupor and Coma, The (Plum and Posner) 3, 5–6, 18, 28–9, 40, 145, 170, 188
diagnostic creep 186–8; *see also* conflation error
Diary 34, 168
DICT; *see* deep insulin coma therapy
Disney
  Dumbo 55
  Sleeping Beauty 1, 182 (*see also* sleeping beauty)
disorder(s) of consciousness
  definition of 1
  as distinct from prolonged disorder(s) of consciousness 1, 4–5, 12, 29–32
divided self, the 59–60, 89
The Divided Self 60, 128
Diving Bell and the Butterfly, The (book) 40, 143, 158
Diving Bell and the Butterfly, The (film) 40
DoC; *see* disorder(s) of consciousness
Dooling, Richard; *see Critical Care*
double, the 43, 53, 60, 91, 135–6
Draper, Derek 183
Driver: San Francisco 49–50, 60, 94
Dystopia 85–6, 89, 93, 166

Eagleman, David 112–13, 116
Eaglestone, Robert 65
Echo Maker, The 134–7, 139, 142–3, 188–9
Eco, Umberto
  The Mysterious Flame of Queen Loana 108–10, 112, 116, 118, 131, 133
  'Travels in Hyperreality' 133–4
ego-identity 128–9, 134, 136
eidola 85–6, 90–7
eidolon; *see* eidola
Englaro, Eluana 178
ethics 4–5, 31–3, 39, 65, 137, 164–5, 169, 177–8, 184–7
Eurydice 93
Everyman, the 76, 94

Evolution 67, 84, 87–8
exile 37–69, 178; *see also* memory

fairy tale 1–2, 24, 43, 95, 167, 169–70; *see also* sleeping beauty
Falconer, Rachel 70, 74, 76, 87, 93, 96–7
Fast, Omer; *see Remainder* (film)
feedback loop 115, 119–20, 128, 154–5
Ferrier, David; *see* animal experimentation
fetishization 1–2, 8, 43, 50, 58, 65, 83
Fins, Joseph J. 9, 29–31, 177, 179, 186, 190
Fisher, C. M. 28–30
fMRI; *see* functional Magnetic Resonance Imaging
Frank, Arthur 101, 103, 148; *see also* restitution narrative
Frankenstein 38, 79
Freud, Sigmund 41–4, 47–9, 57–8, 61–2, 74, 83–6, 98–9, 151–3; *see also* trauma
  Beyond the Pleasure Principle 41, 44, 66–8
  Civilization and Its Discontents 106
  condensation 55–6, 63
  death drive 67, 123, 125
  displacement 55–6
  the ego 106
  free association 21, 62
  hypnosis 20, 62
  the id 59, 84, 95, 106
  The Interpretation of Dreams 13
  with Joseph Breuer 20
  latency (*see* nachträglichkeit)
  Moses and Monotheism 44
  mystic writing pad 115
  remembering, repeating, working through 44, 57, 76, 100, 103, 151
  screen memories 47, 55–7, 95
  split subject 106
  the superego 106
  the uncanny 42, 49, 56, 69 (*see also,* uncanny, the)
  via regia 86, 88
'Freud's Master Plot'; *see* Brooks, Peter
Frost, Mark; *see Twin Peaks: The Final Dossier*

Frye, Northrop   71, 77–8, 84, 86, 90, 99–100
functional brain injury; *see under* brain injury (BI)
functional Magnetic Resonance Imaging   32, 180–1, 183, 186–7; *see also* Owen, Adrian

Gage, Phineas   139–42
Galen   14–16, 18–19
  animal experimentation   15–16
  diagnosis of brain injury   15–16
Garland, Alex; *see The Coma*
Garland, Nicholas   63–4
Garraway, Kate; *see* Draper, Derek
Gaylin, Willard   163–5; *see also* bioemporium
geology   86–93, 96
German expressionism   21, 64; *see also Cabinet of Dr Caligari, The*
Ghost Stories   94–5
Giacino, Joseph   31–2, 166
Girlfriend In A Coma   165–73, 184
Glamour, The   188
Glasgow Coma Scale; *see under* coma
glorification of the body   43, 162
Good Bye, Lenin!   167
Gospel of Nicodemus, The   71–3, 76
Gowers, William   19–20, 28
Grant, Gwynfa   154–5, 157
Grant, Steph   153, 173
  'Blue Polystyrene Shoes'   144, 152–3
  'Unremembered Memoirs'   154–7, 176–7
Gray, Alisdair; *see Lanark*
Greenberg, Judith   98
Grzebski, Jan   167, 169–70, 186
Guardian, The (newspaper)   6, 33, 67, 167, 170, 177
Guignon, Charles   106

Hable con Ella   1–2, 4–6, 8–9, 23, 43, 105, 182; *see also* Almodóvar, Pedro
Halbwachs, Maurice   49
hallucination   34–6, 39, 86, 109, 120, 145–6, 149–50, 173
Hamlet   119
Harlow, John (Dr)   140, 142; *see also* Phineas Gage

Harrison, Robert Pogue   101–2
hauntings; *see under* trauma
Hawkins, Anne Hunsaker   26–7, 37–9, 69, 81, 84, 94, 98–100, 150, 159–61
Head/Case   109, 111
Head-lines   139, 153; *see also* Cox, Laurence; Grant, Gwynfa; Grant, Steph; Waugh, Caroline; Wilde, Joel
Hell   191 n.1 (ch.3); *see also* katabasis
  in Christianity   17, 70–1, 74–5, 77, 80, 91, 94–6
  Hades (god)   16, 71–2, 81
  Hades (place)   16–17, 73, 75–6, 81–3, 88, 91–7, 102, 191 n.1 (Ch. 3)
  harrowing of   70–1, 80, 95, 102
  hell-time   97
  punishment   91, 93, 95, 97, 106
  Sheol   17
  Tartarus   16–17, 91–2, 94, 102
  topography of   83–90, 96, 102
Heracles   71, 81, 95
Hercules; *see* Heracles
Hillman, James   70–1, 84–6, 91, 96; *see also* archetypes; Jung, Carl
Hippocrates   14–15
Hogancamp, Mark   129–34, 136, 173
Holland, Stephen   5, 31
Hollander, John   34–5
Hollyman, Steve; *see Lairies*
Homer   17, 102, 147
  the *Odyssey*   81–2
hope economy   169, 180, 182–4
Hutchence, Michael   175
Hutchinson, Roy; *see Head/Case*
hypnos   14, 16, 77
hypnosis
  developing from mesmerism   20–2
  hypnoanalysis   62
  hypnotherapy   20, 35 (*see also* Freud, Sigmund)
  James Braid   20
  John Elliotson   20
  neurohypnology   20
hypogeusia; *see* ageusia; loss of taste
hysteria   20–1, 25, 119, 181

I Feel Pretty 110, 182
If Only It Were True 43–5, 60, 162, 185
Inferno, the; *see* Aligheri, Dante
innovation 99, 102; *see also* Ricoeur, Paul
Irving, Washington; *see Tale of Rip Van Winkle, The*

James, William 106
Janet, Pierre 20–1
Jennett, Bryan 5, 29–31; *see also* Glasgow Coma Scale; Teasdale, Graham
Jensen, Liz; *see Ninth Life of Louis Drax, The*
Jian, Ma; *see Beijing Coma*
Johansen, Ruthann Knechel 50, 143, 145, 149, 152, 156, 158
Johnny Got His Gun 39–40, 73
Joker 35–6
Jonah 71, 80, 90
Jones, Duncan; *see Source Code*
Journeyman 188–9
Journeys In Dream and Imagination 146
Jung, Carl 84–6, 94, 98–100; *see also* archetypes; Hillman, James
  collective unconscious 84, 88, 99
  individuation 98
  the shadow 95–6
  the wise old man 84, 96
Just Like Heaven 45, 185

karos 15–16; *see also* carus
katabasis 17, 69–103, 135, 147–9, 158–61, 169, 181; *see also* quest narrative
katalepsis 15, 22
Kazantzakis, Nikos; *see The Last Temptation*
Kennedy, A. L. 36
Kill Bill Vol 1 1–2, 6, 23
King, Stephen 76–85, 105, 108, 169–71; *see also Dead Zone, The*
  influence of Baby Boomer generation 78–9
Kristeva, Julia 96; *see also* abjection

Lacan, Jacques 50–2, 54, 61–3, 86
LaCapra, Dominick 8, 65, 150

Laing, R. D. 60, 128; *see also* the divided self
Lairies 50–2, 76, 135, 143, 158, 168
Lanark 89, 93
Lancet, The 25, 30, 122
Laplanche, Jean 44; *see also* nachträglichkeit
Last Temptation, The 73–5, 77–9, 181
Last Temptation of Christ, The 73
Lawrenson, Mark 36
Lazarus 39, 64–83, 98, 121, 147, 181; *see also* Plath, Sylvia; Redgrove, Peter
Lazarus Child, The 69
lethargia; *see* lethargy
lethargy 15, 18–19
Lethe 17, 102
leviathan 80, 90
Life On Mars 6 -7, 49, 92
life support technologies 4, 31, 43–4, 70–1, 92, 171–2, 185
Lifton, Robert Jay 67, 103
limbo 8, 37, 48, 52, 77, 90, 101, 168
liminal states 8–9, 20–1, 24, 34, 43, 71–2, 80, 93, 146, 171
living dead 35, 73, 78, 80, 165
locked-in syndrome 40, 95, 143
long-term neurological condition; *see under* brain injury
loss of taste 25, 142, 175; *see also* ageusia
Luckhurst, Roger 44, 47, 56, 65, 120, 157
Lumet, Sydney; *see Critical Care* (film)
Lundkvist, Artur; *see Journeys In Dream and Imagination*
Luria, A. R. 26–8, 108, 149, 153; *see also* Zasetsky
Lyman, Sandra; *see Waking Up: Memoirs Of A Coma Recoverer*
Lynch, David; *see Twin Peaks: The Return*

McCarthy, Tom; *see Remainder*
McClure, John 174–7
McCormack, Mike; *see Notes On A Coma*
magical realism 110
Malabou, Catherine 11, 107, 111–12, 114–15, 123, 157
  shredded psyche 8, 151–53 (*see also* psyche)

Man With a Shattered World, The; see
    Luria, A. R.; Zasetsky
Marabou Stork Nightmares   46, 54–60,
    63–9, 82, 86
  authenticity of selfhood   106–8
  coma as hell   82, 89–92, 97
  as marvellous fiction   169–71
Marwencol   129–34, 136, 173
Mason, Michael Paul   107–8
Mawson, Robert; *see Lazarus Child, The*
MCS; *see* minimally conscious state
Memento   119–20, 127–8, 139
'Memento Mori' (story)   119–20
memory
  collective memory   156
  coma 'islands'   144–5 (*see also* coma)
  in exile   40–68 (*see also* exile)
  false memories   48, 58, 113, 116–19,
    121
  memory edits   47, 116, 131
  memory loss   3–7, 27, 105, 108–10,
    143–4, 150–1, 156 (*see also*
    amnesia)
  post-coma   105–38, 174
  rememory   156
  traumatic memory   40–68 (*see also*
    trauma)
messianic trope   76–7, 79, 169, 171,
    182
metamorphosis   75, 87–9, 93, 112, 115,
    134, 151, 158
Metaphors We Live By (Lakoff and
    Johnson); *see* Conceptual
    metaphor theory
minimally conscious state   170, 177–9,
    181, 183, 186–8
  definition of   5, 31
  MCS+ and MCS-   31–2
mise-en-abyme   132, 173
mise-en-page   58, 63, 65, 176
models   129–30, 132, 173
Montreal Neurological Institute   15
Morpheus   16, 87–8
MotherFatherSon   188–9
Mott, Frederick   25–6; *see also* shell
    shock
muscle atrophy   1, 6, 35, 38, 79–80, 105,
    157–8, 166, 171
Muybridge, Edweard   141–2

Myers, Charles   25, 27, 122; *see also* shell
    shock
Mystify; see Michael Hutchence
myth-making   57, 100, 160–1

nachträglichkeit   43–4, 58, 148; *see also*
    afterwardsness
narrative identity   69, 184; *see also*
    Ricoeur, Paul
Narrative Prosthesis (Mitchell and
    Snyder)   12, 158, 161, 172–3
  narrative prosthesis in fiction   159–90
NDE; *see* near-death experience
near-death experience   7, 34, 74, 101,
    145–51
  white tunnel trope   7, 34, 101
nekyia   70–1, 81–2, 90
  as distinct from nekyomanteia   81
  in the *Odyssey*   81–2, 90
neomort   11, 162–9, 171, 178, 181, 185
neurology   9, 11, 13, 20, 25–6, 127, 189
neuronovel   11, 127, 137, 169
Ninth Life of Louis Drax, The (film)   88
Ninth Life of Louis Drax, The (novel)
    82–7, 89–90, 92, 97, 162
Niven, John; *see Amateurs, The*
Nolan, Jonathan; *see* 'Memento Mori'
Norman, Tom   21
Notes On A Coma   38–9, 54–5, 58, 178
nuclear winter; *see* apocalypse

OBE; *see* outer-body experience
Odysseus   81–3, 85, 90, 97, 181
organ donation   163–5
organic brain injury; *see under* brain
    injury (BI)
Orpheus   81, 93, 95, 98, 161
Other, the   60, 62–3, 87, 96
Ouroboros, the   117–18, 120–1, 124–5,
    127–8
outer-body experience   47, 146–7,
    149–51
Owen, Adrian   1, 10, 114
  fMRI studies   180–1, 187–8 (*see also*
    functional Magnetic Resonance
    Imaging)

Palahniuk, Chuck; *see Diary*
Panorama   180–1

Parkinson's disease   191 n.1 (ch.6)
parosmia   122
paternalism   73, 165
Patrick   182
Patrick: Evil Awakens   182
patterns   63, 107, 115, 124, 128, 131–2, 159; *see also* circuits
Paul, St.   17
Paula; *see* Allende, Isabel
PDoC; *see* prolonged disorder(s) of consciousness
Penfield, Wilder   15
permanent vegetative state   6, 29, 32, 172
persistent vegetative state   37, 145, 166, 170, 174, 178–80, 185–8; *see also* chronic vegetative state; continuing vegetative state
   definition of   4–5, 29–32
   the Multi-Society Task Force on PVS   5, 29–30
   and unresponsive wakefulness syndrome (UWS)   32
phrenology   20–1, 140
   Franz Joseph Gall   20
Plath, Sylvia   72–7, 82; *see also* Lazarus
Plato
   the allegory of the cave   82, 85
   authenticity   106
   the Myth of Er   17
Platts-Mills, Ben   107, 109, 135, 144, 155–6, 161
postmodernism   106–8, 113, 117, 119, 126–7, 137, 166–8
Potter, Dennis; *see Cold Lazarus*
Powers, Richard; *see Echo Maker, The*
Priest, Christopher; *see The Glamour*
primal self   58, 62, 84, 86, 96
Pritchard, Paul   145, 157
prolonged disorder(s) of consciousness   158, 170, 172, 177–81, 184–90
   definition of   1, 4–5, 19, 28–32
   as distinct from disorder(s) of consciousness   1, 4–5, 12, 29–32
   in fiction   80, 100–1, 166–7, 171
Proof Of Heaven; *see* Alexander, Eben
prophetic knowledge   80–3, 105, 166, 168–9, 172; *see also* second-sight

psyche   22, 53, 59, 69–71, 82–6, 91, 96, 100, 127–8
   goddess   88
   shredded psyche   8, 151–3 (*see also* Malabou, Catherine)
psychiatry   11, 13, 20, 26, 32, 36
psychic shift   49, 56, 60; *see also* astral projection
psychology   52, 57, 61–2, 85, 88, 102–3; *see also* archetypal psychology; depth psychology
   neuropsychology   27
purgatory; *see* limbo
PVS; *see* persistent vegetative state

quest narrative   7, 37, 50, 54–9, 63
   and katabasis   69–71, 78–83, 86–7, 91–2, 95–8, 147, 161 (*see also* katabasis)
Quinlan, Karen   171–2, 184; *see also* right-to-die cases

Raising the Dead; *see* Selzer, Richard
Ramachandran, V. S.   135–7
rape   1, 2, 9, 54–7, 66
realism   65, 80, 131, 137, 172
Redgrove, Peter   84, 100, 110, 121, 135, 188
   interview with   76
   'Lazarus and the Sea'   74–7, 79, 84, 143, 147–9 (*see also* Lazarus)
re-enactment   54, 83, 117, 121–32, 137
'Reflections On Exile'; *see* Said, Edward
Regicide   85, 89–90, 92–3, 108, 111, 115, 122
reincarnation   75, 89
Remainder (film)   112–13, 116, 121, 128
Remainder (novel)   105–33, 136–9, 142–5, 154–6, 176, 188–9
repression   56–9, 61–2
restitution narrative   101–3, 148; *see also* Frank, Arthur
resurrection   17, 39, 69–78, 80, 89, 94, 110, 133–5, 168, 171
revenge   1, 66, 96, 119–20, 128
Ricoeur, Paul   98–102, 183–4; *see also* innovation; narrative identity; sedimentation

right-to-die cases 11, 31, 184–7; *see also* Quinlan, Karen
Rip Van Winkle 167–70; *see also* Tale of Rip Van Winkle, The
ritual 75, 81–2, 96, 160
Roberts, Neil 74
Rosen, Michael 144
Rousseau, Jean-Jacques 106–7
Royal College of Physicians 1, 32
Royle, Nicholas; *see* Regicide

Sacks, Oliver 26, 108, 136, 149–50
Said, Edward 40–2, 45–7, 50
same-but-different, the 114, 117, 155; *see also* Derrida, Jacques
Satan 71–2, 94, 96
Schiavo, Terri 178–9, 184–7
Schnabel, Julian; *see* Diving Bell and the Butterfly, The (film)
Schumacher, Michael 5–6, 183
Scorsese, Martin 73, 113
Scotland
    Caledonian anti-syzygy 60, 89
    dialect 59, 191 n.2 (ch.3)
    housing redevelopment 54, 56
    identity 56, 59–60, 63, 90, 93, 95
    independence vote 89
    oneiric motif in literature 89
second-sight 79–80, 83; *see also* prophetic knowledge
sedimentation 99, 102, 183–4; *see also* Ricoeur, Paul
Selzer, Richard 146–9, 152
sexual abuse 1–2, 23, 55–7
sexual violence; *see* sexual abuse
shell shock 24–8, 122, 188–9; *see also* Mott, Frederick; Myers, Charles
Sherry, Mark 111, 148–50, 153, 156–7
Sisyphus 91, 95, 97
skull imagery 70, 83, 92, 134, 140–1
sleeping beauty
    in Disney 1, 182
    exhibits 9, 22–3
    fairy tale 2, 43, 95, 185 (*see also* fairy tale)
    in John Collier's 'Sleeping Beauty' (short story) 23–4
    phenomenon/motif 1, 38, 43, 77, 83, 95, 167

Price's 'Sleeping Beauty' 23
Prince Charming 2, 23–4, 43–4, 185
    in *Some Call It Loving* 24, 85
    subversion of trope 43, 45, 134, 157–8, 162, 165–6, 169, 182
sleep-wake cycle 3–4, 29, 44–5
Smith, Zadie 105
soap opera 129
    depiction of coma 8, 174, 185
    paradigm of recovery 8, 35, 109–10
social networking 131
Some Call It Loving; *see under* sleeping beauty
somnambulism 21–4
Sontag, Susan 32–4, 36, 68, 101, 159–61, 174
Sopranos, The 7, 34
Source Code 40, 42
South Africa 55–6
spectrum of consciousness 9, 164, 178, 181
    discovery of 4–5, 15, 18–20, 28–32
stroke 3, 40, 108, 139, 143–4, 180, 189
stupor 3, 13, 16–17, 19–21, 31, 34

Tal, Kalí 57, 72, 78
Tale of Rip Van Winkle, The 167
Tarantino, Quentin; *see* Kill Bill Vol 1
Teasdale, Graham 30–1; *see also* Glasgow Coma Scale; Jennett, Bryan
Telegraph, The 6, 182
telepathy 181–2, 186
Thanatos 16–17, 70–1, 77
Theseus 81, 97
Times, The 81, 97
Todorov, Tzvetan 168–9, 172
Toronto *Globe and Mail* 169, 171
Totem Pole, The; *see* Pritchard, Paul
Townsend, Colonel 22
trace, the 114–17, 122, 125–6, 133–7, 155–6; *see also* Derrida, Jacques
transfiguration 17, 34, 69–70, 73–84, 87–8, 93, 125, 158
trauma 71–89, 95, 103, 109–10, 115–38, 151–7, 175, 181–9; *see also* Freud, Sigmund
    aesthetics 65
    and exile 37–69 (*see also* exile)

repetition compulsion   57, 65–6, 91, 109, 120, 153–4
traumatic departures   44, 58, 74
traumatic hauntings   41–7, 51, 65–6, 74, 151
traumatic memory   40–68 (*see also* memory)
traumatic neurosis   25, 43, 48, 57, 120, 151, 153
traumatic realism   65
the wound   41–2, 152
Trumbo, Dalton; *see Johnny Got His Gun*
Turner, Beverley   143, 154–5, 157
Twin Peaks: The Final Dossier   2–3
Twin Peaks: The Return   2, 6, 8, 23

uncanny, the   7, 48, 52, 56, 68–9, 157, 168; *see also* Freud, Sigmund
unresponsive wakefulness syndrome (UWS); *see under* persistent vegetative state
third person narration   6, 59, 109, 134, 147, 152–3
UWS; *see* unresponsive wakefulness syndrome

Vanishing Waves   181–2
vegetable as diagnostic term   32, 34, 80, 163
vegetative state; *see* chronic vegetative state; continuing vegetative state; minimally conscious state; persistent vegetative state
ventilator   29, 101, 157, 172; *see also* breathing machine; breathing tubes

Virgil
the *Aeneid*   96–7, 102, 147
Virgilian guides   82–3, 85, 91, 95
VS; *see* vegetative state

Wade, Derick   31, 178, 181
Waking Up: Memoirs Of A Coma Recoverer   146
Walking Dead, The (comic)   35
Walking Dead, The (TV series)   35
Wallis, Terry   177–9, 186
Waugh, Caroline   144–6, 157, 173
Welcome to Marwen   129–30, 132, 173–4; *see also* Carrell, Steve, Zemeckis, Robert
Welcome to Marwencol (Shellen and Hogancamp)   129, 133
Welsh, Irvine; *see Marabou Stork Nightmares*
whacky   154–5
Whitehead, Anne   41–2, 65
Wiersema, Robert; *see also Before I Wake*
interview with   169–71
Wilde, Joel   156–7
Williams, Rosalind   86, 97
Willis, Thomas   18; *see also De Anima Brutorum*
worms   72–5, 147, 163
Write Way, The   139, 144, 155, 157, 173

Zasetsky   26–8, 149, 153, 155; *see also* Luria, A. R.
Zemeckis, Robert   129–30, 132, 173–4; *see also Welcome To Marwen*
zombie   35, 73, 114

www.ingramcontent.com/pod-product-compliance
Lightning Source LLC
Chambersburg PA
CBHW072233290426
44111CB00012B/2083